BRENDA ORTIZ
CVM 2000

DR. Ortiz

Small Animal
ORTHOPEDICS

Dr. Ortiz

Small Animal ORTHOPEDICS

with original illustrations by Laura Pardi Duprey

***Robert L. Leighton**, VMD*

Diplomate, American College of Veterinary Surgeons
Emeritus Professor of Veterinary Medicine
The School of Veterinary Medicine
University of California
Davis, California

WOLFE

London • St. Louis • Boston • Chicago • Philadelphia • Sydney • Toronto

Published by Wolfe Publishing, an imprint of Mosby–Year Book Europe, Ltd.

ISBN 1-56375-082-1

LIBRARY OF CONGRESS CATALOGING-IN-PUBLICATION DATA
Leighton, Robert L.
Small animal orthopedics / Robert L. Leighton.
p. cm.
Includes bibliographical references and index.
ISBN 1–56375–082–1
1. Dogs—Surgery. 2. Cats—Surgery. 3. Veterinary orthopedics.
I. Title.
SF991.L43 1993 92–35357
636.7'08973—dc20

BRITISH LIBRARY CATALOGUING IN PUBLICATION DATA
A catalogue record for this book is available from the British Library.

For full details of all Mosby-Year Book Europe, Ltd. titles, please write to Mosby-Year Book Europe, Limited, Lynton House, 7-12 Tavistock Square, London, WC1H 9LB, England.

10 9 8 7 6 5 4 3 2 1

Project Managers: Alison Marek, Tim Condon
Art Director/Designer: Kathryn Greenslade
Illustrator: Laura Pardi Duprey
Editorial Assistants: Jean Unger, Demetrius McDowell
Originated in Singapore by Colourscan Overseas Co.
Produced by Imago
Printed and bound in Hong Kong

DEDICATION

To Dr. Erwin F. Schroeder, one of the pioneer small animal veterinary orthopedists, from whose kindness, instruction, and enthusiasm I developed a lifelong interest in small animal surgery and orthopedics.

PREFACE

It is the hope of every author to produce something that will be useful, practical, and informative. My intent is to provide a concise illustrated description of most of the orthopedic procedures in small animals that the veterinary surgeon is commonly called upon to perform. It is not possible to include all the many variations of techniques that have been developed. It goes without saying that all the criteria for aseptic surgery, maintenance of hemostasis and safe anesthesia are to be observed.

The radiographic illustrations come from the teaching files of the Veterinary Medical Teaching Hospital of the University of California School of Veterinary Medicine. The invaluable assistance of all concerned in the Radiology Department is gratefully acknowledged. Special thanks are extended to the radiologist, Dr. J.P. Morgan, for his discerning eyes in the selection of radiographs.

The drawings have been made from personal sketches, my teaching slides, and instructional models.

I am thankful for the support staff of the Department of Veterinary Surgery, who have so conscientiously typed the manuscript.

If I can provide a working book that will help engender confidence in a surgical procedure that will result in a benefit to the surgeon, the client, and above all to the animals we all care for, I will be most satisfied.

Robert L. Leighton, VMD
Davis, California

CONTENTS

6. VERTEBRAL COLUMN

7. SPECIAL SURGERIES

CHAPTER 1

HEAD

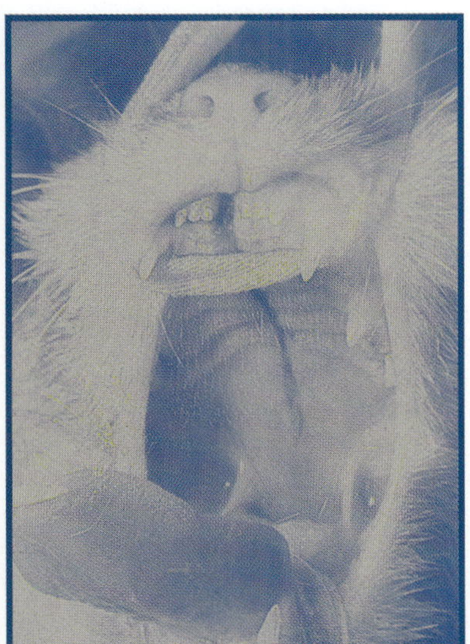
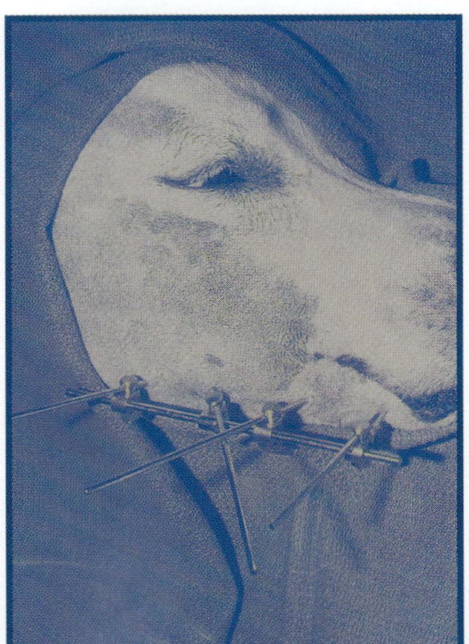
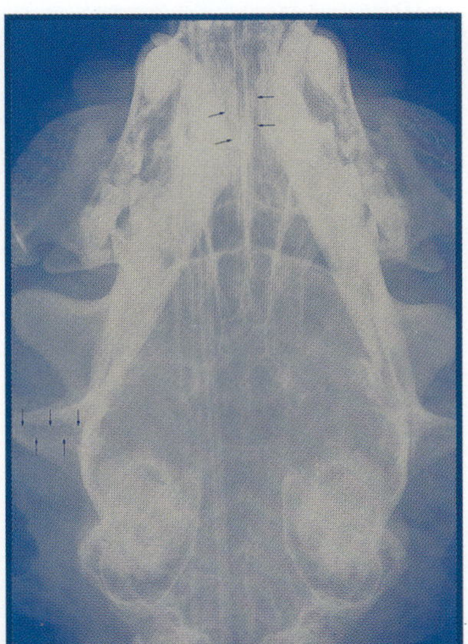

FRACTURES OF THE MANDIBLE

Symphysis

Fractures of the mandibular symphysis are common in both dogs and cats (Fig. 1.1). In the latter they are frequently the result of falls from heights. Although contaminated by the splitting of the overlying gums and frequent eversion of the mentum, there is good tissue resistance to infection. Immobilization is essential and must resist the stresses of eating and chewing. An especially difficult situation is seen in small breeds, such as older Pekingese and poodles, with resorption of the rostral ends of the mandibles, loss of teeth, and lack of healing stimulus (Fig. 1.2).

The fracture may be only slightly displaced with moderate instability, or widely separated and completely unstable, and may occur in conjunction with other mandibular fractures (Fig. 1.3).

SURGICAL TECHNIQUE

Wiring Although a simple figure-8 of wire around the bases of the lower canine teeth is often recommended, it is usually not very effective because the wire slips off and the symphyseal area is not compressed but rather forced apart.

Moderate stabilization can be obtained with orthopedic wire looped around the mandibles caudal to the lower canines (Fig. 1.4). It is introduced with a strong curved needle. A ventral midline incision just caudal to the symphysis exposes the central area. The wire is inserted dorsally on the lateral surface of one mandible, exiting through the gum tissue midway between the canine and first premolar. The wire is brought across to the same area on the opposite side and inserted ventrally on the lateral side of the mandible. The two wire ends are twisted firmly to approximate and compress the symphysis into its normal position. The twisted ends are cut short and bent inwards to project caudally. The incision is closed with catgut and nonabsorbable suture. The wire is removed after healing takes place.

In small dogs and cats, a ventral midline incision is made to expose the separated symphysis. A wire stitch is placed through the rostral mandibular bones and the centers of the symphyseal surfaces. It is twisted tightly, drawing the symphysis together. The twisted wire is cut short and pressed close to the bone. The incision is closed with nonabsorbable suture. The wire remains in place permanently (Fig. 1.5).

Pinning and Wiring Larger animals require additional support to maintain symphyseal alignment. This is done by transfixing the symphyseal area with a small intramedullary (IM) pin inserted caudal to the canines and avoiding the middle mental foramen and the roots of the adjacent premolar.

The pin ends are cut off so as to leave just room enough to offer support to a loop of wire. A figure-8 wire is placed from the

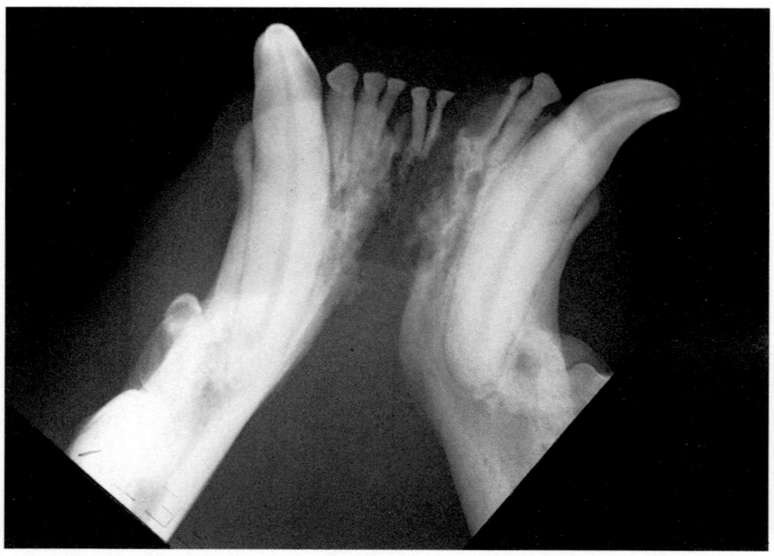

FIGURE 1.1 Radiograph of a fractured mandibular symphysis in a cat.

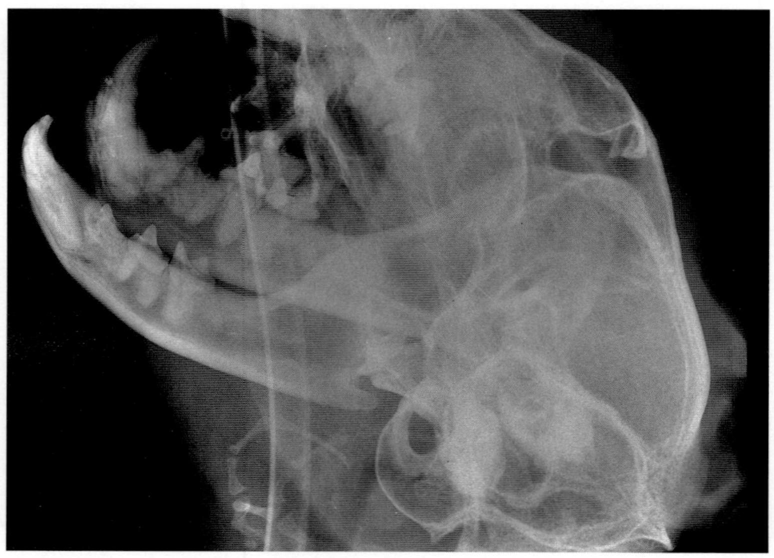

FIGURE 1.2 Radiograph of a Pekingese dog with resorption of the rostral ends of the mandibles.

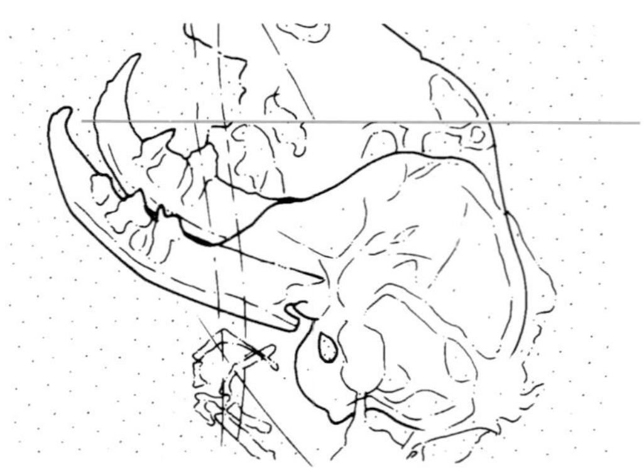

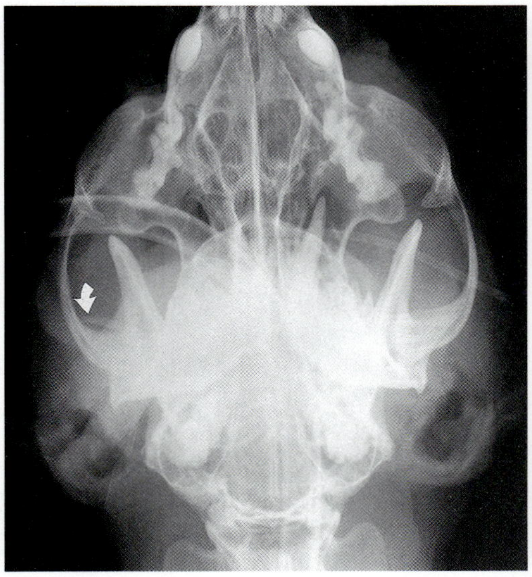

FIGURE 1.3 A slightly displaced mandibular fracture.

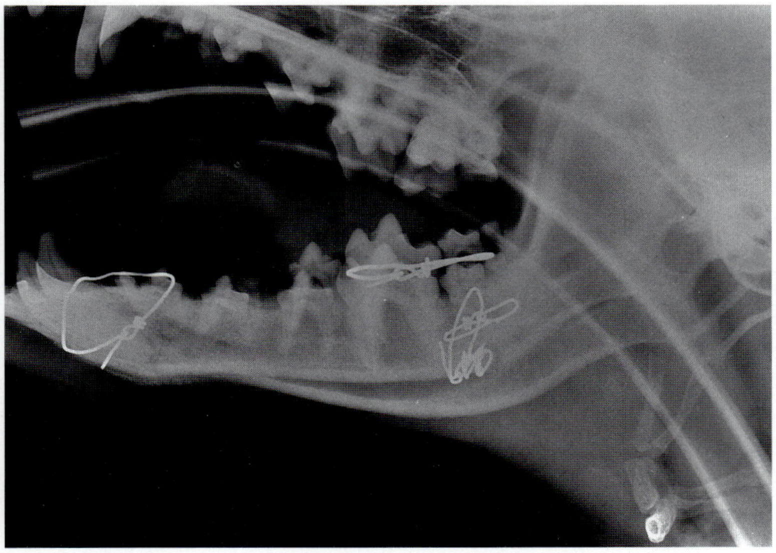

FIGURE 1.4 A mandibular fracture immobilized with wire looped around the mandibles caudal to the lower canines.

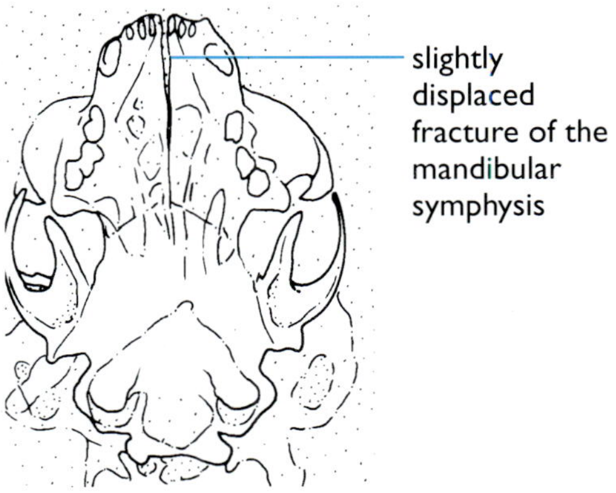

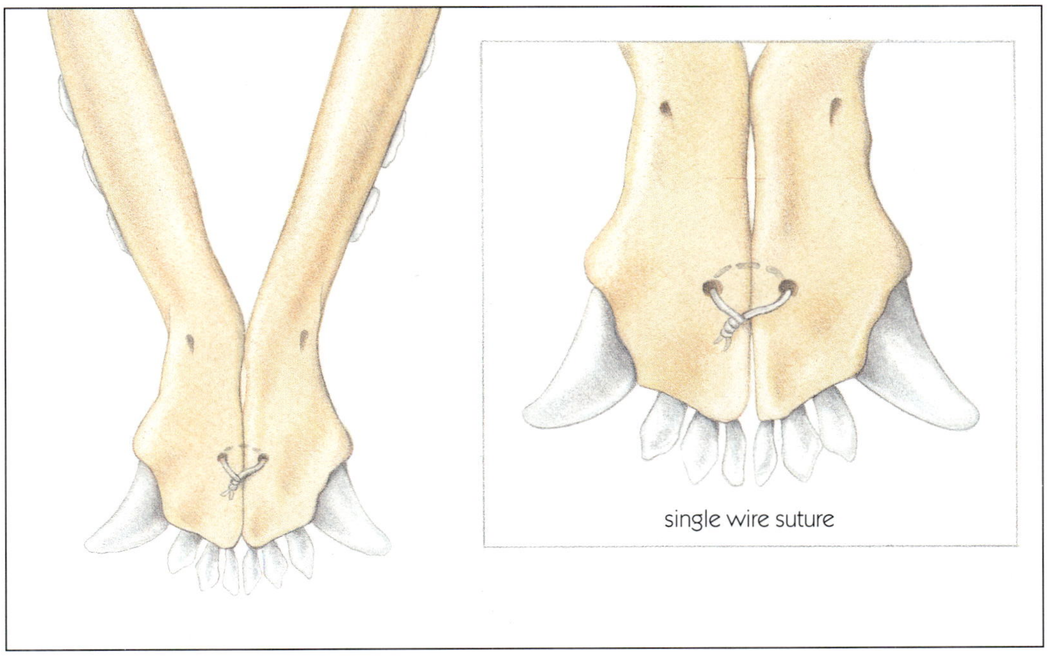

FIGURE 1.5 Ventral view of a fractured mandibular symphysis fastened with a single wire suture, as would be done in a cat.

pin ends to meet rostral to the lower incisors. The wire is twisted tightly to compress the symphysis (Fig. 1.6).

The pin and wire are removed after healing, usually a matter of 2 to 3 weeks.

LAG SCREWS In large dogs, a lag screw is particularly suited to maintain alignment and compress the fracture. A ventral midline incision is made over the symphyseal fracture. The tissues over the adjacent mandibular surfaces are elevated to expose the bone laterally. A hole of the same diameter as the screw to be inserted is drilled transversely just caudal to the symphysis and ventral to the middle mental foramen, avoiding the roots of the first premolars. The first half of the hole is reamed to a size that will not permit the screw to engage the bone. The hole is measured with a depth gauge and the proper size of screw is selected. Using a tap guide, the second half is tapped. The screw is inserted and tightened to lag the two fragments together (Fig. 1.7). The screw is left in place. The incision is closed with chromic catgut and nonabsorbable suture. Occasionally, the oral surface tissues require closure with nonabsorbable suture.

In cats, the torn mentum is replaced by using nonabsorbable sutures that are looped over the ventral canines.

Oral tissues normally heal readily. Thorough debridement of the injury, especially if it is heavily contaminated or infected, is required. A soft diet and antibiotic therapy are instituted.

Body of the Mandible

Fractures of the mandibular body are very common. Accurate alignment and firm immobilization are required. This becomes more difficult when the injury is bilateral, infection is present, there is loss of bone or surrounding tissue, teeth have been loosened or lost, tooth roots are exposed, treatment has been delayed, or previous treatment has failed.

General anesthesia is required. Because it is essential to close the mouth to check for proper occlusion, it is often necessary to introduce a tracheal tube through a pharyngostomy.

SURGICAL TECHNIQUE

WIRING Selected fractures of the body of the mandible, especially those that are unilateral, not severely displaced, and without serious loss of tissue, can be satisfactorily treated by wiring the fragments

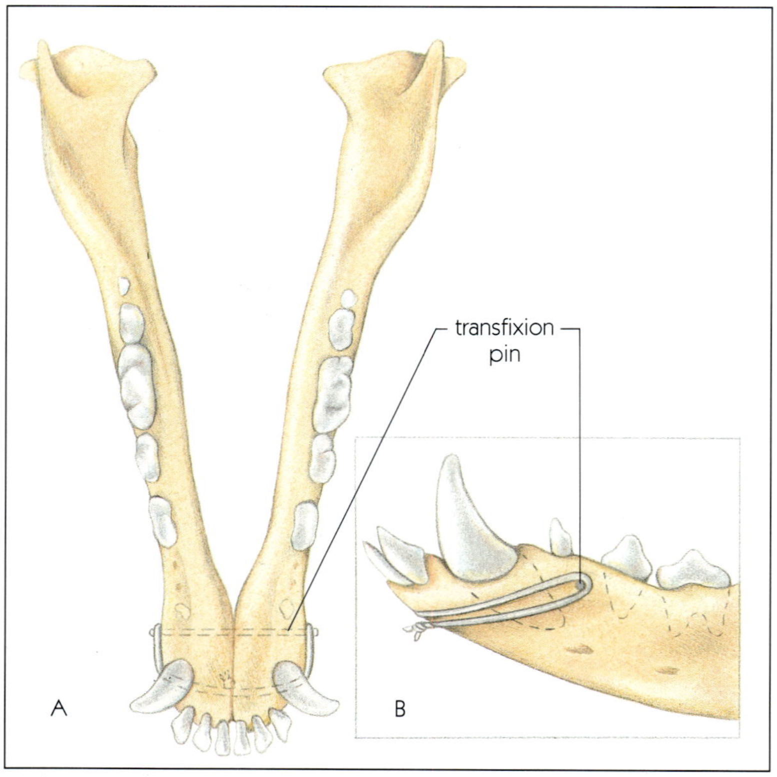

FIGURE 1.6 (A) Dorsoventral view of a fracture of the mandibular symphysis repaired with a transfixion pin. A wire has been looped over the pin ends and twisted tightly just rostral and ventral to the incisor teeth. (B) Lateral view of the same fracture.

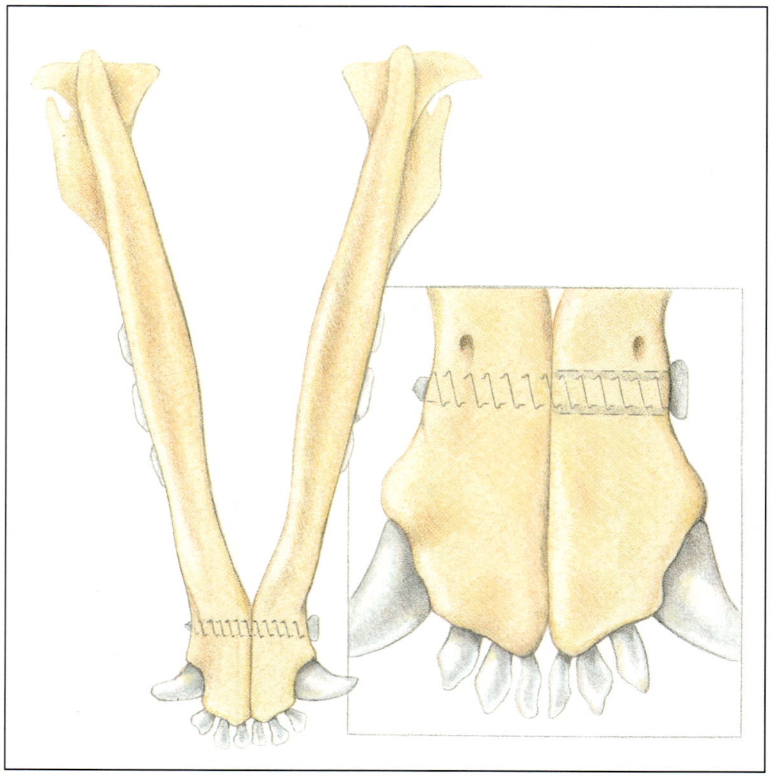

FIGURE 1.7 Ventrodorsal view of a fracture of the mandibular symphysis secured with a lag screw. Note that the hole nearest the screw head is enlarged so that the screw threads do not engage.

together. Simple wiring with a figure-8 around the bases of the teeth is usually ineffective. The wire tends to slip and, when tightened, distracts the fracture. However, it can be used to complement other means of reinforcing the stabilization. With proper precautions, a transverse fracture of the mandibular body can be successfully treated with a cruciate wire pattern. The fracture must be reduced and impacted.

The lips are retracted. Dorsal and ventral holes are drilled transversely through each fragment near the fracture site, but not so close as to fail to provide firm seating for the wire. They must not penetrate the roots of the teeth. From the buccal surface, with a blunt 18-gauge needle as a guide, orthopedic wire is introduced through the dorsal rostral hole, brought over and inserted through from the oral side, the dorsal caudal hole. Here the wire is brought down to the ventral rostral hole and inserted through to the oral side, where it is inserted from the oral side through the caudal ventral hole. The wire ends are twisted together firmly. The twisted ends are cut off short and flattened to the gum surface so that they will not irritate the lip. The wire should present two parallel smooth surfaces against the tongue and a cruciate pattern on the buccal side (Fig. 1.8). Additional control can be obtained by a figure-8 wire applied to the bases of the teeth adjacent to the fracture. In addition, a muzzle is applied for a week or two. It should permit the eating of soft food and drinking. The wire is removed after the fracture heals.

Pins and Wire After wiring, additional stability is provided by inserting a small intramedullary pin at an angle, from caudal to the fracture across the intermandibular space to the cranial aspect of the opposite mandible. Another pin is directed from rostral to the fracture at an angle across the intermandibular space to the caudal aspect of the opposite mandible. The pins are cut off close to the tissues. The tips should completely penetrate the opposite mandible (Fig. 1.9).

External Fixation (K/E Apparatus) In larger dogs, especially when there is marked instability, multiple fractures, loss of tissue, severe infection or contamination, or both mandibles are involved, external fixation offers a means of providing long-term stability, while permitting the animal to eat and drink normally (Fig. 1.10).

The lower jaw is shaved and prepared for surgery. Smooth pins are best inserted with a power drill. Threaded pins inserted in

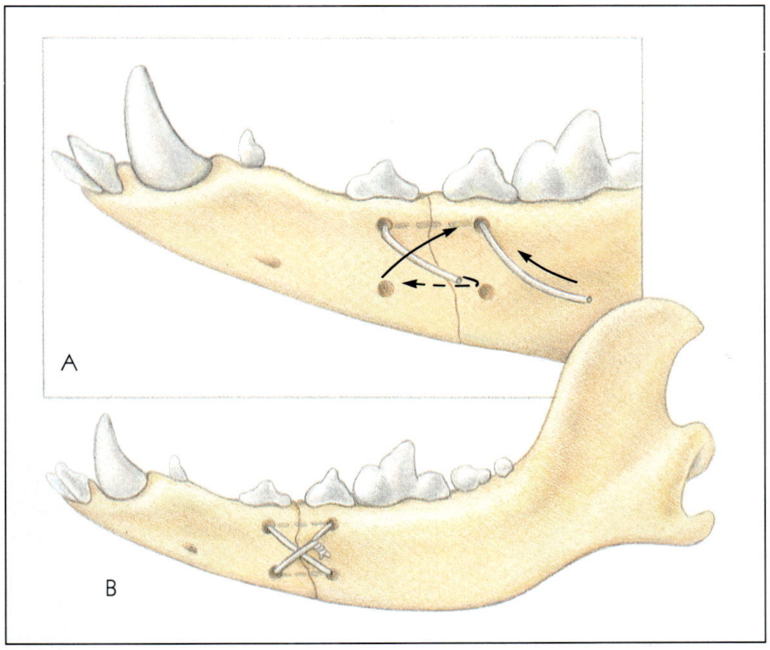

FIGURE 1.8 (A) Lateral view of a fracture of the mandible repaired with wire. Two holes have been drilled in the rostral fragment and two in the caudal fragment. (B) The correct pattern for wire insertion.

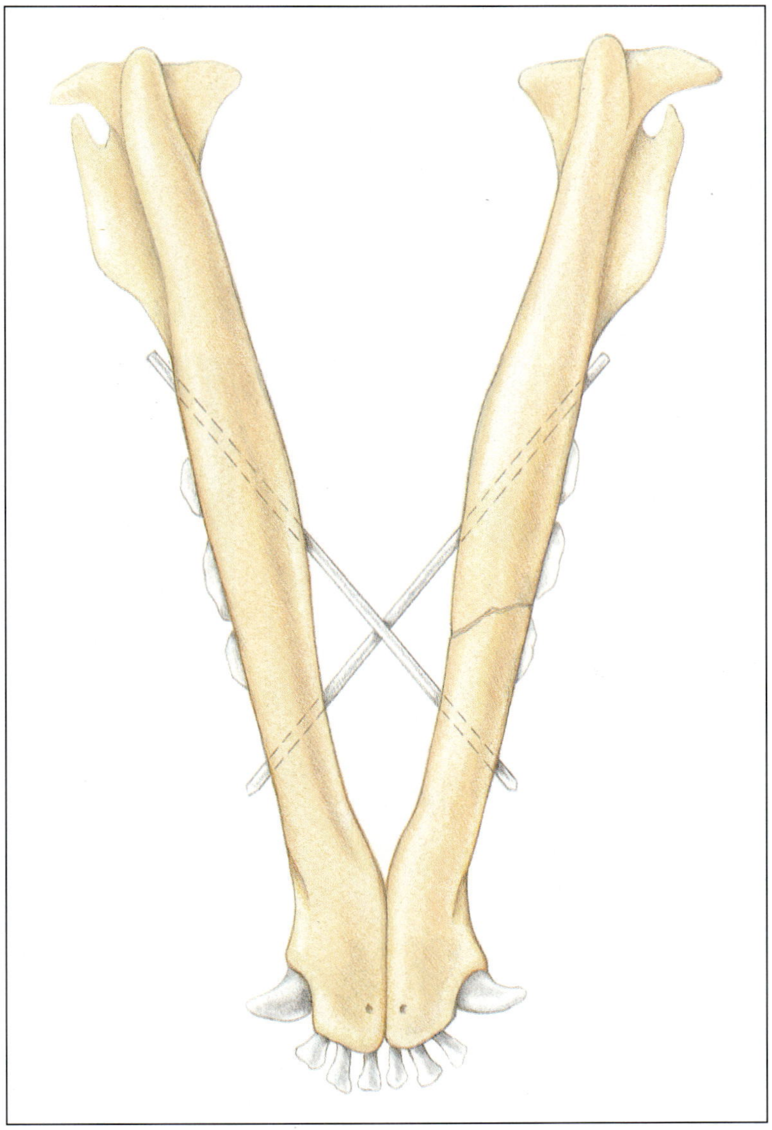

FIGURE 1.9 Ventrodorsal view of mandibular fracture repaired with crossed IM pins.

holes that have been drilled and tapped hold best. The roots of the teeth must be avoided. A single bar is used. The rostral pin is inserted straight through both mandibles. Additional clamps are provided for pins that are driven into the affected mandible only. These are inserted at an angle, with the fracture reduced and adjusted to provide proper occlusion (Fig. 1.11).

In the case of a bilateral fracture, the rostral pin is driven completely through to the opposite side so that it can attach to both apparatuses. Additional pins are placed as needed to control fragments. The mandible is supported by the device where bone is missing or where a graft of iliac crest and cancellous bone has been inserted (Fig. 1.12).

The pins are cut off about 0.5 cm from the clamps. The apparatus is bandaged to protect it from catching on objects and to cover the sharp ends of the cut off pins.

In smaller dogs and cats, where even the smallest version of the K/E device is too large, pins are inserted as for such a device but the connecting bar is replaced by a plastic tube filled with liquid methylmethacrylate. The tube is forced onto the projecting pin ends. The cement soon hardens, providing a light but very strong support, with the pins held very securely. The pins are cut off close to the plastic tube (Fig. 1.13). When there is a bilateral fracture, a separate tube is placed on each side. A single tube curved rostrally will interfere with prehension of food.

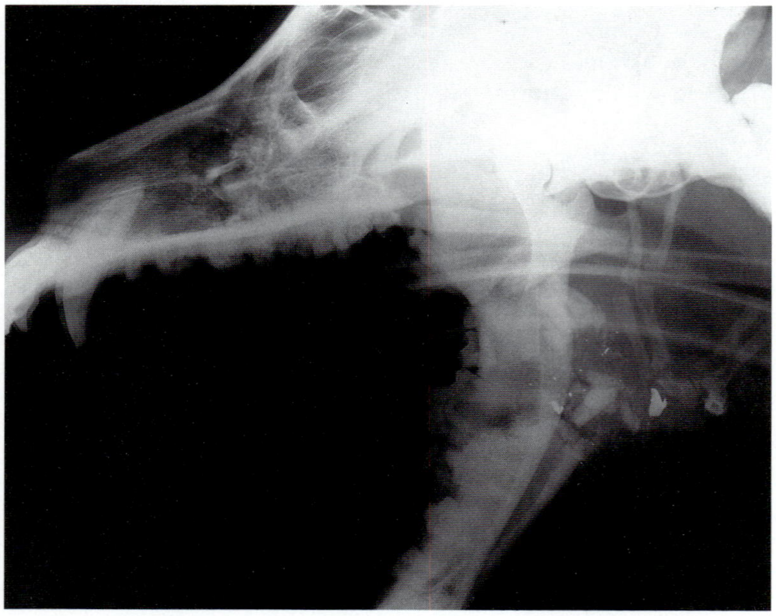

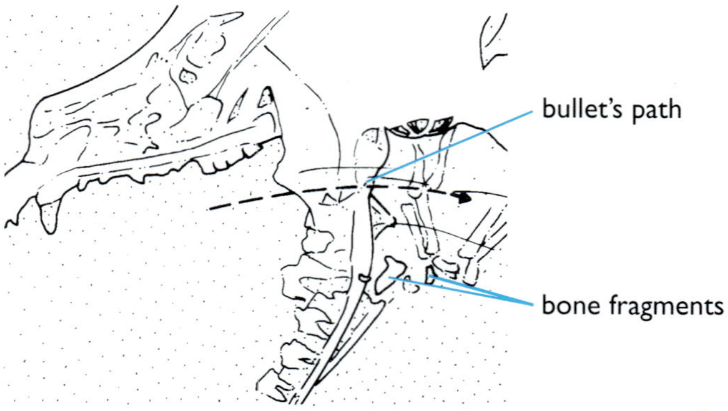

FIGURE 1.10 Radiograph of a gunshot fracture in the mandible of a dog.

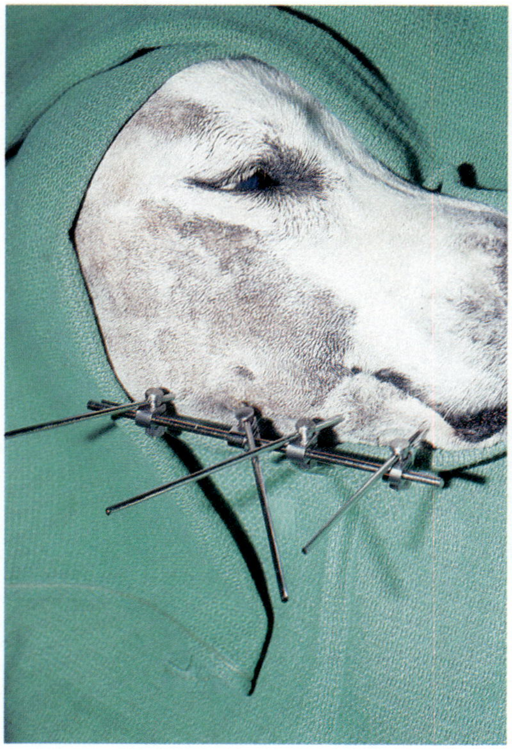

FIGURE 1.11 An external fixation device immobilizes this fractured mandible in a dog.

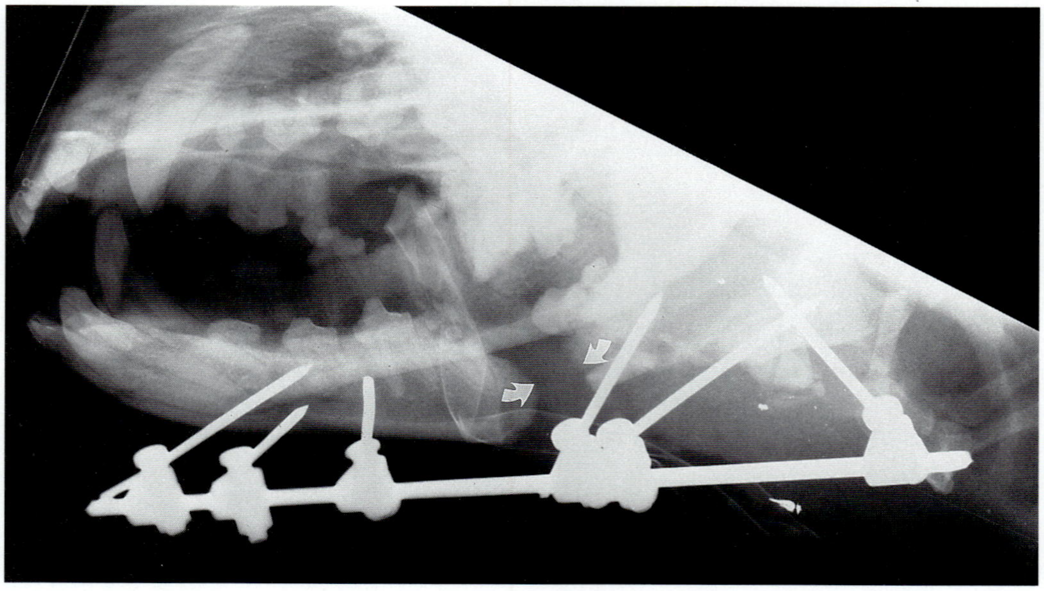

FIGURE 1.12 A fractured mandible with loss of bone in a dog, repaired with an external fixation device.

External fixation splints are very well tolerated. They are removed after the fracture has healed. Some discharge can be expected at the site of entry of the pins through the skin. Tension of the skin against the pin should be relieved by a small incision at the time of insertion.

The pins are cut off in order to remove the methylmethacrylate connection.

Plating Small bone plates offer an excellent means to treat fractures of the mandibular body, especially those that are bilateral or have multiple fragments. They provide excellent immobilization and enable the dog to eat and drink normally. Very small plates can be used in small dogs, especially when there is slow healing. Larger plates provide the rigidity needed in large dogs.

A ventral approach to the mandible is made, exposing a good part of its body. The bone plate is applied to the caudolateral aspect of the bone. The plate should then be contoured for an exact fit to avoid displacing the fracture and causing a malocclusion (Fig. 1.14).

The incision is closed with catgut and nonabsorbable sutures. The plate remains permanently unless the screws loosen and pain is present. Soft food and liquids are fed for a week.

Intramedullary pins should not be inserted in the central canal of the mandibular body. Occasionally a K-wire can be used to stabi-

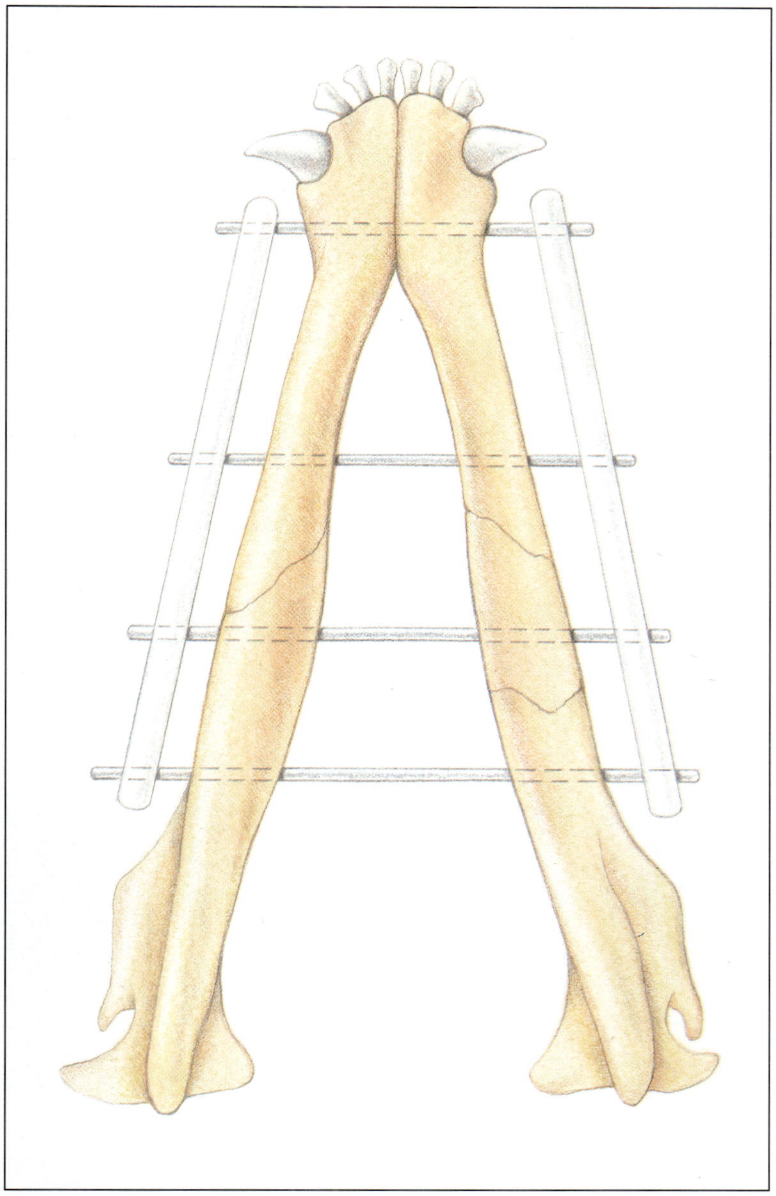

FIGURE 1.13 Dorsoventral view of a bilateral fracture of the mandibles treated with transfixion pins that are secured with tubing filled with methylmethacrylate.

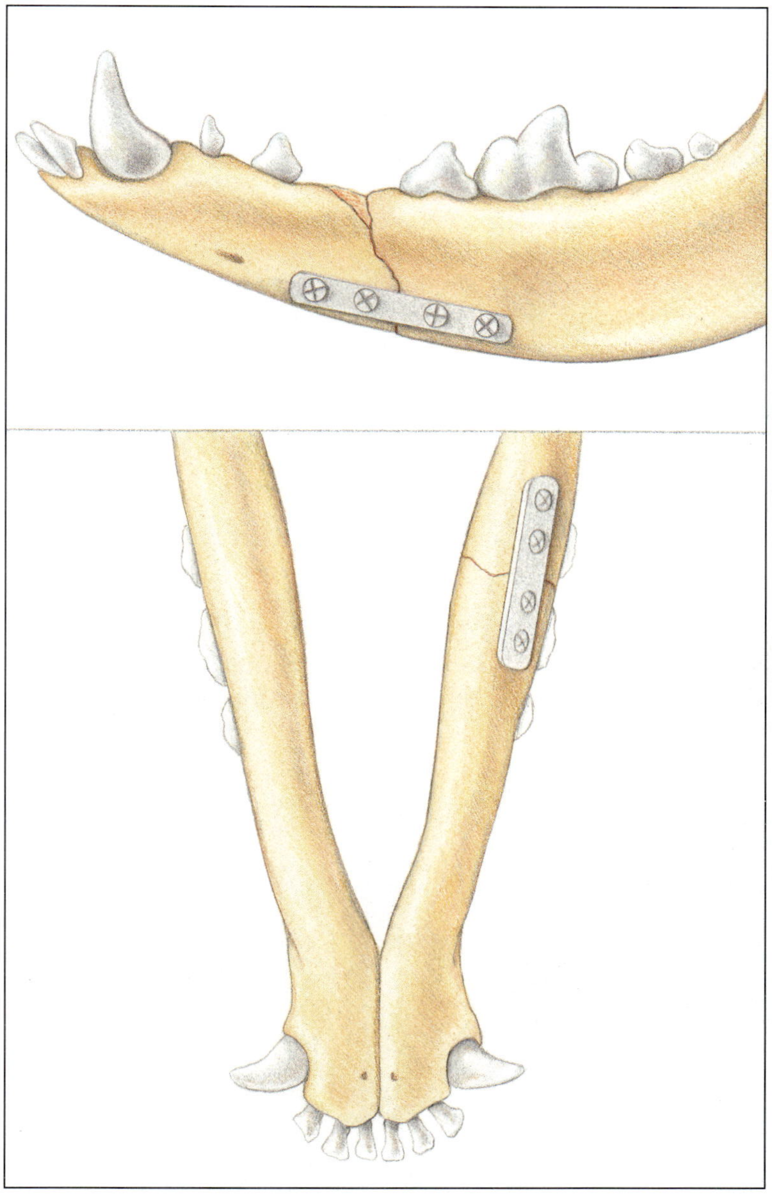

FIGURE 1.14 (A) Lateral view of a mandibular fracture treated with a small bone plate. (B) Dorsoventral view.

lize a fracture by inserting the wire across the fracture in the bone of the ventral portion of the body of the mandible.

Ramus

The ramus is the caudal nontooth-bearing part of the mandible. It is rarely injured, being protected by the overlying musculature. Fractures with minimal displacement are treated by use of a muzzle. When there is considerable displacement and pain, an open reduction is done under general anesthesia. The fragments are usually secured with wire stitches across the fracture edges.

SURGICAL TECHNIQUE

The approach is made along the ventrolateral edge of the mandible. The skin and subcutaneous tissue and the underlying platysma muscle are reflected. The ventral insertion of the masseter muscle is incised. Sharp and blunt dissection elevates it from the underlying bone to expose the fracture. Opposing holes are drilled along the edges of the fracture and orthopedic wire is inserted using a short, blunt 18-gauge needle as a wire guide. The wires are placed before reduction. The handle of a scalpel or a bone hook may be needed to reduce the fracture. The wires are twisted and the ends are cut off short and bent flat to the bone surface. The masseter muscle is replaced by suturing in the covering aponeurosis. The platysma muscle and subcutaneous tissues are closed. The skin is sutured with nonabsorbable suture.

A muzzle is applied that will allow ingestion of soft food and liquids but not firm chewing. It remains on for 2 weeks.

Condyloid Process

Fractures of the condyloid process are rare but they always require immobilization.

SURGICAL TECHNIQUE

A ventral approach is made over the caudal angle of the ramus. The overlying musculature is elevated to expose the fracture. In smaller dogs, a firm wire stitch or two is placed across the fracture line. In larger dogs, a small intramedullary pin is inserted to hold the fragments in place (Fig. 1.15).

Temporomandibular Articulation

The temporomandibular articulation is subject to luxation, fracture, and injuries to the joint meniscus and ligaments. These injuries are occasionally bilateral. Radiographs are needed for accurate diagnosis.

SURGICAL TECHNIQUE

LUXATIONS Luxations are reduced by placing a wooden rod (a piece of dowel) transversely across the mouth at the level of the last molar. A pencil is used in cats. The mouth is forced closed by pressing the muzzle together. In addition, some caudal force is applied to the mandible. Once reduced, a muzzle is applied. Soft food and liquids are fed for a week to 10 days.

FRACTURES Fractures are approached through an incision along the ventral border of the zygomatic arch. The masseter muscle is retracted and the tissues in the area of the joint are bluntly dissected. A wire stitch is placed through the two bone fragments if the fracture is extraarticular. Commonly they are intraarticular and an incision into the joint is made. In large dogs, a K-wire can be used, but treatment is usually with a wire stitch. Very small fragments are removed. The meniscal cartilage may be torn and require suturing. Very severely damaged joints will require excision of the mandibular portion. A pseudarthrosis develops which, although unstable, is functional and pain free. A muzzle is applied and a diet of soft food and liquids is given.

Coronoid Process

The coronoid process of the mandible is rarely fractured. There is, however, a condition in which the process becomes locked in contact with the zygomatic arch. This results in an inability to close the jaw, which is frequently recurrent (Fig. 1.16).

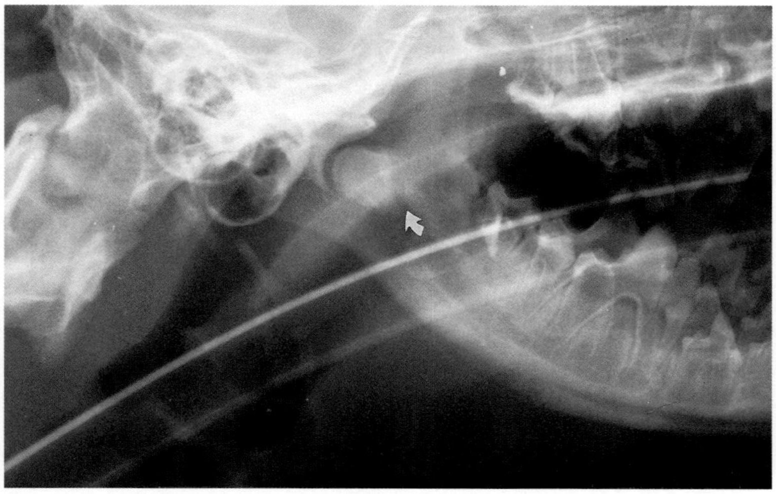

FIGURE 1.15 Radiograph showing a fracture of the condyloid process (arrow).

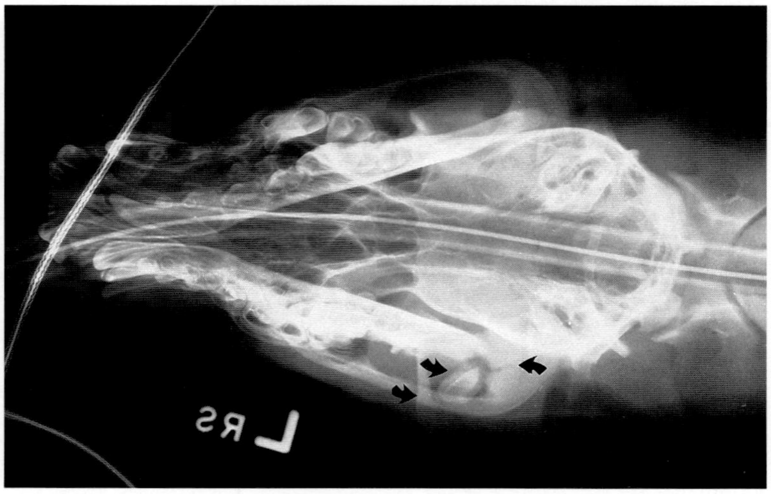

FIGURE 1.16 This locked position of the coronoid process is a result of trauma. Fractures in the area of the left tempero-mandibular articulation are indicated by arrows.

The usual surgery is to remove a portion of the zygomatic arch. Removal of a portion of the dorsal edge of the coronoid process is equally effective and less disfiguring (Fig. 1.17).

SURGICAL TECHNIQUE

An incision is made along the dorsal edge of the zygomatic arch through the fascial attachments. The temporalis muscle is incised and elevated from its insertion on the dorsal edge of the zygomatic arch. Further blunt dissection elevates the temporalis from the lateral surface of the coronoid process. The dorsal edge is exposed and trimmed away with a rongeur. The temporalis muscle is replaced and its fascial attachment is sutured. Closure is performed in the usual manner.

FRACTURES OF THE MAXILLA

The most common maxillary fracture is midline through the roof of the mouth. It is seen most frequently in cats that have fallen from great heights or have been struck by a car (Fig. 1.18). Often these fractures heal by themselves, but if the separation is very large, a loop of wire across the roof of the mouth is placed from around the dorsal fourth premolars.

Fractures across the nasal area with ventral or lateral deviation are reduced and the fragments wired together with simple wire stitches placed in holes drilled in the bone. Incisions are made in the overlying skin and subcutaneous tissues to expose the fracture. It may be necessary to place wires around the bases of the teeth at

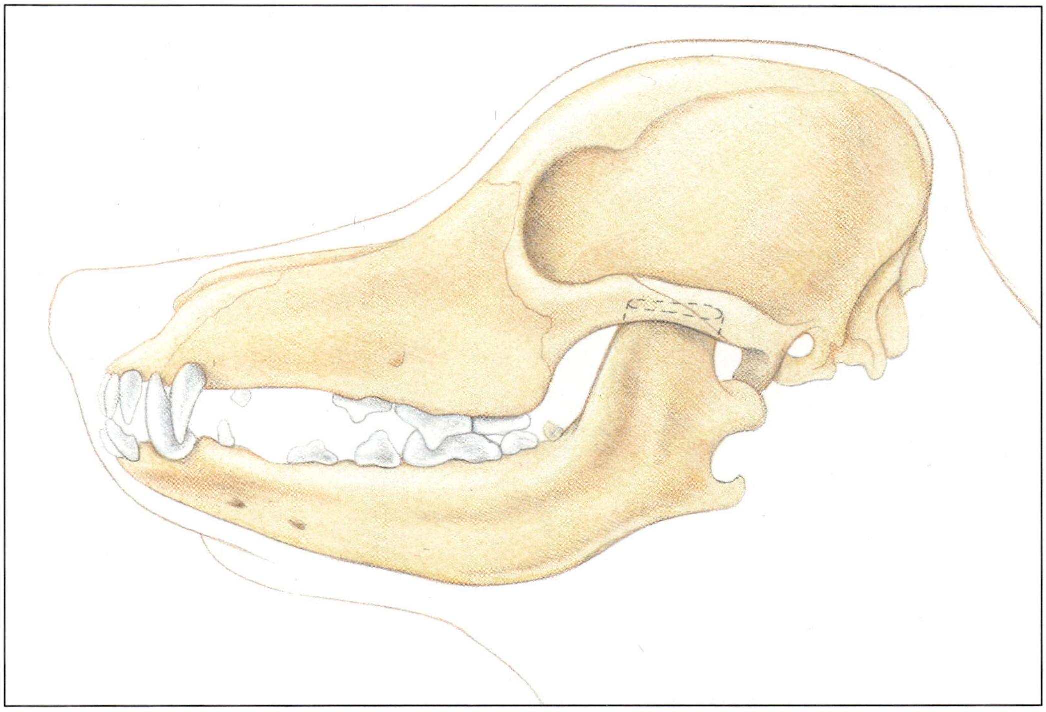

FIGURE 1.17 Sketch of a dog's head showing the removal of the top of the coronoid process for relief of a "locking syndrome."

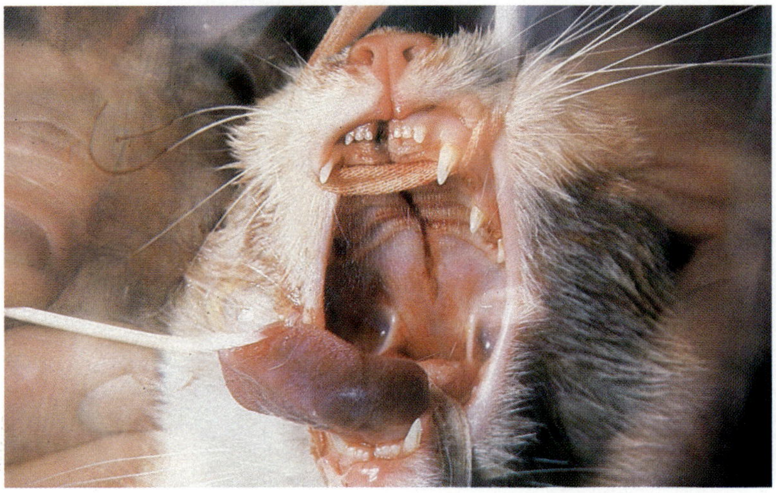

FIGURE 1.18 A maxillary fracture in the cat is evidenced by a longitudinal midline split in the roof of the mouth.

the fracture site in the mouth to ensure proper occlusion. These are removed after healing. The wires in the bone are left in.

A longitudinal nasal split is repaired by introducing a K-wire transversely after reduction, and placing a figure-8 of wire around the ends. The pin penetrates only the most dorsal part of the maxillary or nasal bones.

FRACTURES OF THE ZYGOMATIC ARCH

Fractures of the zygomatic arch are uncommon. Repair is required when the area is contaminated or infected or when a marked cosmetic defect is present. Repair is also necessary when the orbit of the eye is affected (Fig. 1.19).

SURGICAL TECHNIQUE

An approach is made directly over the zygomatic arch. The fragments may resist reduction and care should be taken in levering the fragments because of the possibility of damage to the medially located structures.

The fragments can usually be wired together. Improved stability is obtained by inserting a K-wire longitudinally through the fracture site. The curved formation of the structure will allow both ends of the wire to be free. These ends are cut off, leaving only enough to hold a figure-8 of wire around them. The wires usually remain in place permanently, but can be removed for cosmetic reasons after healing.

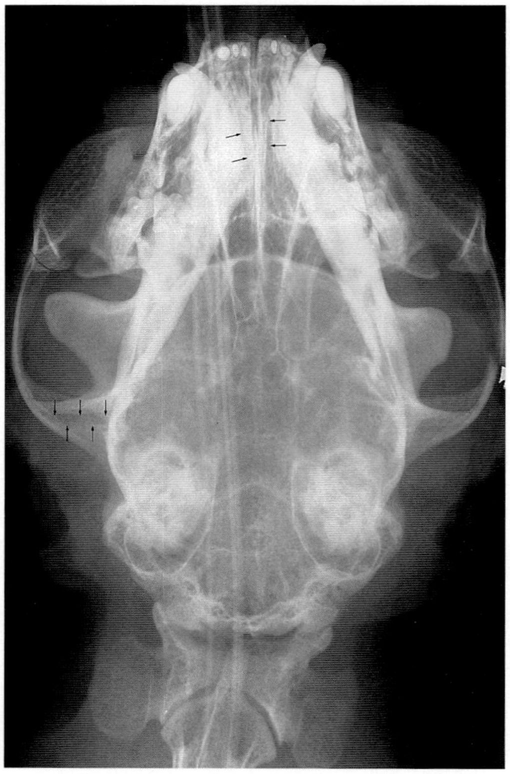

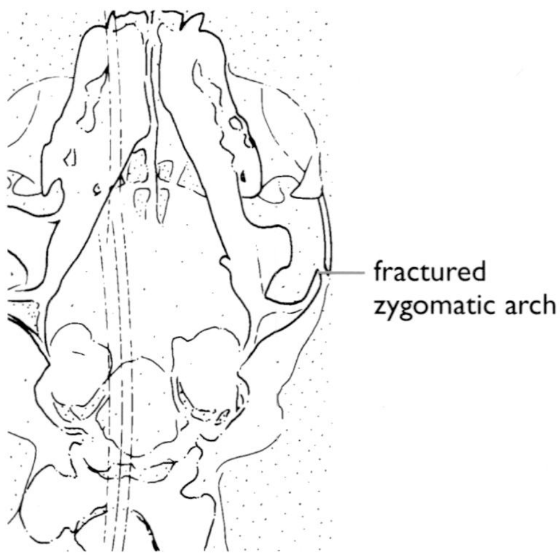

FIGURE 1.19 Radiograph showing a fracture of the zygomatic arch. Small rostral arrows indicate fractured mandibular symphisis. Small arrows to the left show a separation of the temperomandibular articulation.

CHAPTER

2 FORELIMB

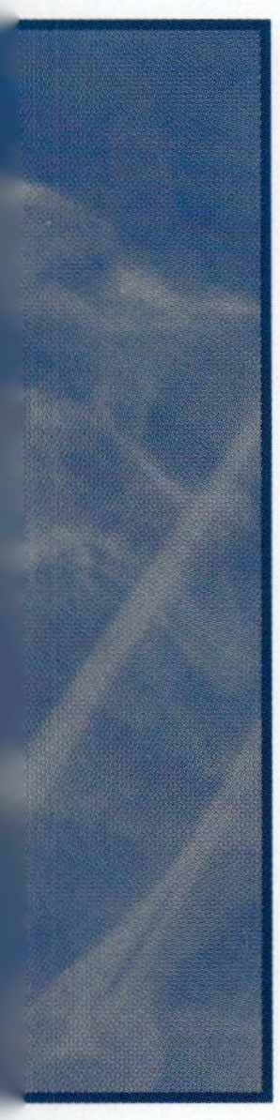
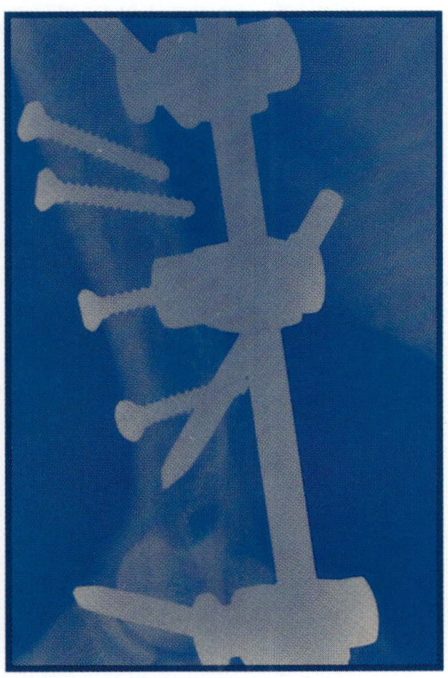
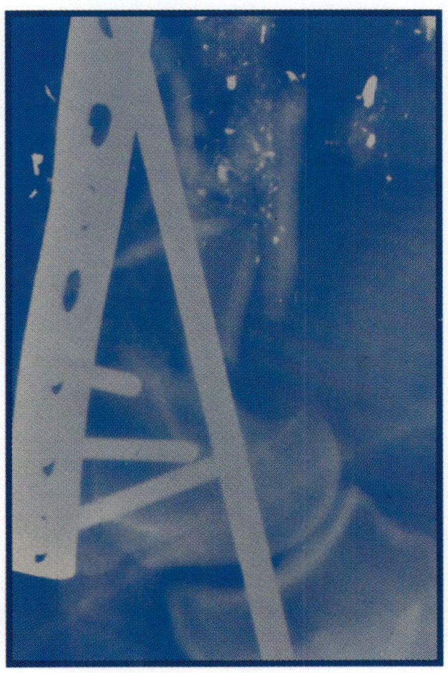
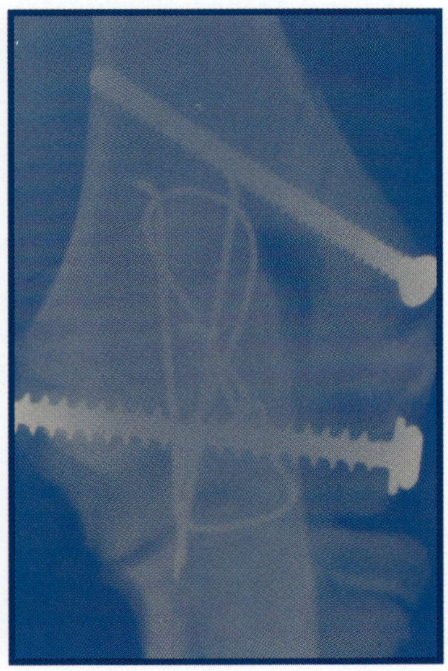

FRACTURES OF THE SCAPULA

Scapular Body

Fracture of the body of the scapula is uncommon. Although usually caused by a car accident, it can also be the result of a gunshot wound (Fig. 2.1A). The protection and support afforded by the underlying musculature and the cancellous nature of the bone will often permit healing with conservative treatment, such as a Velpeau sling used for 3 or 4 weeks. When the fracture is markedly displaced, it is painful and surgical fixation is required to promote adequate healing.

These fractures are usually transverse, with displacement of the lower fragment (Fig. 2.1B). A series of wire sutures is placed across the fracture line or, to ensure greater stability, a small plate is placed along the cranial or caudal aspect of the base of the scapular spine.

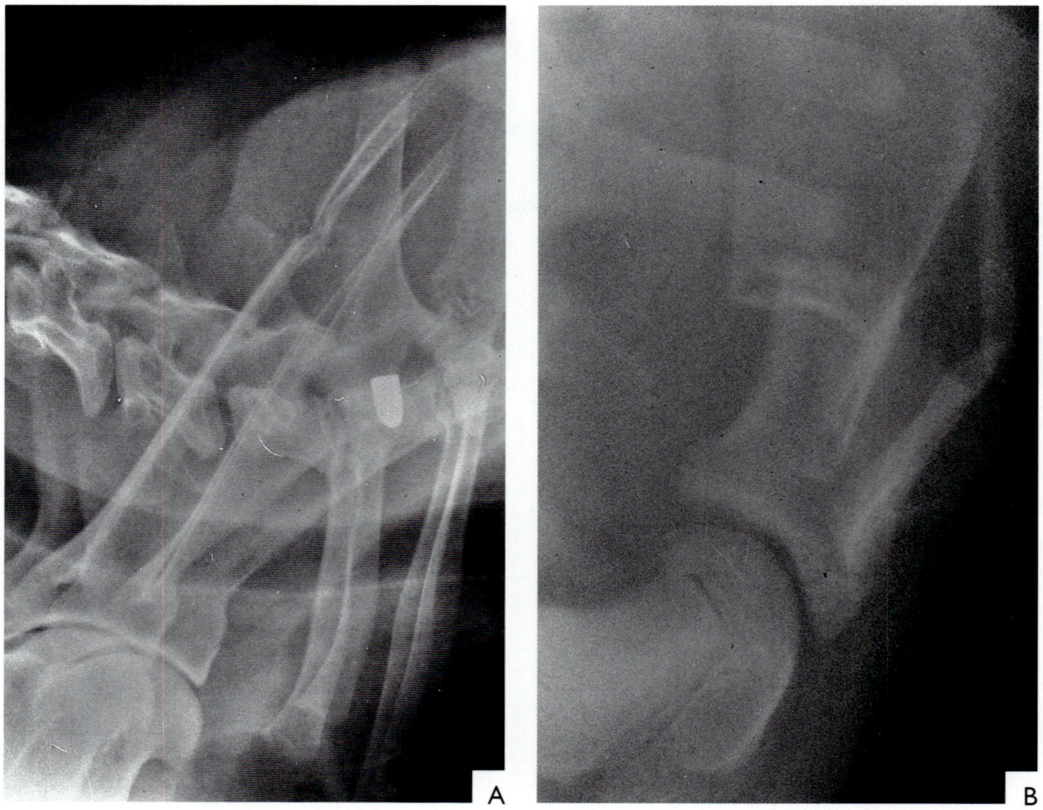

FIGURE 2.1 (A) Radiograph of a gunshot fracture of the scapular body. (B) Radiograph of a fracture of the scapular body.

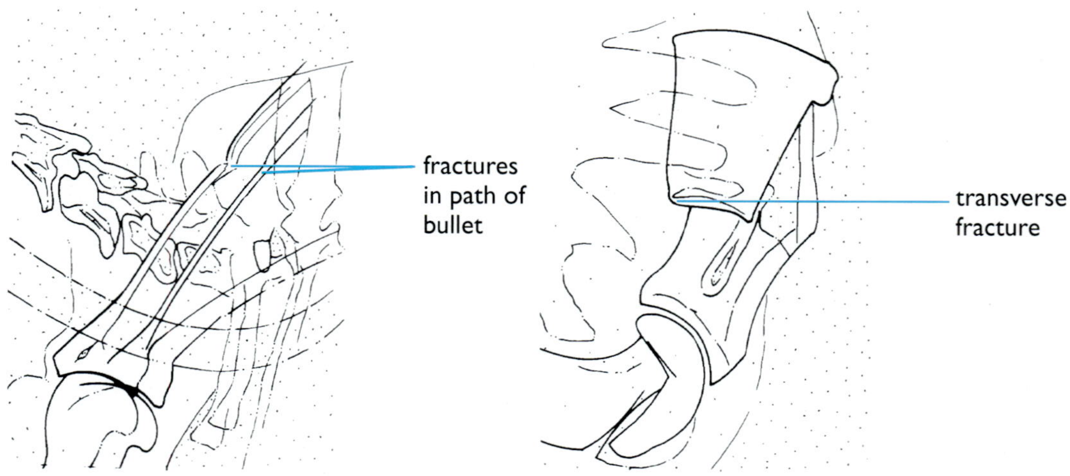

SURGICAL TECHNIQUE

An incision is made directly over the scapular spine. Cranially, the attachments of the trapezius and omotransversarius are severed to reveal the supraspinatus. Caudally, the attachments of the scapular portion of the deltoideus are incised to reveal the infraspinatus. These exposed muscles are retracted to reveal the fracture.

A series of holes is drilled along the fracture line to permit the placement of wire sutures. The fracture is reduced. Some leverage with a scalpel handle or a bone hook is required. The wires are tightened and the twisted ends are cut off and pressed against the bone (Fig. 2.2A). Closure is done by replacing the muscle bodies and suturing the fascial attachments, subcutaneous tissues, and skin. The leg is placed in a Velpeau sling, or a full foreleg wooden splint, for 3 or 4 weeks.

A more satisfactory immobilization is achieved with small bone plates, using either a plate placed cranially at the angle between the spine and the scapular body (Fig. 2.2B) or a semitubular bone plate placed upside down between the spine and the caudal aspect of the scapular body.

The angled position of the plate against the bone at the base of the spine permits the use of longer screws with a more solid seating. The plate should be long enough to accommodate three or four screws above and below the fracture line (Fig. 2.3).

The plate is first secured to the dorsal portion. The fracture is

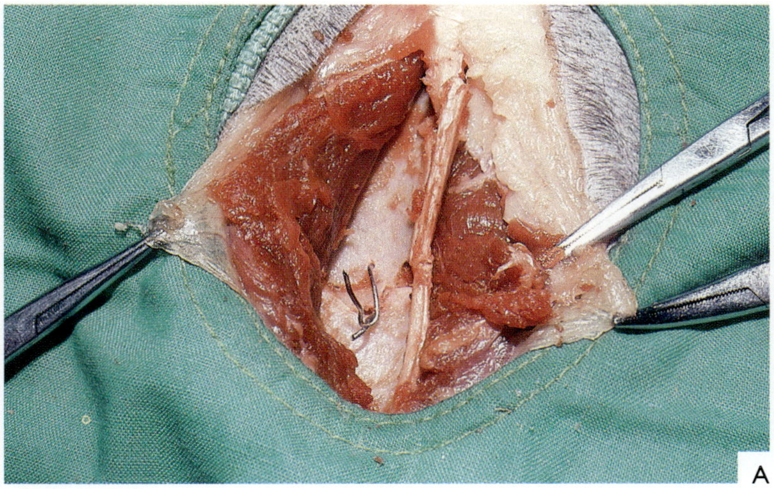
A

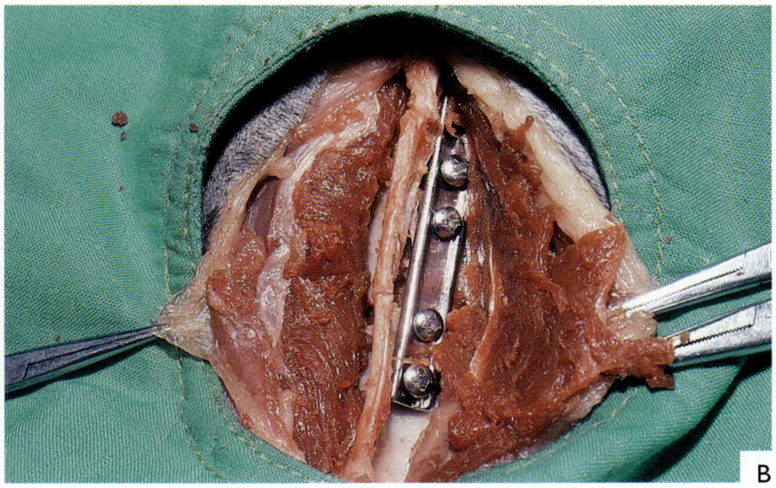
B

FIGURE 2.2 (A) Surgical exposure and wiring of a fracture of the scapular body. (B) Fracture of scapular body treated with a bone plate cranial to the spine.

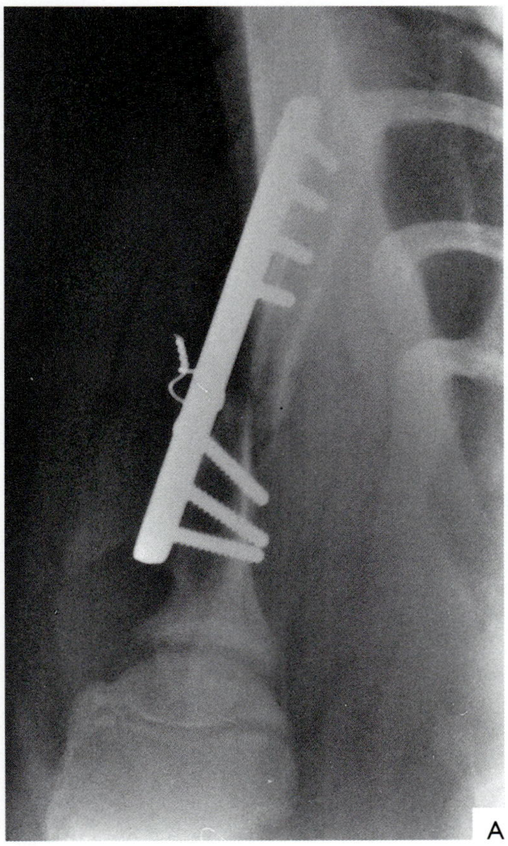
A

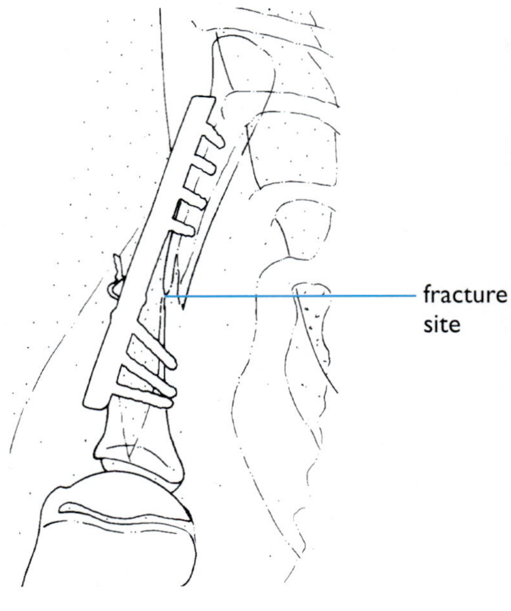

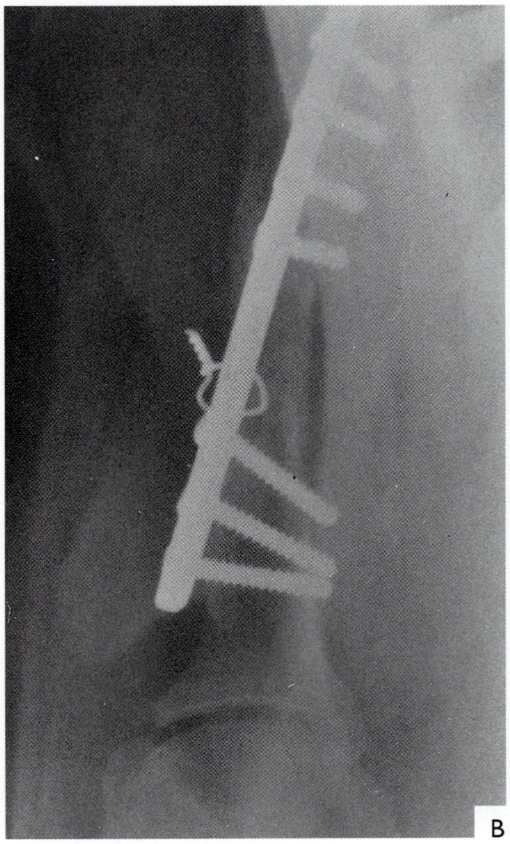
B

FIGURE 2.3 (A) Fracture of the scapular body treated with a bone plate. (B) Healing was complete in 1 month. This fracture of the scapular body was treated with a bone plate.

reduced and the screws set in the distal fragment. Surgical closure is standard. In larger dogs, support with a Velpeau sling or a full foreleg splint is applied for 2 weeks.

Scapular Neck

Fractures of the scapular neck tend to be transverse and may be associated with luxation of the shoulder. The suprascapular nerve may have been injured. Immobilization is obtained by the insertion of two K-wires, angled from both the cranial and the caudal aspects of the distal fragment into the proximal fragment.

SURGICAL TECHNIQUE

An incision is made above the distal third of the scapular spine, curving distally at the shoulder, to the lateral surface of the proximal humerus. The insertions of the deltoid and omotransversarius are severed along the scapular spine, and these muscles are retracted. The acromion deltoid is retracted after osteotomy of the acromion process. Predrilling holes through which two separate wires can be placed to reattach the osteotomized portion will ensure accurate replacement. The insertion of the supraspinatus muscle is osteotomized so that the muscle can be reflected dorsally. The tendon of insertion of the infraspinatus is transected and the infraspinatus muscle is retracted dorsally. The fracture site is exposed and the suprascapular nerve is isolated and protected. A K-wire or small intramedullary pin is inserted from the cranial aspect of the distal fragment and, with the fracture reduced, is driven into the proximal fragment. Similarly, a K-wire is driven from the caudal aspect of the distal fragment into the proximal fragment. The neck is fairly thick at this point and usually provides a solid seating for the pins.

A very secure immobilization is obtained with a small bone plate applied cranial to the scapular spine (Fig. 2.4A). The plate is placed under the suprascapular nerve. Pins and plates are left in place.

Closure is done by replacing the osteotomy of the supraspinatus with K-wires and a figure-8 tension band wire. The transection of the insertion of the infraspinatus tendon is sutured with a mattress suture of nonabsorbable material. The osteotomized acromion process is replaced and secured with two orthopedic wires placed through the previously drilled holes. The rest of the closure is routine. The leg is placed in a full foreleg wooden splint for 3 weeks (Fig. 2.4B).

Scapulohumeral Articulation

Accurate reduction and fixation is essential in these fractures to maintain the congruency of the glenoid joint surface. This requires open reduction with entry into the joint so that the surgeon can visualize the reduction.

Fractures may involve only one portion of the joint. Small chips off the edge of the glenoid that have not become reattached after rest and immobilization of the joint are surgically removed.

Larger fractures are reduced and secured with K-wires. Those involving the cranial portion of the glenoid joint will require additional support with a lag screw.

The glenoid may be split into two or more fragments in addi-

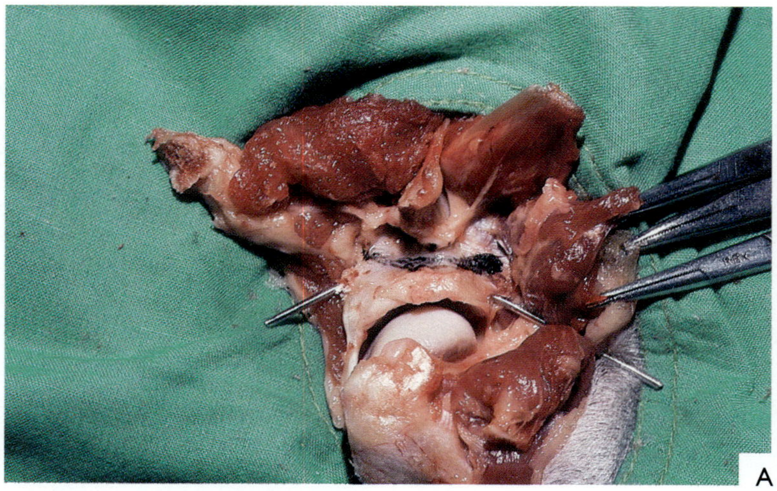

A

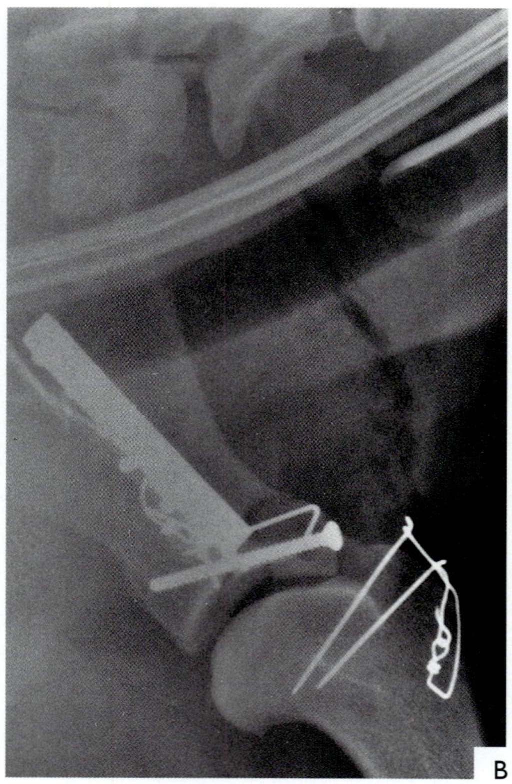

B

FIGURE 2.4 (A) Crossed K-wires inserted for treatment of fracture of the neck of the scapula. (B) Fracture of the cranial glenoid and neck of the scapula, treated with a bone plate and lag screw.

tion to a transverse fracture of the scapular neck (Fig. 2.5). The fragments constituting the joint surface are first reduced and fixed with K-wires. Then a lag screw is inserted to hold and compress them. The reconstituted fragment is secured to the rest of the scapula with K-wires.

SURGICAL TECHNIQUE

The skin and subcutaneous incision is made over the lower third of the scapular spine, directed over the lateral aspect of the joint and extended to the anconeal crest of the proximal humerus. The insertions of the deltoideus and omotransversarius are incised along the scapular spine. These muscles, along with the brachiocephalicus, are retracted to expose the supraspinatus, infraspinatus and acromion deltoid. Osteotomies of the acromion process and the greater tubercle of the humerus permit the acromion deltoid to be retracted ventrally and the supraspinatus dorsally. The tendon of insertion of the infraspinatus is transected about 1 cm from its insertion. The joint capsule is incised, and the suprascapular nerve is identified. The fragments forming the glenoid are reduced and held in place with K-wires. Small bone-holding forceps are used. A lag screw is inserted craniocaudally to secure the glenoid fragments.

After fixation of the glenoid, the combined fragments are secured to the rest of the scapula with K-wires introduced cranially and caudally or with a bone plate (see Fig. 2.4). Closure is done by suturing the joint capsule, reattaching the transected infraspinatus tendon, replacing the osteotomies of the greater tubercle and the acromion process, and suturing the fascial insertions of the deltoideus and omotransversarius. The brachiocephalicus is replaced. Regular closure is performed. The leg is placed in a full-foreleg coaptation splint for 2 weeks.

Avulsion of the Supraglenoid Tuberosity

Avulsion of the supraglenoid tuberosity is not common. It is debilitating and causes chronic lameness that is apparent with exercise and less evident after rest, but does not really improve. When the fragment is large and actually involves the cranial aspect of the glenoid, it must be repositioned. This is usually done with K-wires and, when possible, an added lag screw.

In most cases the tendon of origin of the biceps brachii has pulled away some of the bone at its attachment. Except in a fresh fracture, a lot of scar tissue is present. The avulsed bone may be multiply fragmented. In such cases, the avulsed fragments and the end of the tendon must be excised. The tendon end is secured to the humerus with a metal staple or screw and washer.

SURGICAL TECHNIQUE

The skin and subcutaneous incision is made from the acromion process, curving over the point of the shoulder to the deltoid tuberosity. This incision is undermined and retracted to expose the brachiocephalicus. Its lateral fascial edge is incised and the muscle is retracted medially. The superficial pectoral is incised at its insertion on the humerus, avoiding the distally located communicating vein. The deep pectoral is transected at its insertion on the humerus and is then separated from the suprascapular nerve. The superficial and deep pectorals are retracted medially and the belly of the supra-

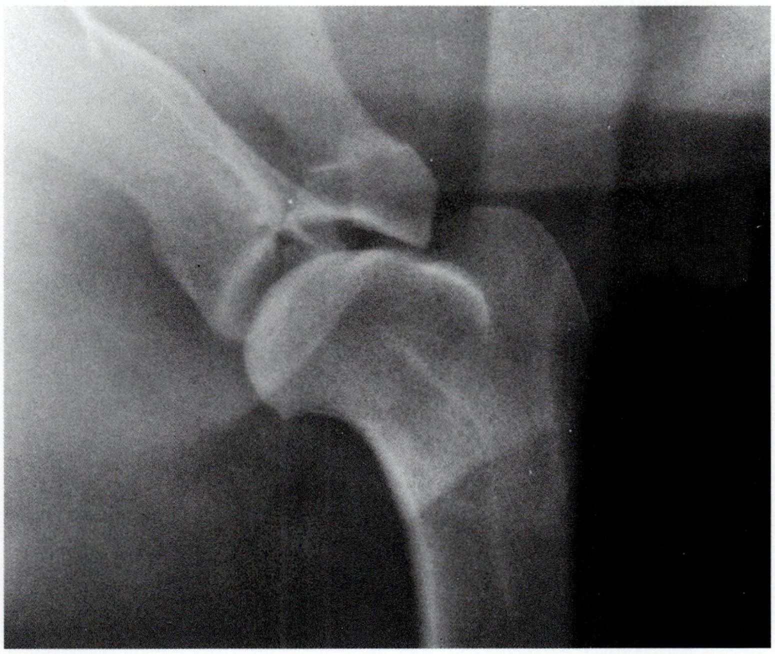

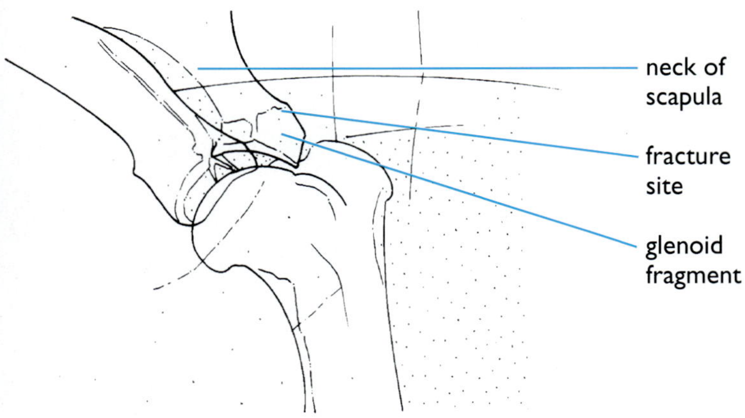

FIGURE 2.5 Radiograph of a fracture of the cranial glenoid and scapular neck.

spinatus is retracted laterally. The origin of the biceps brachii at the supraglenoid tuberosity is exposed. Fragmented pieces of bone and the involved portion of the tendon are cut off. The tendon end is secured to the head of the humerus with a staple or screw and washer at the intertubercular groove (Fig. 2.6).

Closure is done by suturing the deep and superficial pectorals to the humerus at the anconeal crest. The brachiocephalicus is replaced and the fascial incision is sutured. The rest of the closure is routine.

Fracture of the Scapular Spine

Fracture of the scapular spine is uncommon and is often quite painful. Immobilization is achieved by a series of wire sutures that secure the long fragment to the body of the scapula.

SURGICAL TECHNIQUE

The skin and subcutaneous tissues are incised over the spine of the scapula. The edges are retracted to expose the insertions of the trapezius and omotransversarius cranially and the deltoideus caudally. These are incised and the muscles are freed from underlying tissues and retracted to expose the fracture. Opposing holes are drilled in the bone of the scapular body and in the loosened fragment. A number of wires are placed and tightened to immobilize the fracture. The twisted ends are cut short and bent close to the bone (Fig. 2.7).

At closure, the supra- and infraspinatus muscles are released, the trapezius, omotransversarius, and deltoideus are resutured to the spine, and the rest of the incision is closed routinely. A Velpeau sling is used to rest the leg for a week.

FRACTURES OF THE HUMERUS

Proximal Physis

Fractures of the proximal humeral physis are uncommon and occur only in young animals before physeal closure takes place. Closed reduction can sometimes be accomplished, but is often unstable. Surgical replacement and fixation with two parallel small intramedullary pins or K-wires is preferred. The danger of premature fusion is reduced by use of pins driven straight through the epiphysis rather than crossed pins or a lag screw, both of which compress the physis and promote fusion.

SURGICAL TECHNIQUE

A craniolateral incision is made from the point of the shoulder to mid-humerus. The brachiocephalicus muscle is exposed, the deep fascia on its lateral border is incised, and the muscle is isolated and retracted cranially. The fracture site is exposed.

Leverage and angulation are required to replace the epiphysis onto the blocklike end of the humerus. One or (preferably) two small intramedullary pins or K-wires are driven from the cranial aspect of the greater tubercle across the physis and into the humeral diaphysis. The pin ends are bent at right angles, cut off, and driven close to the bone.

Closure consists of suturing the fascia of the brachiocephalicus back into place. The skin and subcutaneous tissues are closed in the usual manner.

Diaphyseal Fractures of the Humerus

All diaphyseal humeral fractures have the potential for injury to the radial nerve (Fig. 2.8), which can be either temporary or permanent. The animal's neurologic status should be established before extensive surgery is performed.

Transverse or Short Oblique Fractures

Transverse or short oblique fractures respond well to intramedullary pinning. Increased stability is obtained by external fixation with a K/E apparatus, consisting of a single connecting bar with single pins inserted proximally and distally. Increasing the number of pins provides a marked improvement in stability.

SURGICAL TECHNIQUE

A craniolateral approach is made by an incision through the skin and subcutaneous tissue slightly lateral to the cranial midline. It can

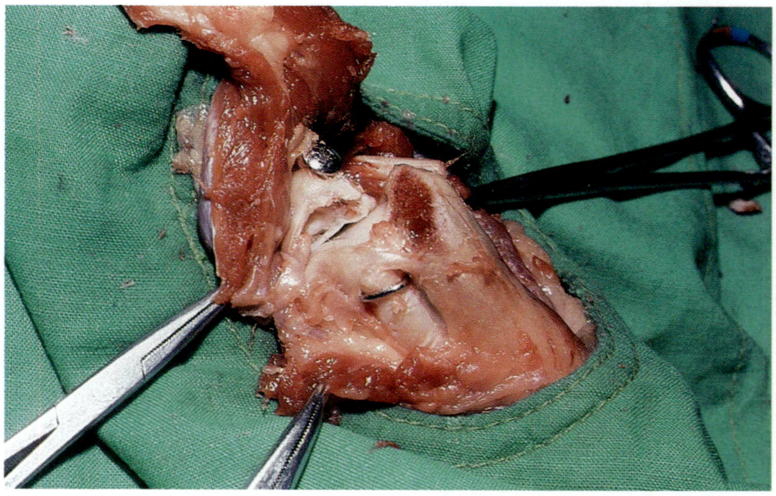

FIGURE 2.6 Tendon of origin of the biceps brachii secured to the humerus with a staple.

three, or four pins are inserted (Fig. 2.10). An additional connecting bar will provide further strength and stability.

In larger dogs, the fragments are reduced, held with small K-wires, and secured with two or more lag screws. External fixation (Fig. 2.11) or a neutralizing bone plate is applied to the cranial surface of the bone (Fig. 2.12). This location requires less contouring and decreases the risk of injury to the radial nerve.

Closure is done by reattaching the insertions of the brachialis and the lateral head of the triceps. If other, more cranial, muscles had to be elevated, they are also re-placed and sutured. The deep fascia of the brachiocephalicus is sutured. Standard closure of the skin and subcutaneous tissues is performed.

Comminuted Fractures

Comminuted fractures, especially of the more distal diaphysis, are extremely common. A lateral or medial surgical approach can be taken. In the lateral approach, the incision avoids the cephalic vein, which is retracted and preserved. The radial nerve is carefully protected. It can be retracted either dorsally or ventrally as required.

SURGICAL TECHNIQUE

A craniolateral approach is made through the skin and subcutaneous tissues from the midshaft to the lateral condyle. The cephalic vein is isolated and retracted cranially. The deep brachial fascia is incised along the insertion of the lateral head of the triceps, preserving the cephalic vein. Distally, the radial nerve is isolated and retracted. The fascia between the brachiocephalicus and the brachialis is incised and the muscles are retracted to expose the fracture site. Blood and clots are flushed away with Ringer's solution or saline. All possible fragments are preserved. The fragments are fastened into position by use of a power drill and short K-wires. Cerclage wires are applied at strategic locations. Where possible, lag screws are inserted. The major fragments are attached to either the proximal or distal portion. Traction and angulation are used to achieve final reduction, which is held in place with bone forceps until the K-wires can be inserted. Cerclage wires or lag screws are applied.

A bone plate is contoured to fit craniolaterally and is applied in the neutralization mode. Cancellous bone grafts are placed to stimulate healing.

When there is insufficient solid bone caudally to provide seating for a bone plate, an external fixation splint, consisting of a single connecting bar and several clamps, can be applied. The first pin is inserted perpendicular to the condyle from the lateral epicondyle to the medial epicondyle. The second pin is inserted into the proximal and distal fragments at an angle in the most proximal portion. Several other pins are placed into the proximal and distal fragments at strategic angles.

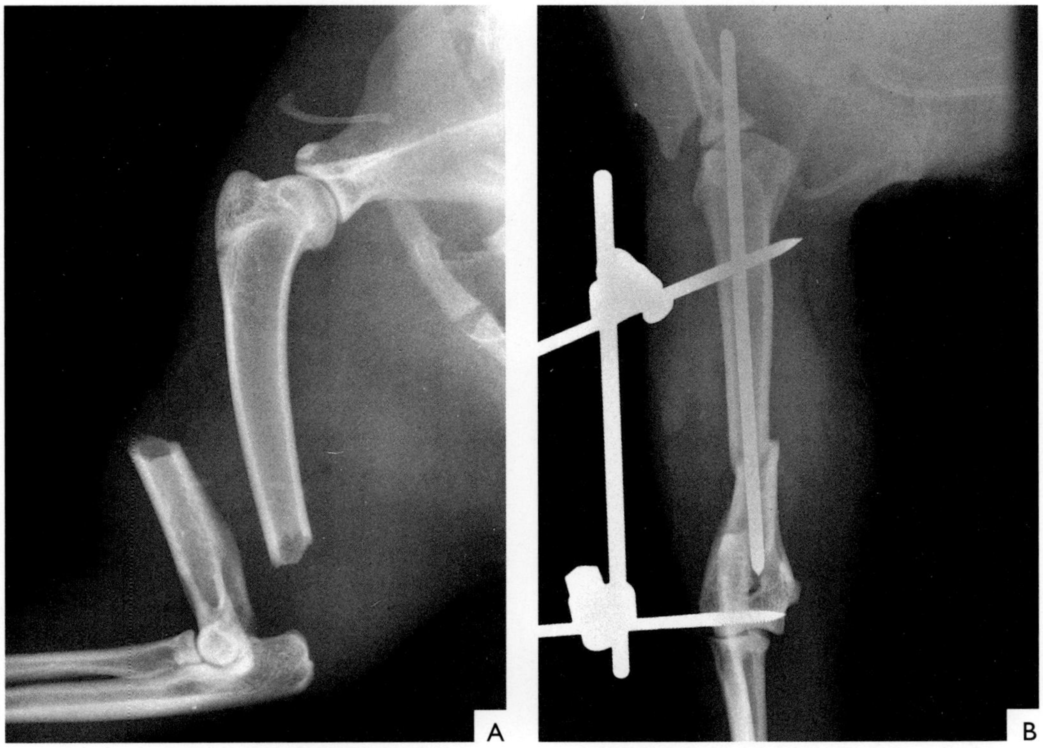

FIGURE 2.10 (A) Transverse midshaft fracture of the humerus in a cat. (B) Transverse midshaft fracture of the humerus treated with an IM pin and ancillary external fixation.

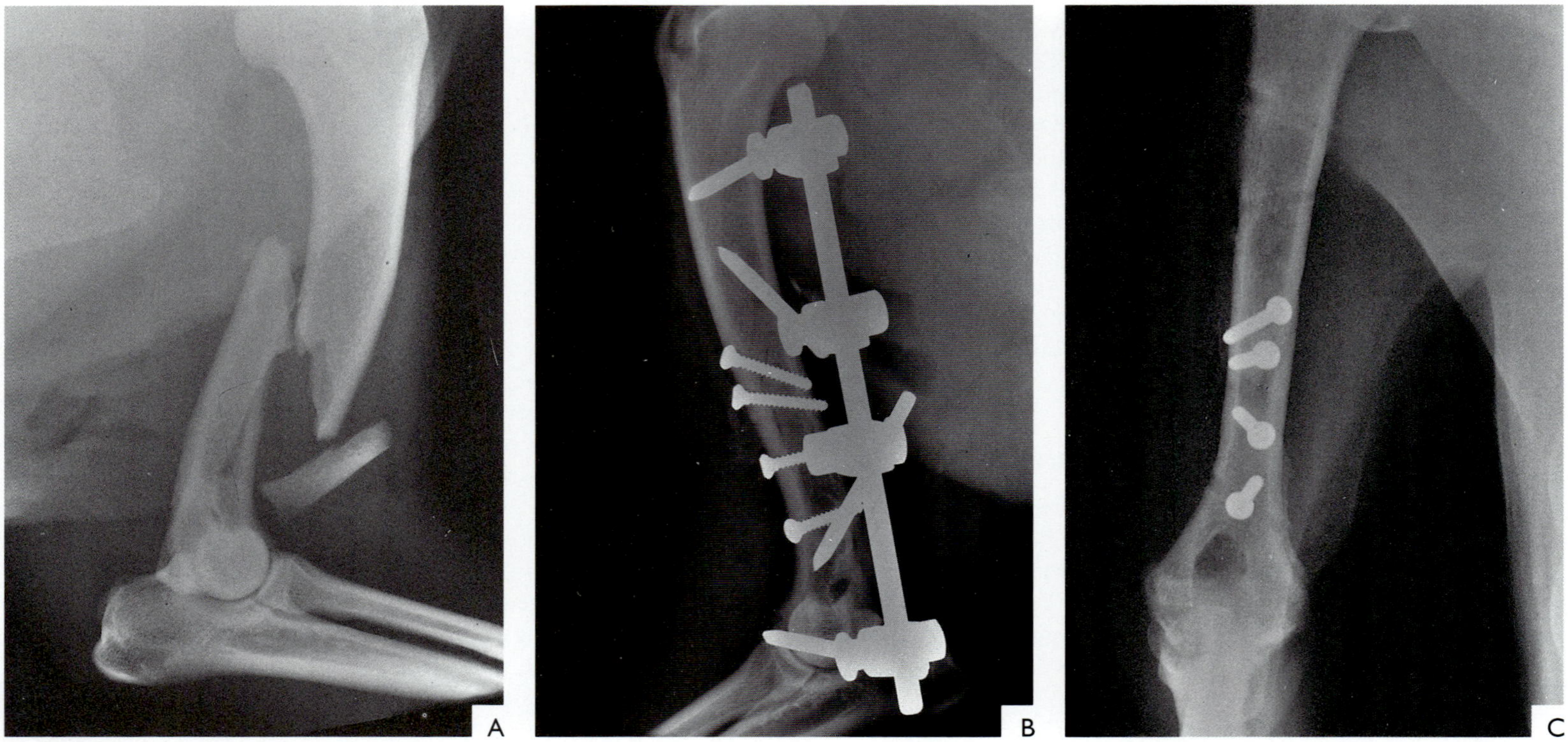

FIGURE 2.11 (A) This oblique fracture of the humerus shows a large loose fragment. (B) An oblique fracture of the humerus with a large loose fragment is treated by multiple lag screws and an external fixation splint. (C) An oblique fracture of the humerus with a large loose fragment after removal of the external fixation splint. The lag screws will remain.

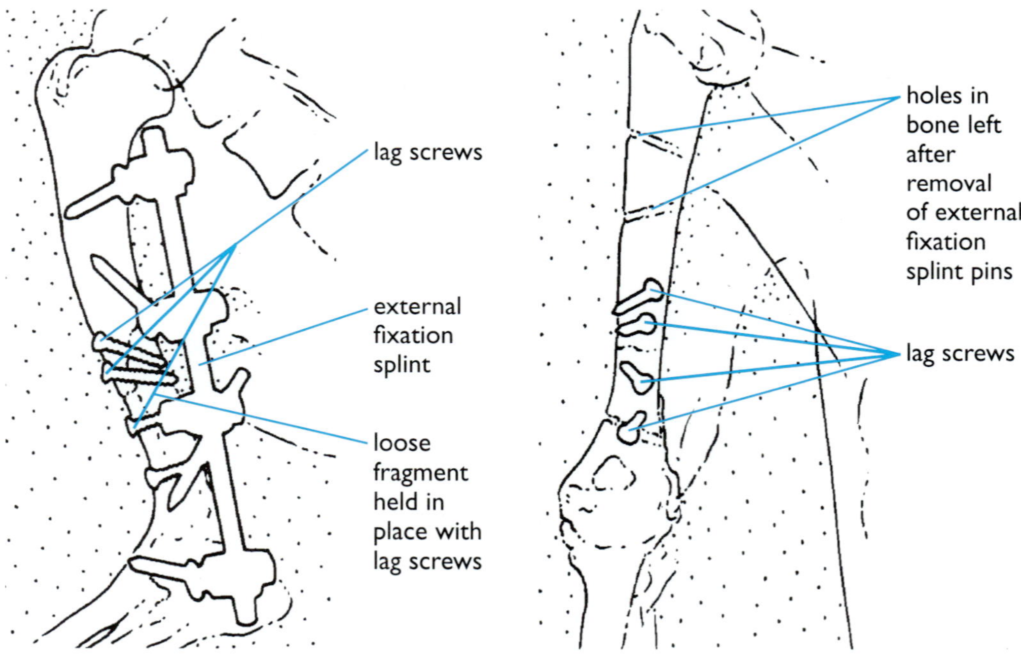

A second connecting bar above the first adds to the fixation's strength. Threaded pins in predrilled and tapped holes offer the best security and protection against loosening.

External fixation devices must not contact the body, and the skin at the sites of pin entry must not be under tension. The apparatus is wrapped in cotton and bandaged for protection.

Closure is performed by suturing the deep fascial attachment of the lateral head of the triceps and the fascial attachments of the brachialis and brachiocephalicus. Skin and subcutaneous tissues are closed in the usual manner.

Gunshot Fractures

Gunshot fractures are unfortunately rather common. The bone is markedly fragmented and the wounds are contaminated. Air pellets cause less severe damage and can be removed. Bullets of larger caliber can cause severe injury (Figs. 2.13, 2.14). Thorough debridement is needed. Immobilization of the fracture with external fixation permits stabilization, some joint-sparing use of the limb, and the opportunity to treat the soft tissue injuries (Figs. 2.15, 2.16).

Distal Condylar Fractures

Distal condylar fractures are probably the most common fractures of the humerus, frequently involving the supracondylar portion of the shaft. The most serious aspect of such fractures is the involvement of the elbow joint. The articular surfaces must be congruent to avoid osteoarthritis. In almost all cases open reduction must be performed, although in some fractures of the lateral condyle closed reduction and immobilization are possible.

Fractures can involve either medial or lateral parts of the condyle, or both. When combined with a fracture of the distal

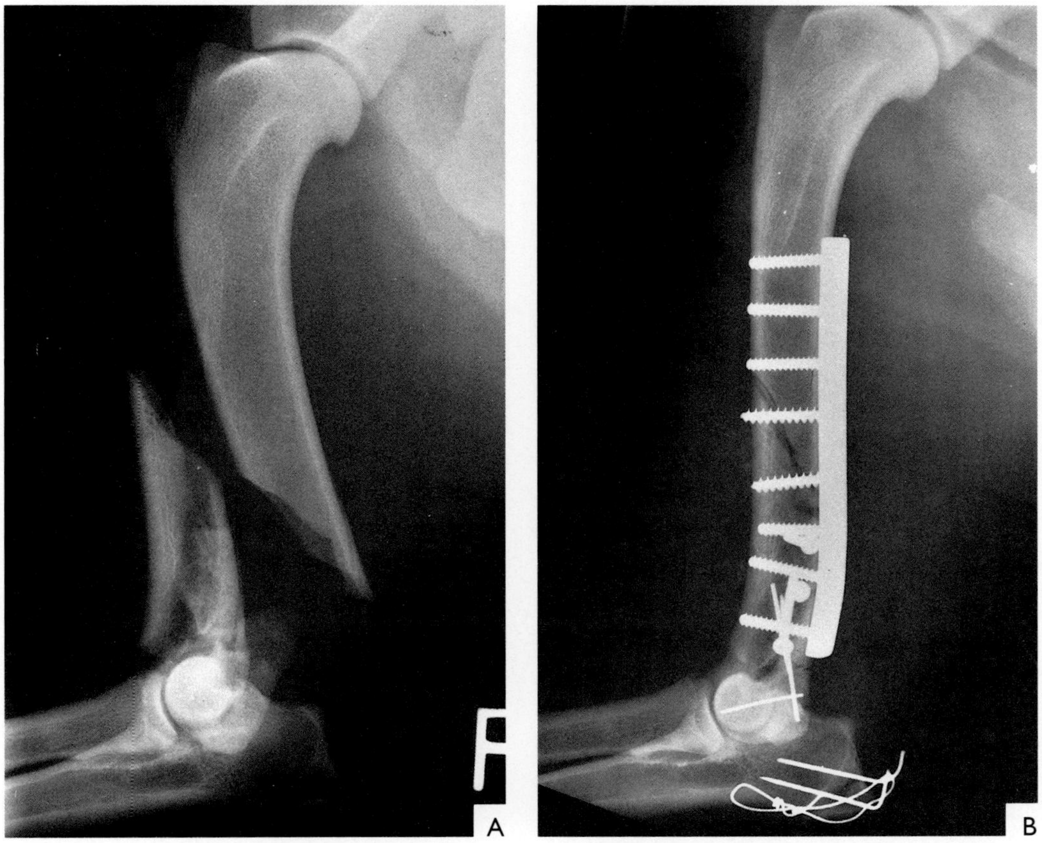

FIGURE 2.12 (A) Radiograph of oblique distal third and distal fractures of the humerus. (B) Radiograph of the surgical repair of oblique distal third and distal humeral fractures with K-wires and lag screw. A bone plate in the neutralization mode has been applied.

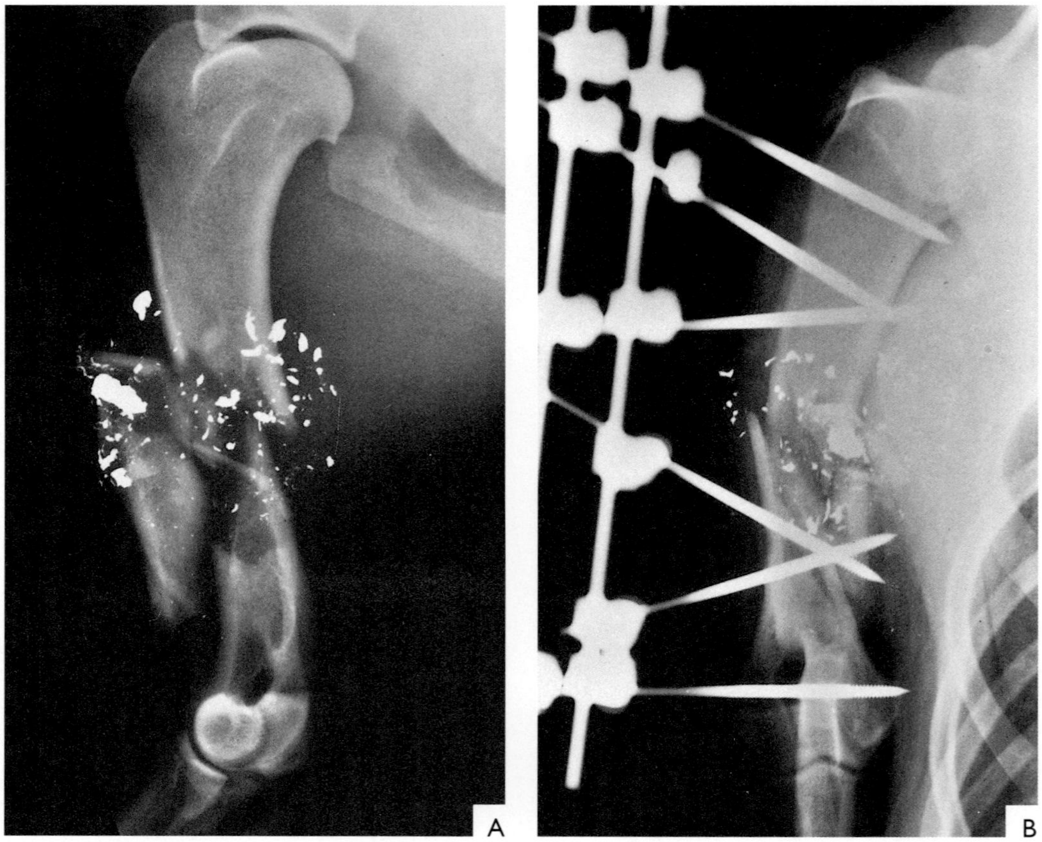

FIGURE 2.13 (A) Gunshot fracture of the humerus. (B) Same fracture, treated with an external fixation splint.

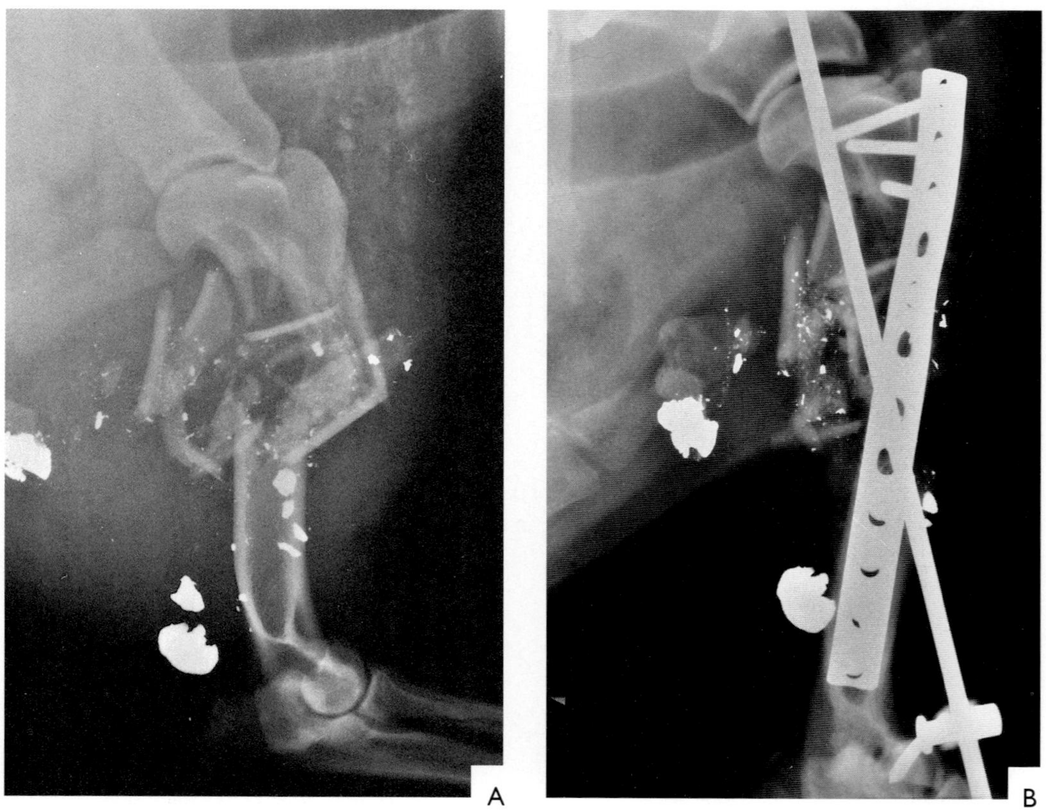

FIGURE 2.14 (A) Gunshot fracture of the humerus. (B) Gunshot fracture of the humerus treated with a bone plate and external fixation. Insufficient solid bone in the proximal fragment required placement of the external fixation device in the neck of the scapula.

humeral shaft they form a T- or Y-fracture. The condylar fragments must be exactly aligned and held by pins or a lag screw. The reconstructed condyle is then secured to the humeral shaft by intramedullary pinning, pinning through the condyle into the humeral shaft (Figs. 2.17, 2.18), a modified Rush pin technique, or bone plating.

An intramedullary pin is driven through the entire medullary cavity and is seated in the area of the medial condylar fragment. In addition, a small pin is inserted through the bone constituting the epicondyloid crest of the lateral condylar fragment and is seated in the medial cortex of the distal humeral shaft. For larger dogs, a lag screw is used at this location.

Flexible pins are inserted from the medial and lateral condylar fragments into the medullary cavity of the humeral shaft, similar to placement of Rush pins.

In some cases, small bone plates can be used. Open reduction of the elbow for a lateral condylar fracture is performed by a simple craniolateral approach. Almost all more complicated fractures require open reduction with an osteotomy of the olecranon.

SURGICAL TECHNIQUE

For the approach to the lateral condyle, an incision is made through the skin and subcutaneous tissues over the distal fourth of the humerus, just caudal to the lateral epicondyle. Further dissection reveals the lateral edge of the triceps. The deep fascia is incised along the border of the muscle to expose the lateral condylar bone underneath. The radial nerve lies cranially and must be protected. The loose condylar fragment is reduced and held in place with a vulsellum forceps or other bone forceps (Fig. 2.19). A transcondylar pin or K-wire is inserted through the bone of the epicondyloid crest and into the medial cortex of the humeral shaft (Fig. 2.20).

A lag screw is now inserted across the condylar fragments. The transcondylar K-wire can be retained or removed (Fig. 2.21). In large dogs, a lag screw is used to secure the condylar shaft in position (Fig. 2.22). Closure is done by suturing the deep fascia, subcutaneous fascia, and skin in layers.

Fractures of the medial portion of the condyle can be repaired similarly to those of the lateral portion but using an approach over the medial condylar area. This is an extension of the medial approach to the distal humeral shaft.

The skin and subcutaneous tissues are incised from the medial epicondyle to the distal third of the humerus. The brachial artery and vein are identified and retracted. The deep fascia is carefully incised over the bone between the biceps brachii as well as the long and medial heads of the triceps. The median nerve is isolated and retracted.

The loose condylar fragment is reduced and secured in place with a transcondylar K-wire, and a lag screw is inserted. A K-wire is inserted caudally and driven through the medial condylar shaft into the humeral shaft to stabilize the fracture. In large dogs, a lag screw is placed at the cranial fracture site.

Fractures involving both condylar fragments and the distal humerus are called T- or Y-fractures, depending on their location. An open reduction with osteotomy of the olecranon must be performed.

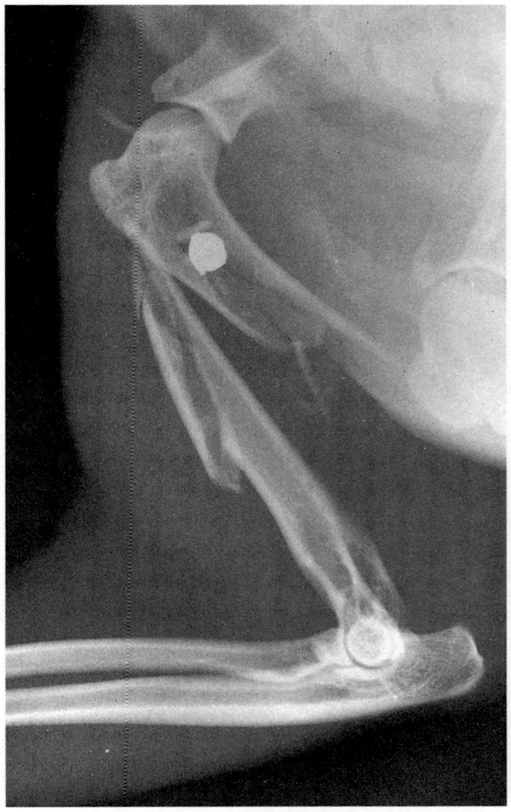

FIGURE 2.15 Radiograph of a gunshot fracture of the humerus of a cat.

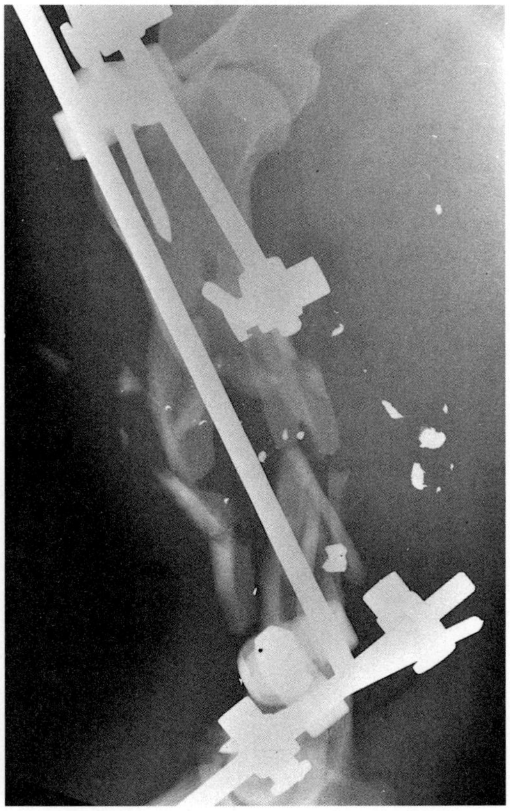

FIGURE 2.16 This gunshot fracture of the humerus was treated with an external fixation splint.

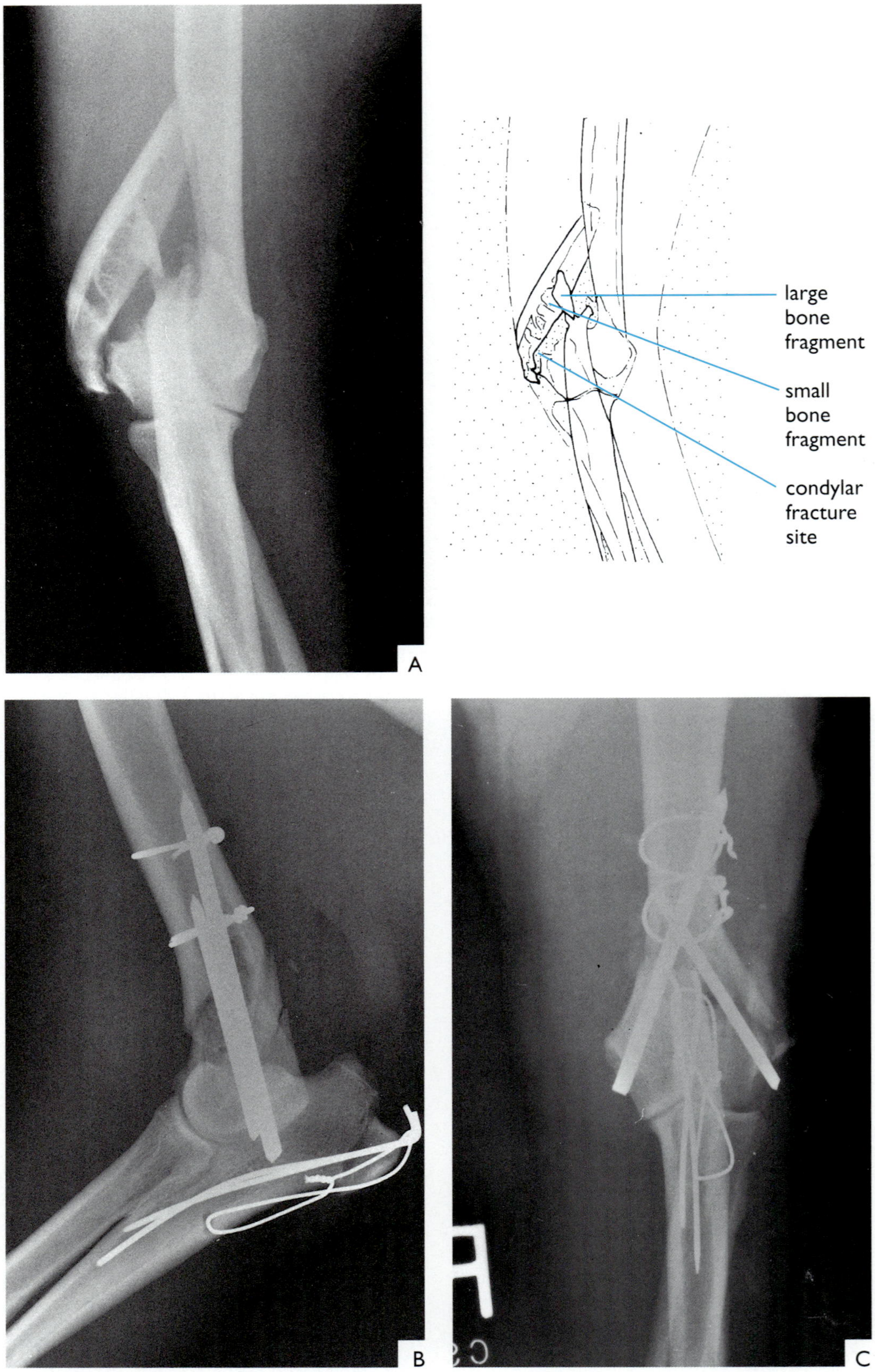

FIGURE 2.17 (A) Distal humeral and condylar fracture with a large loose fragment. (B) Lateral radiograph of a distal humeral and condylar fracture with a large loose fragment treated with short IM pins inserted from the caudolateral condylar surfaces to insert in the distal humeral medullary cavity. Fragment control was obtained with cerclage wires. (C) The distal humeral and condylar fracture shows good healing 8 weeks after surgery.

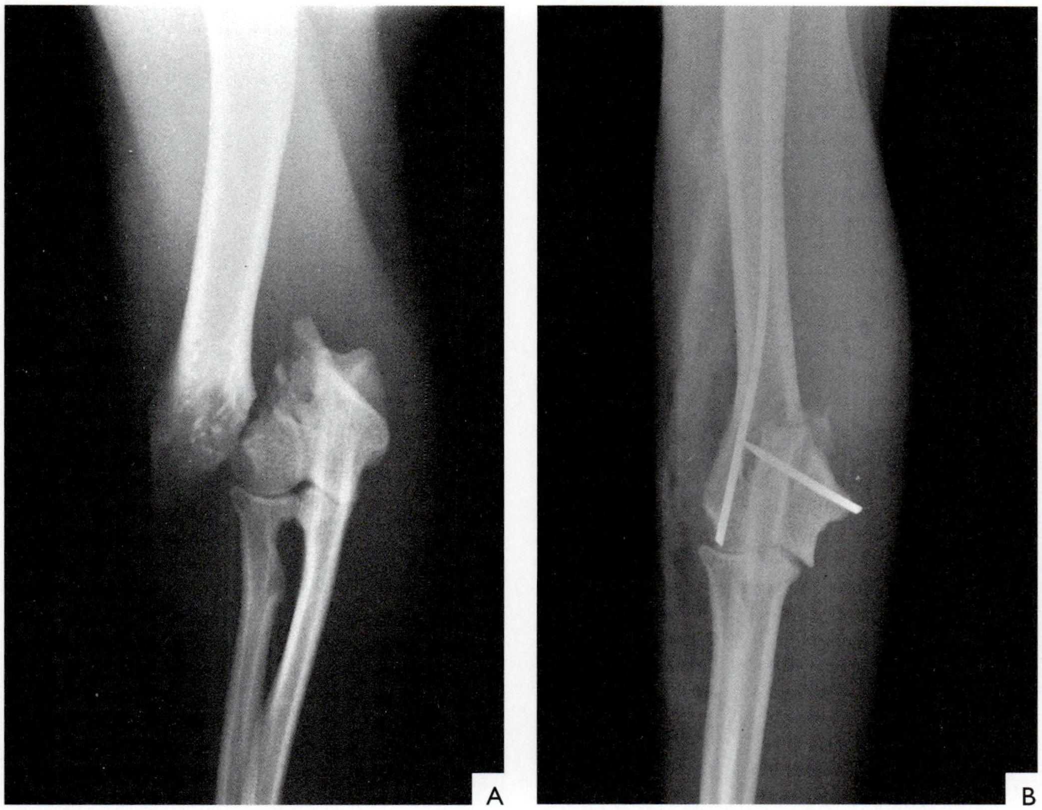

FIGURE 2.18 (A) Distal humeral and condylar fracture in a cat. (B) Distal humeral and condylar fracture treated with a long flexible pin inserted up the humeral medullary cavity from the medial condyle and a short K-wire in the lateral condylar portion.

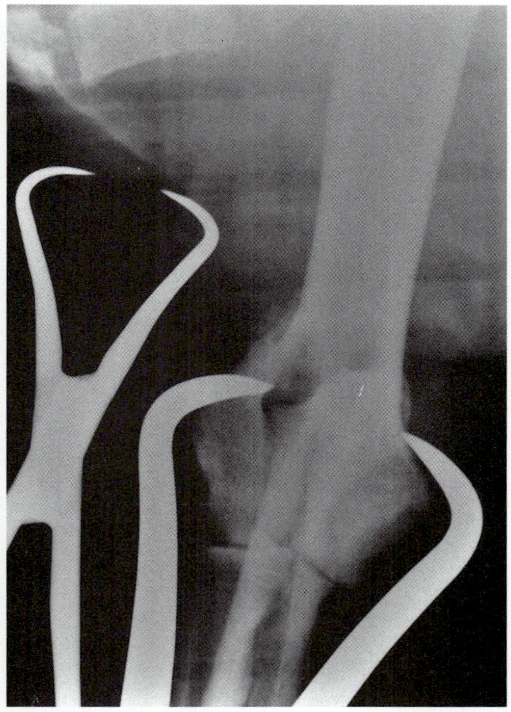

FIGURE 2.19 This condylar fragment is held in position by forceps.

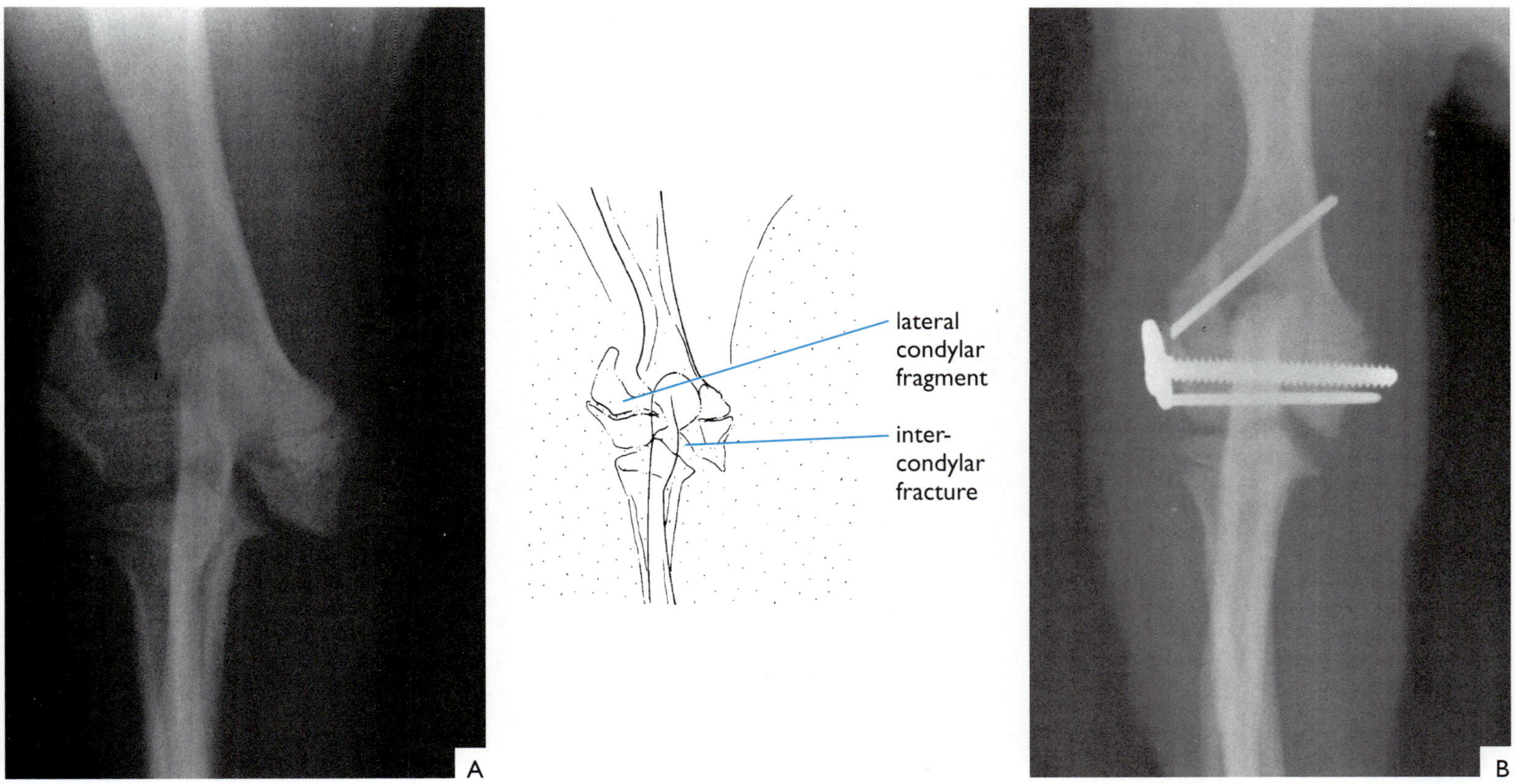

FIGURE 2.20 (A) Lateral condylar fracture. (B) Lateral condylar fracture treated with a K-wire and lag screw in the lateral epicondylar ridge. In this case it was not necessary to osteotomize the olecranon.

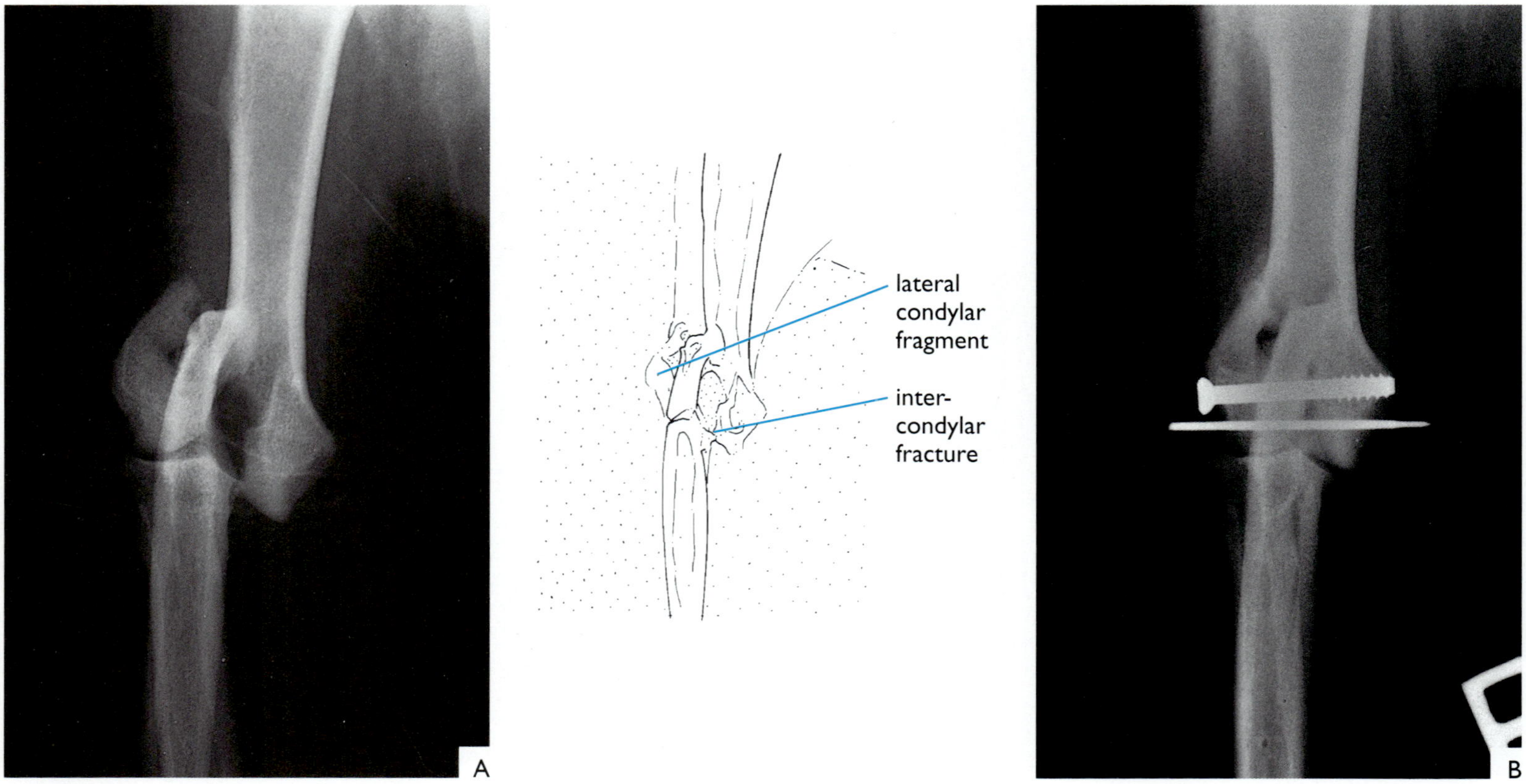

FIGURE 2.21 (A) Lateral fracture of the humeral condyle. (B) Lateral fracture of the humeral condyle treated with a K-wire and lag screw.

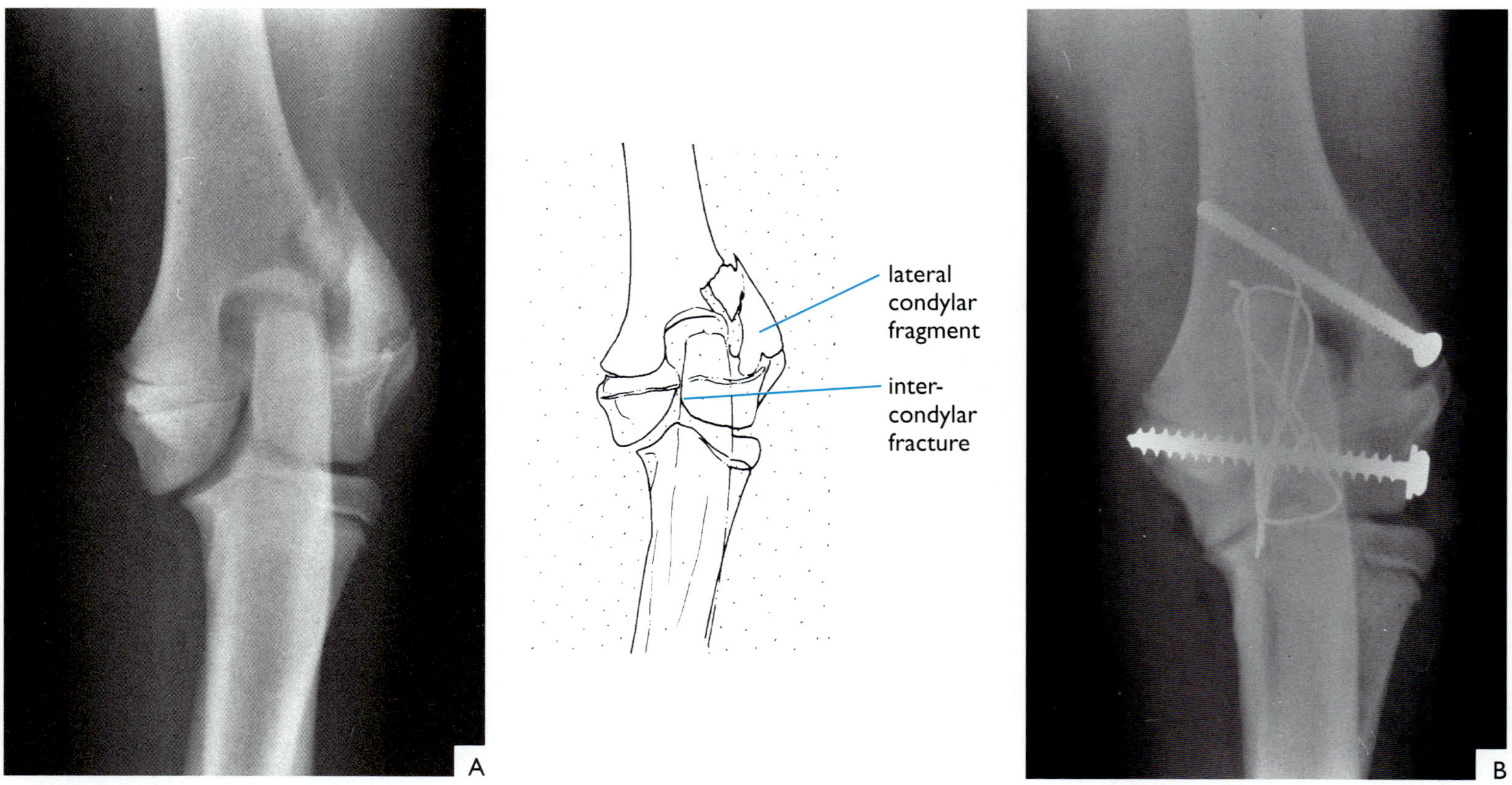

FIGURE 2.22 (A) A large dog suffered a fracture of the lateral condyle of the humerus. (B) Same fracture, treated with two lag screws and osteotomy of the olecranon.

A caudally curved incision extending from the caudal midline of the humerus to the proximal ulna is made, passing midway between the olecranon and the lateral epicondyle. The skin and subcutaneous tissues are reflected and an incision is made through the anconeal attachment to the olecranon, entering the joint. The skin is further undermined to enable it to be retracted and reflected over the olecranon as far as the medial epicondyle. The triceps fascia is exposed. The ulnar nerve lies medially under this fascia.

To provide accurate repositioning of the olecranon that is to be osteotomized, it is predrilled with a small intramedullary pin. A Gigli wire bone saw is inserted above the anconeal process and a straight caudal cut is made. The triceps and the surrounding fascia are elevated and retracted to permit visualization of the joint. The joint is flushed with saline and the fragments are identified. Flexion of the joint permits inspection of the articular surface under the anconeal process.

An elbow clamp, bone clamp, or vulsellum forceps is used to hold the condylar fragments in apposition. A transcondylar K-wire is inserted. The area just below the lateral and medial epicondyles is the site for a lag screw. Once the two fragments are secured, the reconstituted condyle is reattached to the distal humerus. A double-pointed intramedullary pin is run retrograde up the humeral shaft to exit beneath and somewhat lateral to the greater tubercle. The fracture is reduced and the pin is driven into the medial condylar portion and seated firmly. The pin is cut off under the skin.

A smaller intramedullary pin is introduced from the caudolateral aspect of the lateral condylar surface and driven through the length of the lateral condylar shaft into the humerus. It is usually at an angle so that it penetrates the distal medial humeral cortex. The pin is cut off close to the bone. In larger dogs, a lag screw is used (Figs. 2.23, 2.24).

Another method is to insert flexible, small-diameter intramedullary pins from the caudolateral and caudomedial surfaces of the condyle to pass across the fracture site and impinge on the cortical bone of the humeral shaft. The pins are, in effect, used as Rush pins. They do not penetrate the cortices but slide along them internally. The spring tension secures the pins (Fig. 2.25).

In larger dogs, the most secure control is obtained by placing small bone plates on the medial and lateral condylar shafts. This requires a larger amount of exposure and careful dissection.

Closure is performed by replacing the osteotomized olecranon fragment and placing a small intramedullary pin or K-wire in the previously drilled location. This ensures accurate replacement. A second pin is inserted cranial to the first to control rotation. A figure-8 tension band wire is placed over the caudal pin and through a transverse hole drilled through the ulna a few centimeters below the osteotomy site. Each pin is bent at a right angle and cut off. The ends are turned cranially and tapped in close to the bone (Fig. 2.26).

In closure, the anconeal incision needs no sutures. The skin and subcutaneous tissues are brought back over the olecranon and sutured in the usual manner.

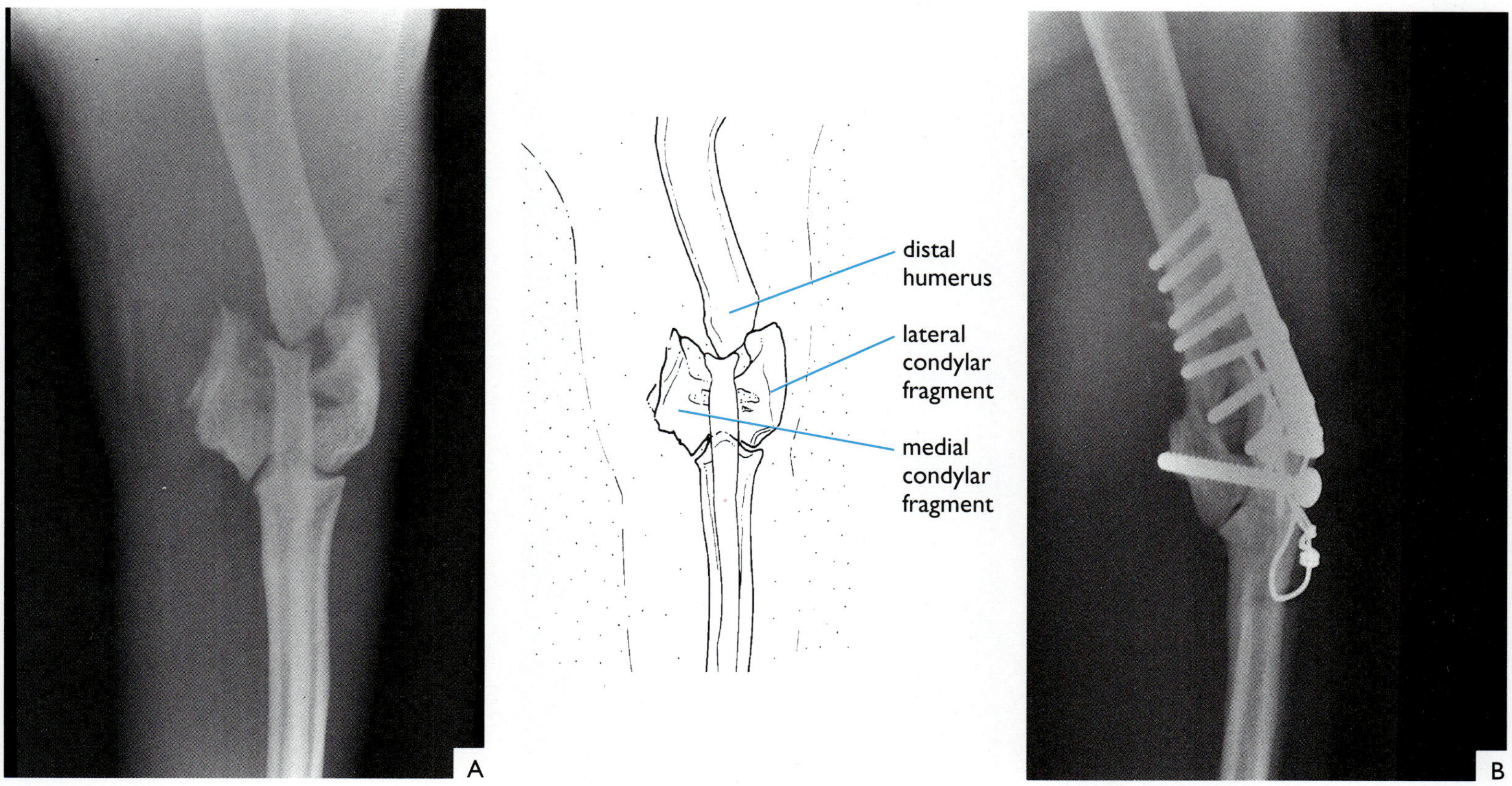

FIGURE 2.23 (A) AP lateral radiograph of a distal humeral and condylar fracture. (B) Radiograph of a distal humeral and condylar fracture treated with a bone plate and a lag screw. An olecranon osteotomy was done.

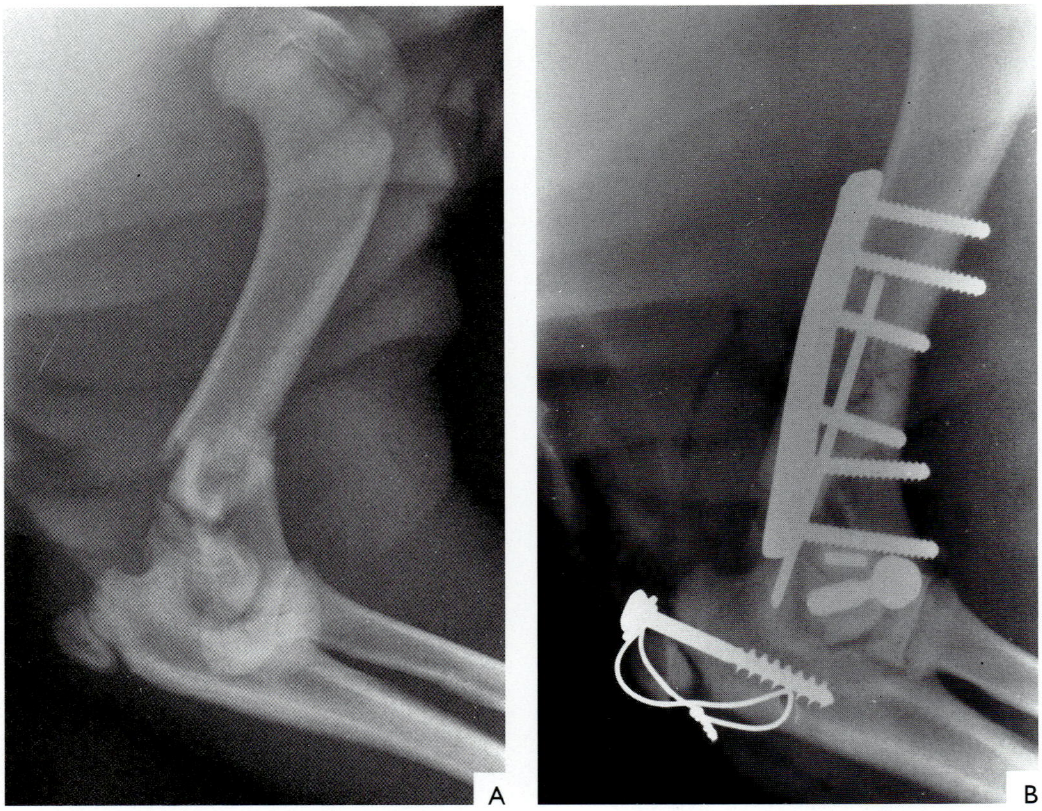

FIGURE 2.24 (A) Lateral radiograph of a distal humeral and condylar fracture. (B) Lateral radiograph of a distal humeral and condylar fracture treated with a bone plate, lag screw, and a small IM pin in the lateral condylar shaft.

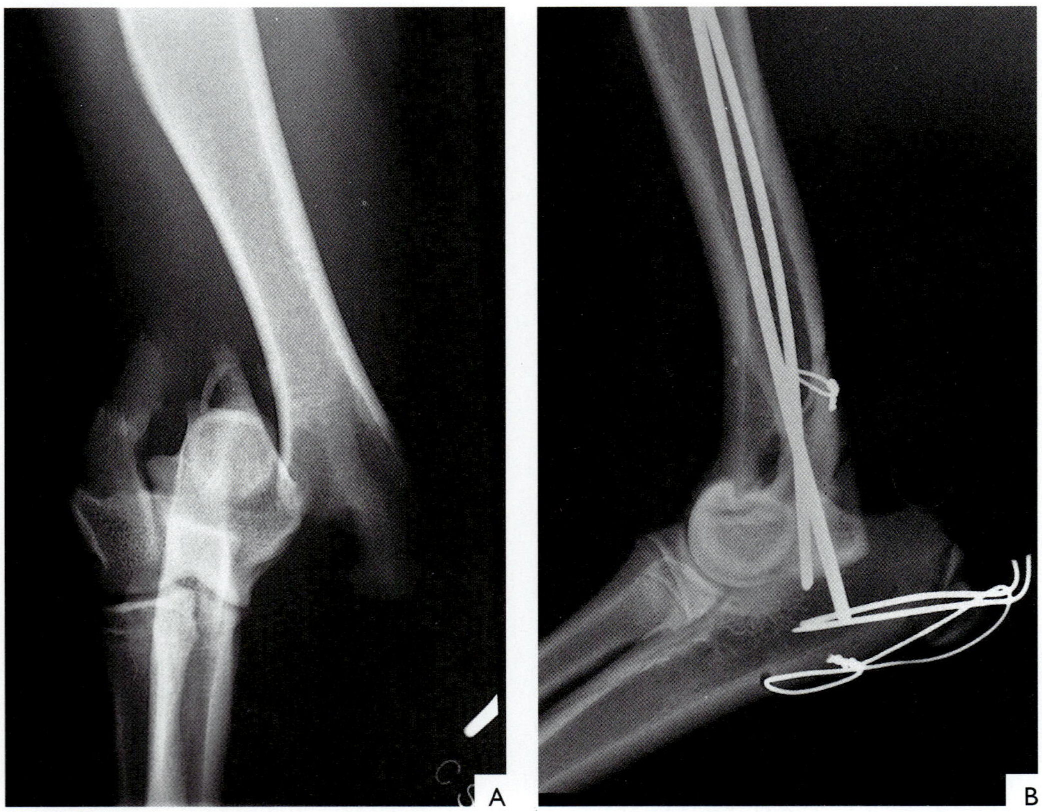

FIGURE 2.25 (A) Distal humeral fracture. (B) Distal humeral fracture treated with flexible IM pins inserted from the caudolateral surfaces of the condyle in the Rush pin mode.

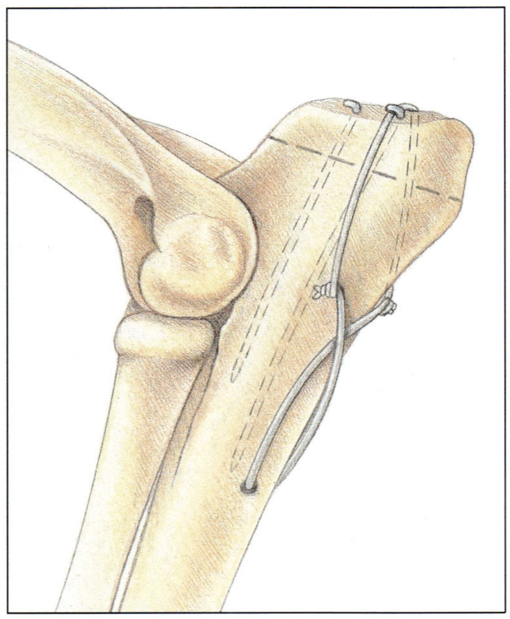

FIGURE 2.26 Location of cut and placement of pins and figure-8 tension wire in osteotomy of the olecranon.

A modified Robert Jones splint is applied for a few days. The dog's activity is restricted, but some use of the limb is allowed to ensure recovery with a good range of motion. A certain degree of osteoarthritis is expected where any joint has been affected, especially as the animal becomes older.

An alternate method of placing a lag screw can be used to reposition a split between the medial and lateral portions of the humeral condyle: a hole is drilled from the center of the fracture site of the lateral fragment to exit on the lateral epicondylar surface. The drill is reversed and, with the fragments approximated, the hole is drilled further through the medial condylar fragment. The hole in the lateral fragment is overdrilled.

A screw inserted in the lateral epicondylar hole will turn freely. It will seat in the hole in the medial condylar fragment, lagging the two together.

FRACTURES OF THE RADIUS AND ULNA

Fractures of the radius and ulna are very common in the dog and cat, and can occur anywhere along the length of the bones. Fractures that involve articular surfaces must be realigned to preserve the congruity of the joint. The pull of the triceps distracts fractures of the olecranon and proximal ulna. Opposition to this force is obtained by the use of tension band wires and plates. Surgical exposures of fractures that involve the head of the radius require special care to avoid injury to the radial nerve.

The most common fracture sites are the midshaft and the distal third. Fractures involving the distal epiphyses and carpal joint usually require open reduction and secure fixation.

In all immature patients, there is the possibility of epiphyseal injury with premature fusion, causing interference with growth and subsequent articular damage. Premature fusion of the distal ulnar epiphysis results in radius curvus (Fig. 2.27). Complete or partial fusion of the distal radial epiphysis leads to marked deviational deformities (Fig. 2.28). Premature fusion of the distal radial epiphysis results in progressive damage to the elbow joint (Fig. 2.29). The primary injuries may be subtle and not immediately recognizable. All owners should be warned of this possibility.

There is a tendency to use casts and splints for reasons of expense or expediency. Some simple greenstick fractures of the

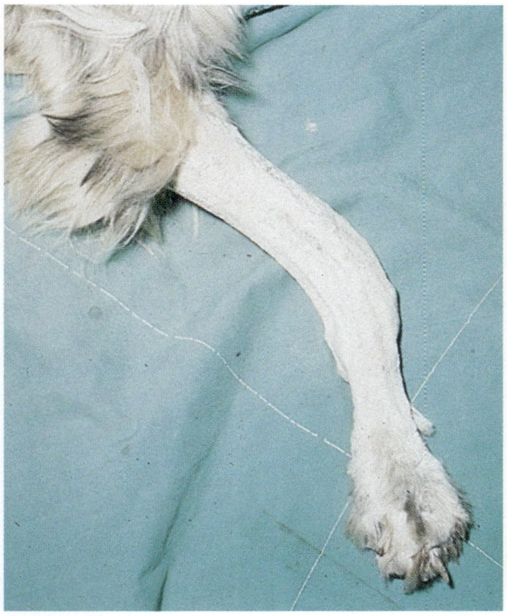

FIGURE 2.27 Radius curvus in a dog, the result of premature fusion of the distal ulnar epiphysis.

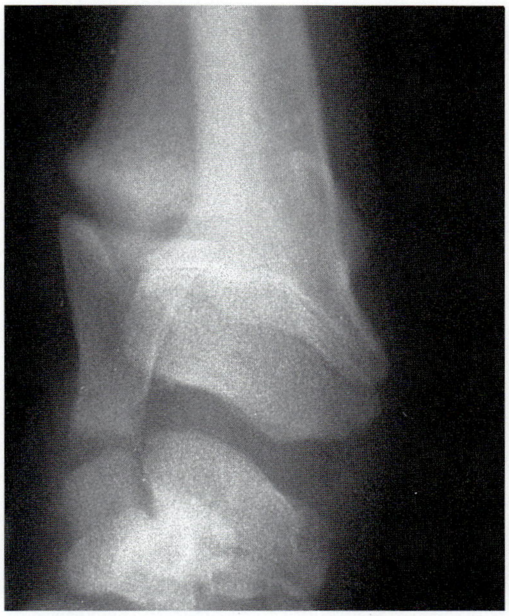

FIGURE 2.28 This radiograph of the distal radius shows the deformity resulting from a partial lateral fusion of the distal radial epiphysis.

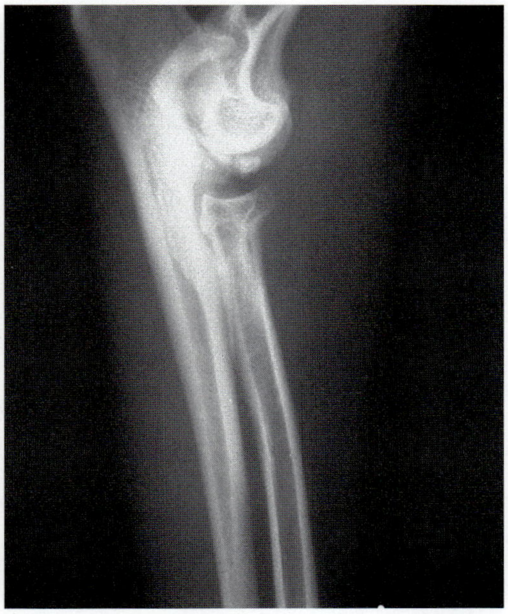

FIGURE 2.29 This dog had elbow joint deformity and ulnar coronoid fracture resulting from premature fusion of the distal radial epiphysis.

radius can be successfully treated in this way (Fig. 2.30). These older methods require expertise in their application and constant supervision of the patient to achieve reasonably good results. More modern methods, using bone plates and other forms of internal fixation, and external fixation have less potential for complications such as malunion, nonunion, delayed healing, stiff joints, pressure, sores, pain, and discomfort to the patient.

A particularly disturbing problem is the development of atrophic nonunion in the toy breeds and in cats. Distal fractures of the radius and ulna in these little animals cannot be satisfactorily treated with casts and splints (Fig. 2.31) because the necessary immobilization is not obtained and the small distal fragments are absorbed. Open reduction with adequate fixation by means of small bone plates (Fig. 2.32), or external fixation plus a cancellous bone graft at the fracture site, is required. Delay in treatment can be disastrous.

Olecranon/Proximal Ulna

Anatomically, the olecranon is that part of the proximal ulna above a line drawn transversely through the middle of the trochlear notch. Fractures can range from avulsion at the insertion of the triceps to multiply fragmented fractures. It is much more common for the

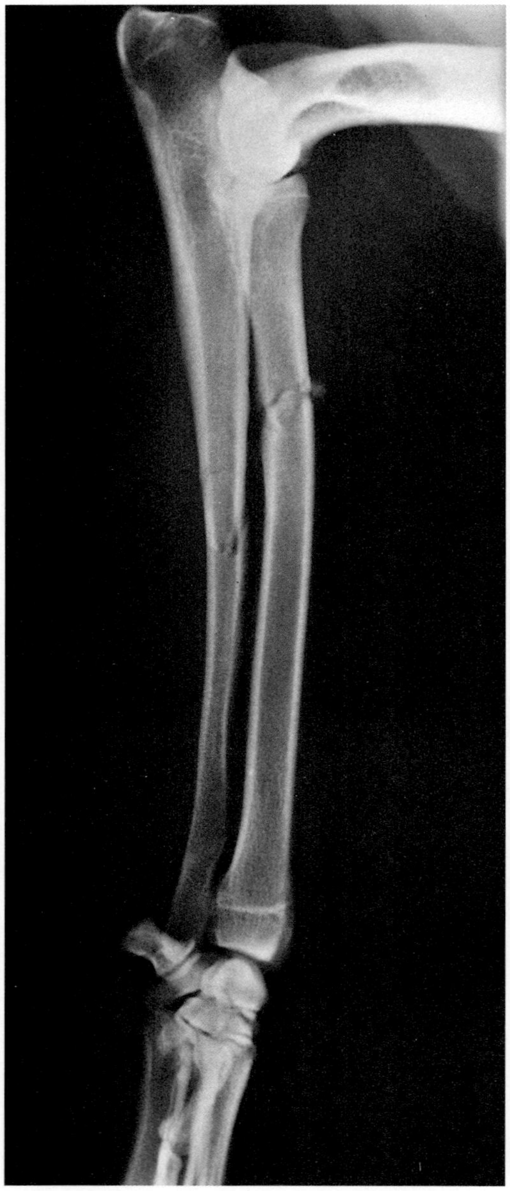

FIGURE 2.30 Simple stable fracture of the radius and ulna.

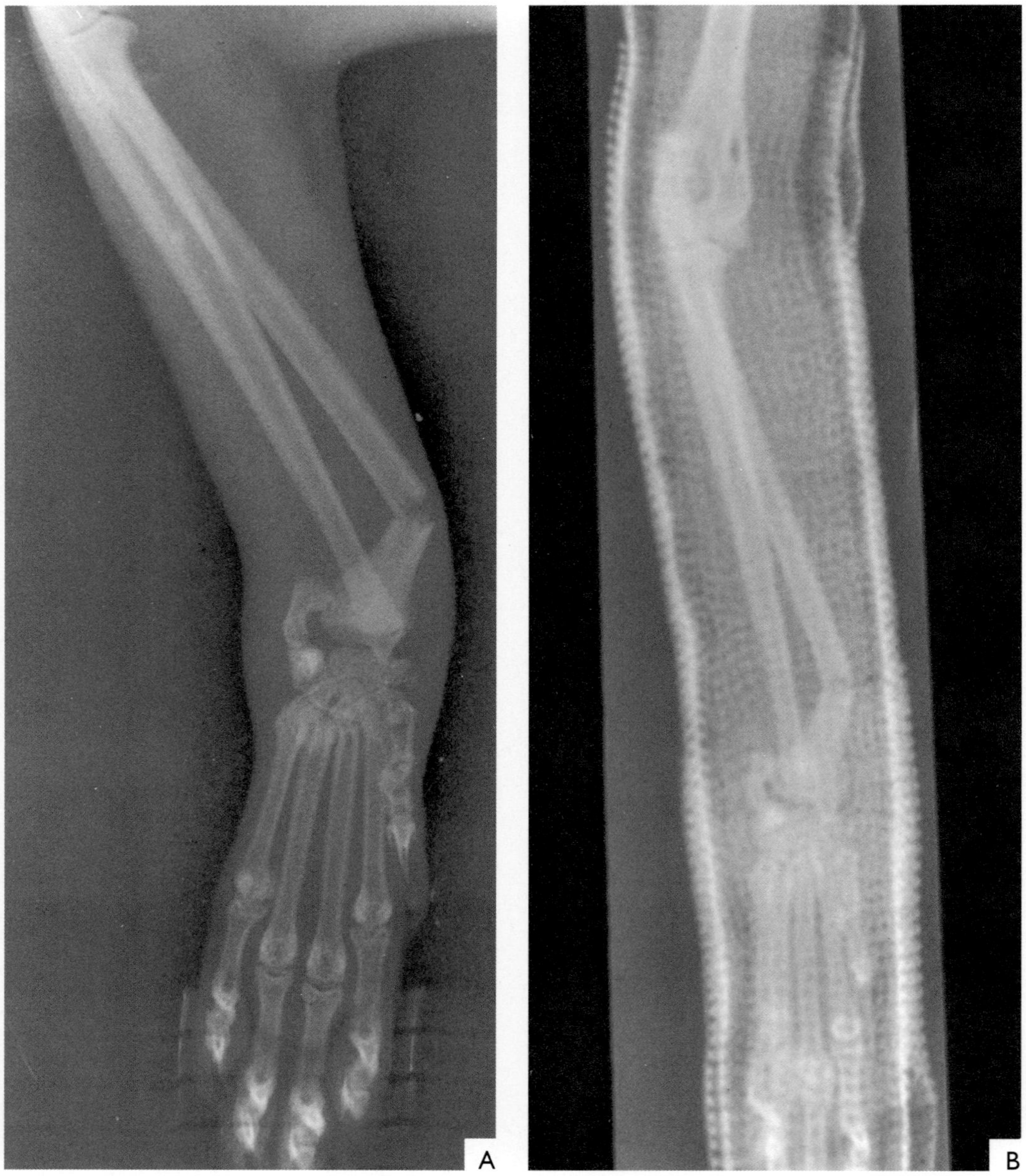

FIGURE 2.31 (A) A distal fracture of the radius and ulna in a cat. (B) Inadequate reduction of a distal fracture of the radius and ulna with a cast.

fracture to be in the proximal ulna and to involve the articular surface of the trochlear notch (Fig. 2.33). Congruency of this surface must be obtained and maintained to avoid posttraumatic joint disease. The pull of the triceps separates these fractures. A single intramedullary pin or bone screw may be subjected to enough cyclical strain to break it. Tension band wires or bone plates help to counteract the distractive forces and thus permit healing.

SURGICAL TECHNIQUE

It is convenient to have the animal in dorsal recumbency. A caudolateral incision through the skin and subcutaneous tissues extends from the olecranon so that it can be exposed, to a level well below the fracture site. The underlying fascia is incised close to the bone so that the extensor carpi ulnaris on one side and the flexor carpi ulnaris on the other can be exposed and elevated from the bone. With a single fracture, extension of the limb and digital pressure can bring about reduction. Two K-wires are introduced from the proximal end of the bone to pass across the fracture and insert into the cranial cortex of the distal ulnar fragment. Two pins help prevent rotation. A transverse hole is drilled through the bone distal to the fracture and orthopedic wire is inserted through the hole to loop over the caudal K-wire in a figure-8 (Fig. 2.34). It should be in-

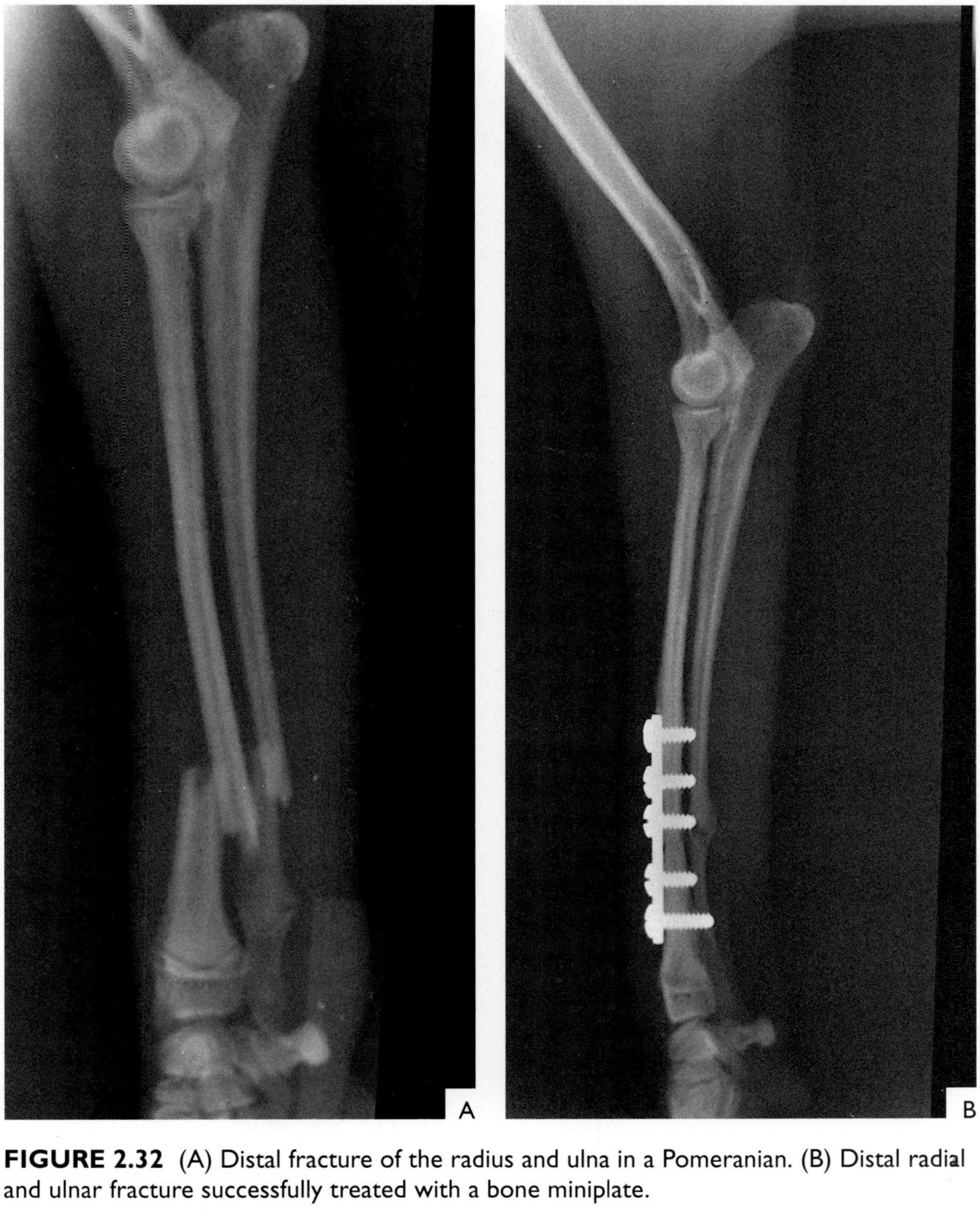

FIGURE 2.32 (A) Distal fracture of the radius and ulna in a Pomeranian. (B) Distal radial and ulnar fracture successfully treated with a bone miniplate.

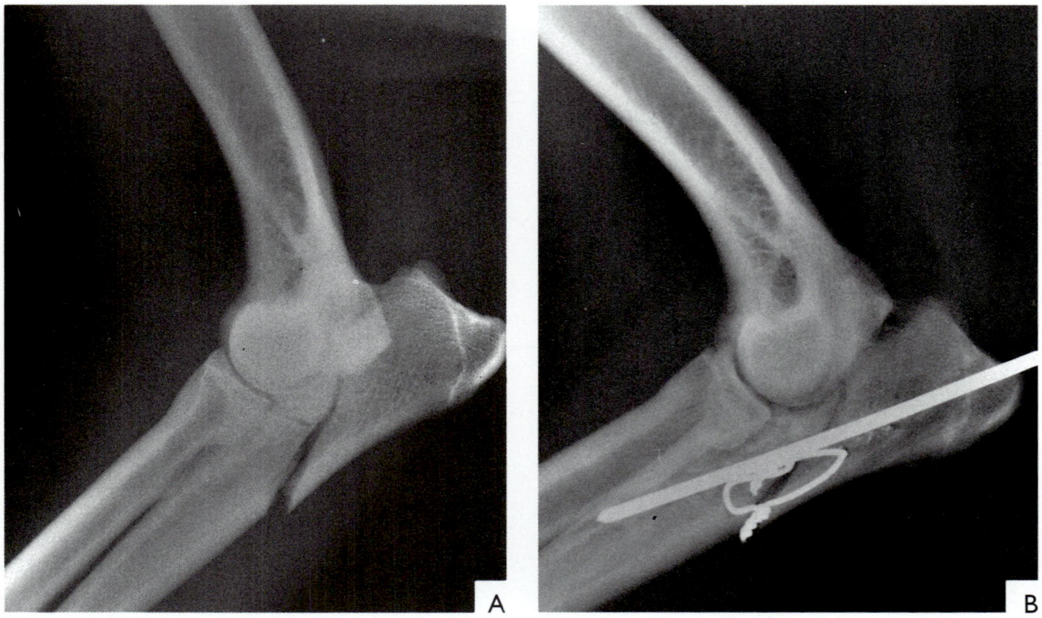

FIGURE 2.33 (A) This proximal ulnar fracture involved the trochlear notch. (B) Radiograph of a proximal ulnar fracture treated with an IM pin and a small tension band wire. (It is more effective to loop the wire proximally around the base of the IM pin.)

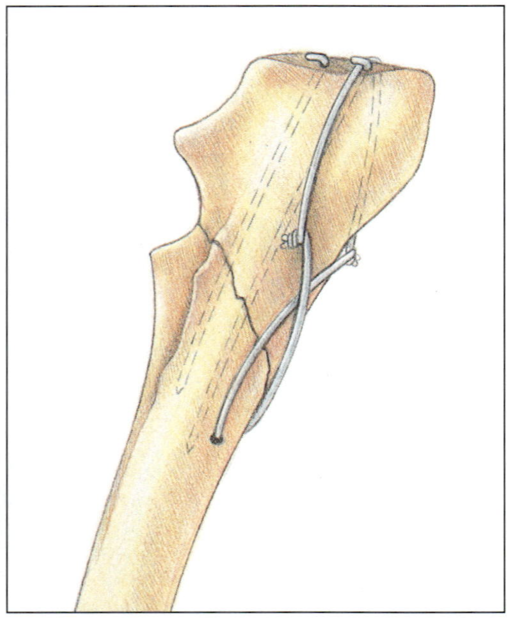

FIGURE 2.34 The use of two K-wires and figure-8 tension band wire for treatment of a proximal ulnar fracture.

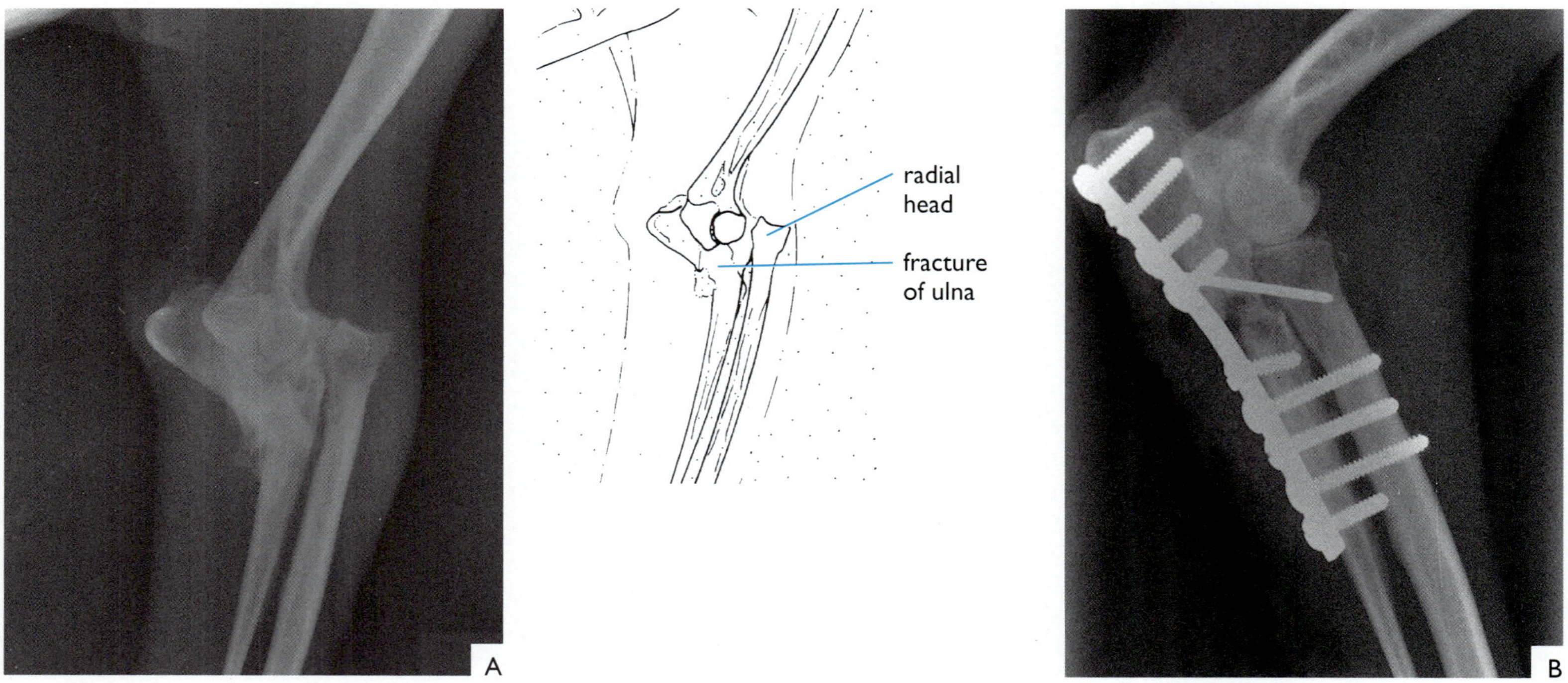

FIGURE 2.35 (A) Monteggia fracture in a Shetland sheep dog. (B) Monteggia fracture treated with a bone plate on the ulnar fracture and a K-wire to retain the head of the radius.

serted through the fibrous insertion close to the bone. The wire is tightened to put tension on the fragment, compressing the fracture site. Each K-wire end is bent at a right angle, cut off leaving a short hook, turned cranially, and seated by blows from a small mallet. This form of treatment is used if there are multiple fragments that can be lined up in a stable manner.

Unstable multiple fractures require a plate, which is usually located laterally but can be placed caudally (Fig. 2.35). Dynamic compression plates are used in the neutralization mode.

It may be necessary to remove the K-wires or the tension band wire after healing if a reaction to them occurs. Ordinarily the pins, wires, and plates remain. The skin and subcutaneous tissue are re-placed over the olecranon and the incised tissues are closed in the usual manner.

A modified Robert Jones splint is applied for a few days. The animal's activity is restricted for 2 weeks. Healing is usually uncomplicated.

Monteggia Fracture

Fractures of the ulna just below the elbow joint with cranial or lateral luxation of the radial head are referred to as Monteggia fractures (Fig. 2.36). Such fractures, although not common, necessitate surgery. The annular ligament is usually torn as the head is luxated.

It is possible to reduce the luxation manually if the injury is recent. Usually the radius and ulna are held together by the interosseus ligament. When the head is re-placed, the ulnar fracture is reduced. It is immobilized with K-wires or intramedullary pins with a tension band figure-8 wire or, in large dogs, a bone plate.

When the radius is torn free of the ulna, it may have to be fastened to the ulna with a lag screw introduced either from the radius into the ulna or vice versa. This procedure is not performed in cats, since they have need of pronation and supination.

In some cases, it is not possible to reduce the radial head and surgical exposure must be done. The head is levered into place, tak-

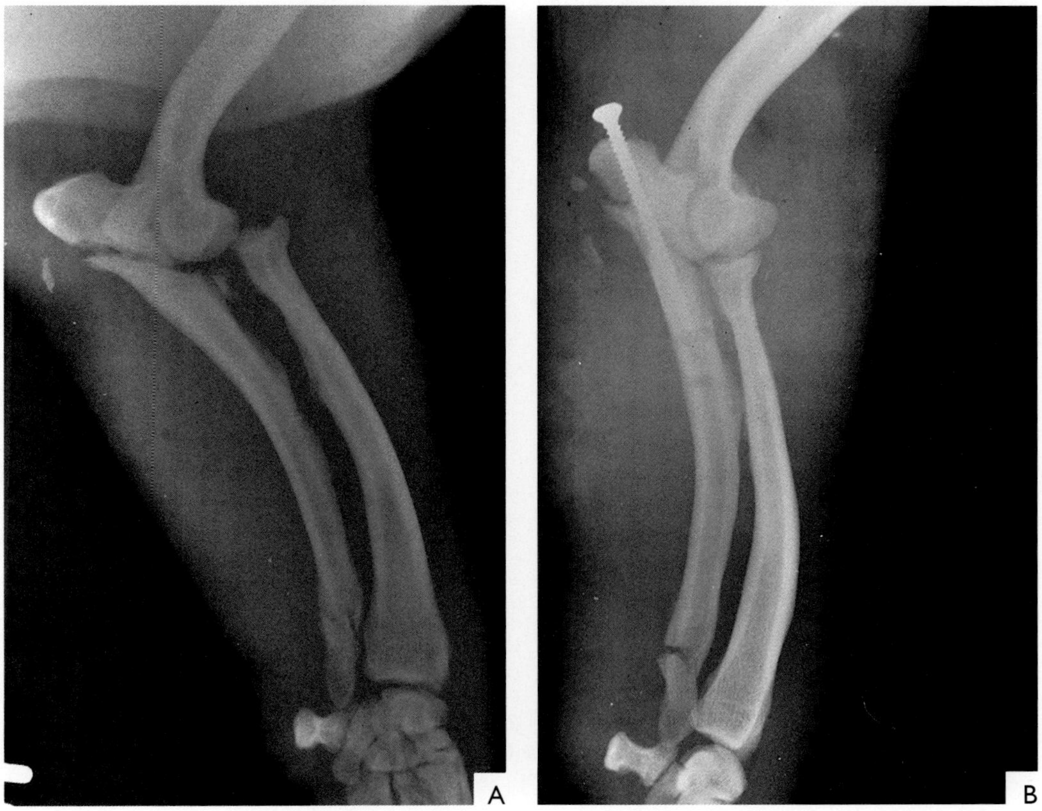

FIGURE 2.36 (A) Monteggia fracture in a Lhasa Apso. (B) Monteggia fracture treated with a lag screw in the proximal ulnar fracture. A figure-8 tension band wire and a screw in the radius have been removed.

ing care not to injure the joint surface of the radial head or to damage the radial nerve. The torn annular ligament is repaired with silk sutures.

SURGICAL TECHNIQUE

The ulnar fracture is usually located just distal to the elbow joint. A caudolateral incision through the skin and subcutaneous tissues is made near the caudal edge of the ulna. The tissues are reflected over the top of the olecranon. The extensor carpi ulnaris is elevated and retracted at the site of the fracture. An intramedullary pin can be driven retrograde up the proximal fragment to exit on the dorsal aspect, or the pin can be driven normograde. The fracture is reduced at the same time the luxated radial head is re-placed. The pin is deeply seated and cut off close to the fibrous insertion of the triceps (Fig. 2.37). A figure-8 tension band is applied from a transversely drilled hole below the fracture to loop over the proximal end of the pin. The wire should pass through the insertion of the triceps close to the bone, next to the pin. A smaller pin is driven from the olecranon through the fracture site to seat into the cranial aspect of the distal fragment of the ulna to control rotation. In large dogs, a small bone plate is applied across the fracture.

If the radial head cannot be re-placed, an open reduction is done. The brachial and antebrachial fascia are incised from just cranial to the lateral humeral condyle and extended across the joint along the lateral surface of the radius to about its proximal fourth. The lateral edge of the triceps is retracted to expose the fascial

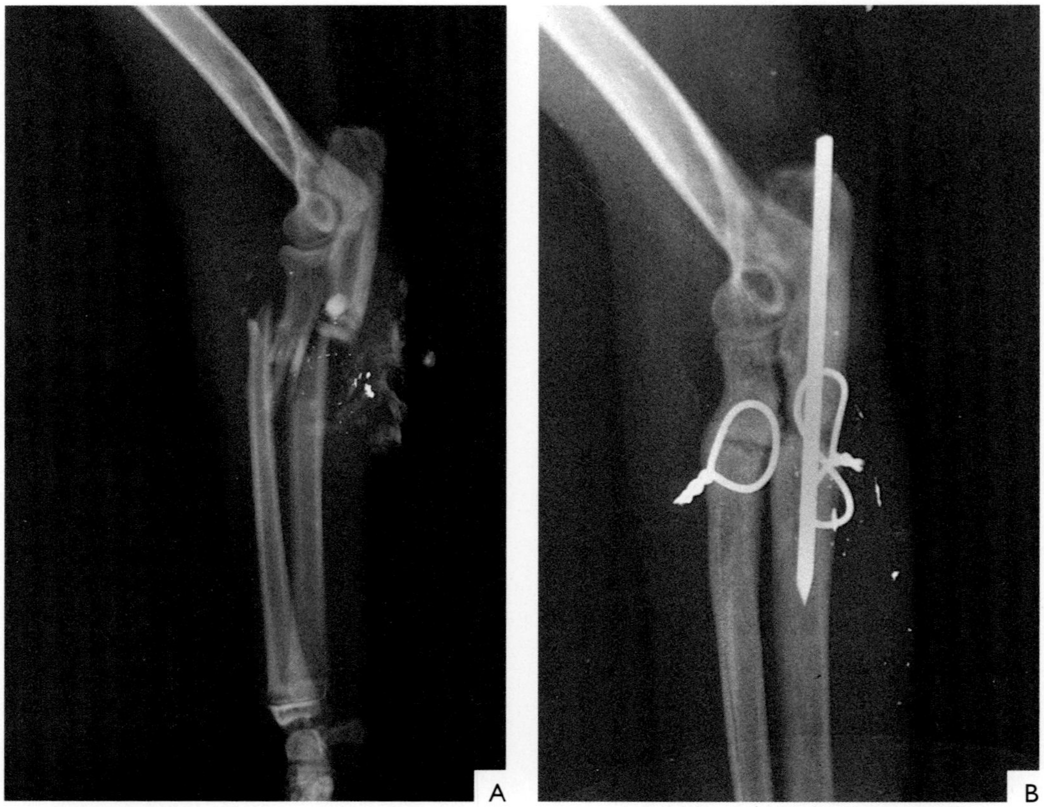

FIGURE 2.37 (A) Proximal radial and ulnar gunshot fracture in a cat. (B) Proximal gunshot fracture of the radius and ulna treated with an IM pin in the ulna with a figure-8 tension band wire and an interfragmentary wire in the radius.

attachment of the anconeus on the lateral humeral condyle, which is incised so that the muscle can be retracted.

An incision is made between the lateral digital extensor and the ulnaris lateralis at their origins. The latter muscle is identified and transected, leaving about 1 cm for reattachment. The lateral digital extensor and the other extensors are retracted cranially. The transected ulnaris lateralis is retracted caudally. The cranial and caudal crura of the radial collateral ligament are isolated and the caudal crura is elevated at its radial insertion. This exposes the area of the radial head, which is pried into place. Care must be taken not to damage the radial nerve, which is located just cranial to the radial head.

Closure consists of suturing the tenotomy of the extensor carpi ulnaris with nonabsorbable sutures. The reflected skin and subcutaneous tissues are re-placed over the olecranon. The usual closure of the skin incision is made.

The leg is immobilized in a modified Robert Jones splint for a week, followed by 2 weeks of restricted activity. Healing is usually satisfactory. Some degenerative changes may develop at the radial head as the result of trauma.

Shaft of the Radius and Ulna

The middle and distal third of these bones are the areas most commonly involved. Rarely, only one bone is affected (Fig. 2.38). These fractures can occur at all levels and range in severity from a simple

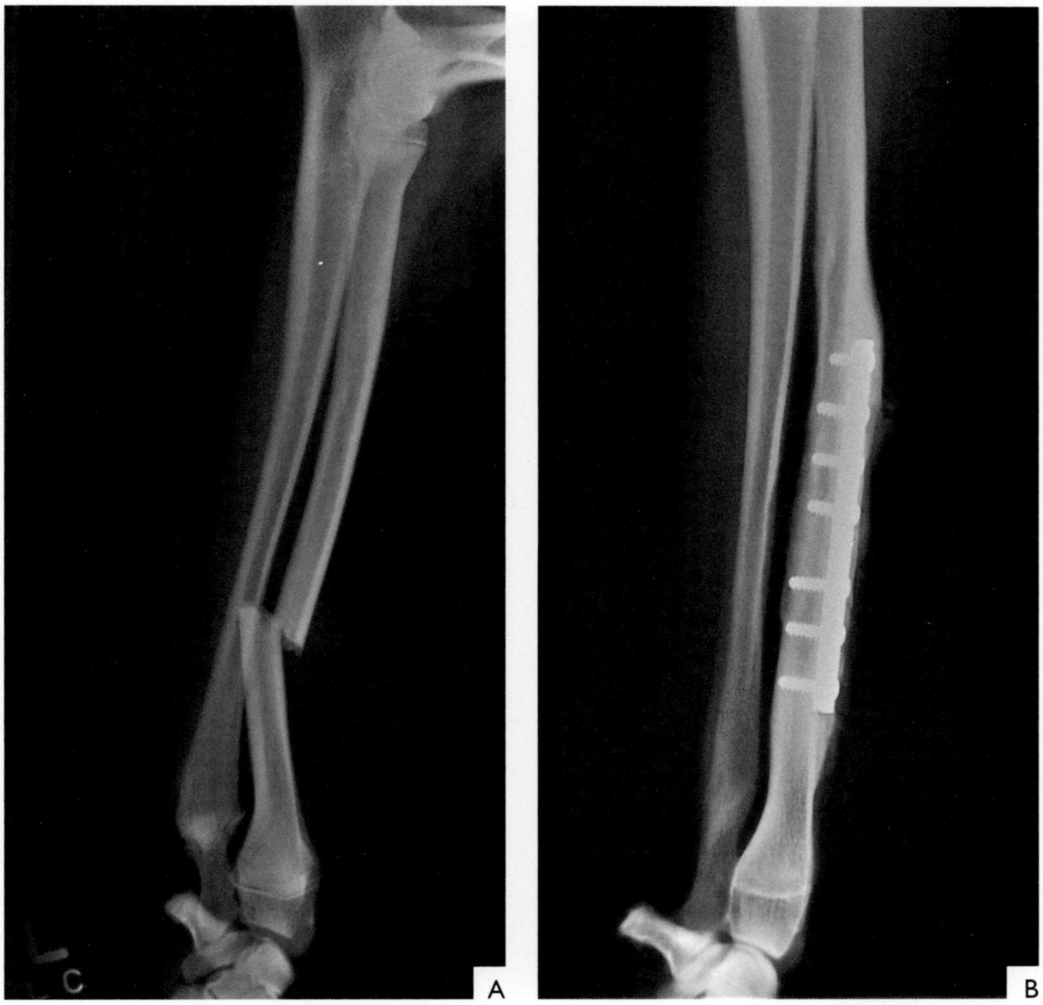

FIGURE 2.38 (A) Fracture of the radius. (B) Fracture of the radius treated with a bone plate. It is unusual that the ulna was not also affected.

greenstick fracture to one that is massively comminuted and infected (Fig. 2.39).

Proper selection and application of the fixation method are imperative. Malunion, nonunion, or delayed union can occur with inadequate control of motion and rotation or when the device is removed too soon.

Coaptation splints and casts do not eliminate internal movement or rotation well enough to be relied on as the primary treatment, especially in upper third fractures. They can be used satisfactorily in greenstick and stable fractures, especially in young animals (Fig. 2.40). External fixation and bone plating are the most commonly used methods of treatment.

Some radial and ulnar fractures can be reduced in a closed manner by traction, angulation, and manipulation. In many cases the process is excessively traumatic or the reduction cannot be maintained. An open reduction is preferable. Even an apparently good closed reduction is often a disappointment when radiographed (Fig. 2.41). Fractures of the distal third, in particular, will develop a valgus deviation and lateral rotation when they are splinted or placed in a cast. To counteract this, the foot must be held in a slight varus and inward rotation. This is best done with a cast of plaster of Paris or moldable plastic.

Greenstick and intraperiosteal fractures can be treated with coaptation splints, such as the Mason metasplint or similar plastic

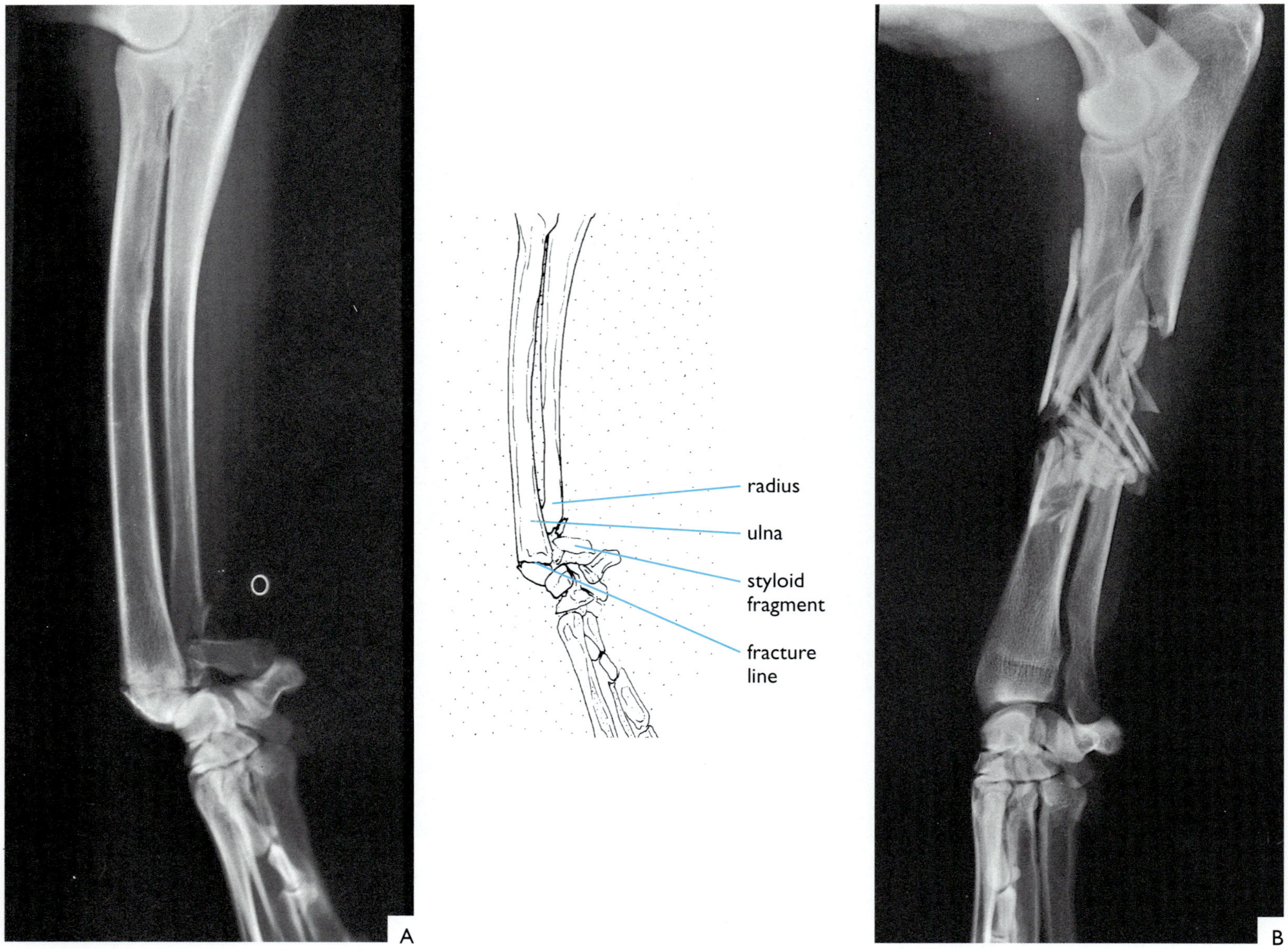

FIGURE 2.39 (A) Very distal left radial fracture and a fracture of the styloid process of the ulna. (B) Massive comminuted fracture of the right radius and ulna in the same dog.

devices. The Schroeder–Thomas splint is not as satisfactory and is outmoded.

All casts and splints require a good deal of care in application and maintenance. It is often difficult to immobilize the joint above the fracture. Prolonged immobilization of joints is harmful, and pressure sores, loss of toes, or even loss of the limb can result from inadequate application and supervision.

SURGICAL TECHNIQUE

APPLICATION OF A COAPTATION SPLINT The leg should be relatively clean and trimmed of excess hair. Wisps of cotton are placed between the toes and the dew claw. A strip of adhesive tape is placed on the dorsal and volar surfaces of the lower leg and foot. A thin wrap of cotton covered with bandage and some tape will keep the tape from slipping off. The adhesive surfaces of the tape strips are stuck together below the foot. An assistant holds the leg at the axilla and maintains traction on the tape while the surgeon manipulates the fracture into reduction. With the leg held in reduction by the assistant, a half-thickness single strip of roll cotton is applied to the caudal surface of the leg, extending from above the elbow to below the foot. It is folded cranially to cover the leg. This wrapping can be covered with rolled bandage to hold it in place. The metasplint or plastic splint must not press on the foot. Padding is placed over the carpal pad and the caudal aspect of the olecranon. The splint is

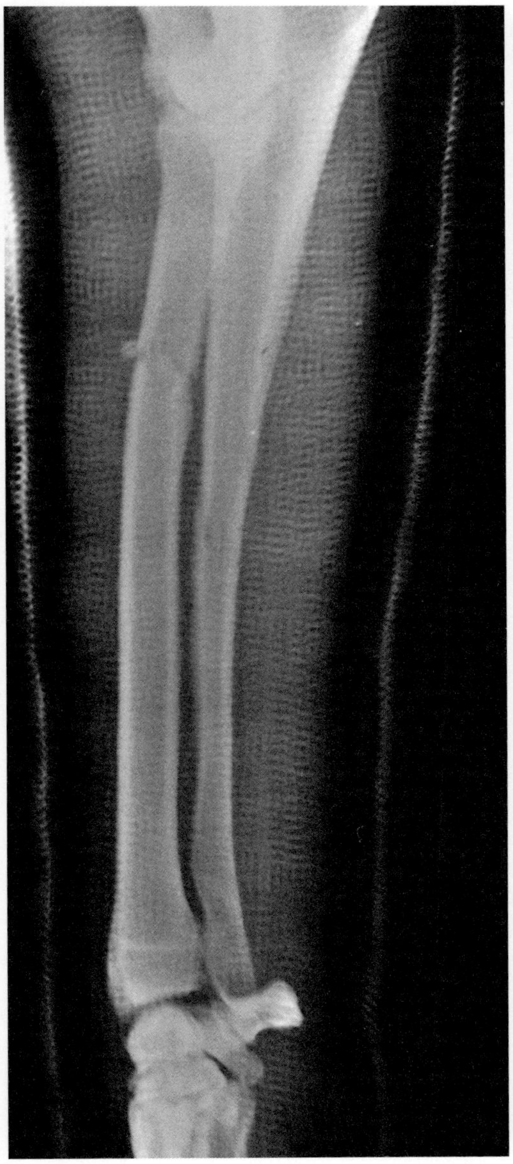

FIGURE 2.40 Stable fractures of the radius and ulna successfully treated with a cast.

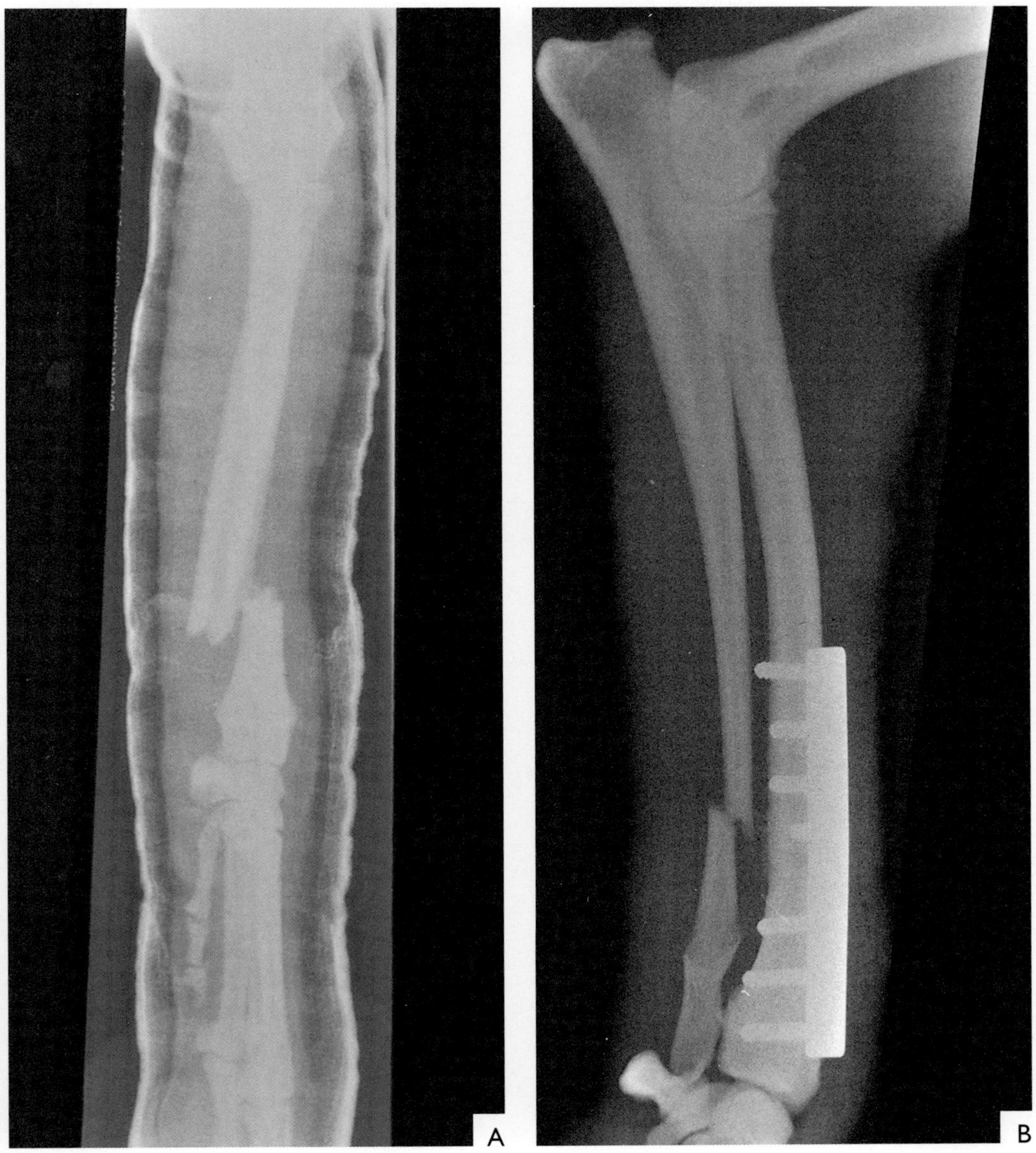

FIGURE 2.41 (A) Distal fracture of the radius and ulna in a dog, showing an unsatisfactory reduction with a cast. (B) Successful reduction and fixation with a bone plate of a fracture of the distal radius and ulna in a dog.

applied to the caudal aspect of the leg. The tape end is placed on the caudal distal end of the splint. The splint is secured with bandage applied from the foot upwards to an area above the elbow. The foot is covered, and the entire cast is protected with overlapping 1" adhesive tape. A notch is cut on the cranioventral edge of the cotton and bandage cranial to the elbow. This will prevent irritation of the underlying skin and musculature.

The foot of the splint can be covered temporarily with a waterproof covering if the dog is to be exercised outdoors. This covering is then removed when indoors. Frequent inspections must be made, since a splint that is loose, ill-smelling, chewed by the patient, or wet requires an immediate change. A comfortable splint is usually well tolerated.

Application of a Molded Cast The leg should be clean and dry. Excess hair is trimmed away. A strip of adhesive is applied to the medial and lateral sides of the distal third of the limb, extending about 10 cm beyond. The adhesive edges are applied to a tongue depressor so that they will not become entangled as the cast is put into place.

A smooth-fitting stockinette is drawn over the limb. The assistant maintains traction on the limb by holding the stockinette at the axilla and the tape and stockinette beyond the foot as the surgeon manipulates the fracture into reduction. While this is maintained by the assistant, circular wraps of cast padding are placed from the toes to the elbow. Each wrap advances one half the width of the material. Extra padding is placed at the caudal olecranon and the carpal pad. A thin, smooth application is required.

Moldable plastic or plaster of Paris strips are wrapped circularly around the leg from the toes to the elbow and a bit beyond. Reinforcing strips are applied caudally. When the material has set enough to hold its shape, adjustments for rotation and valgus are

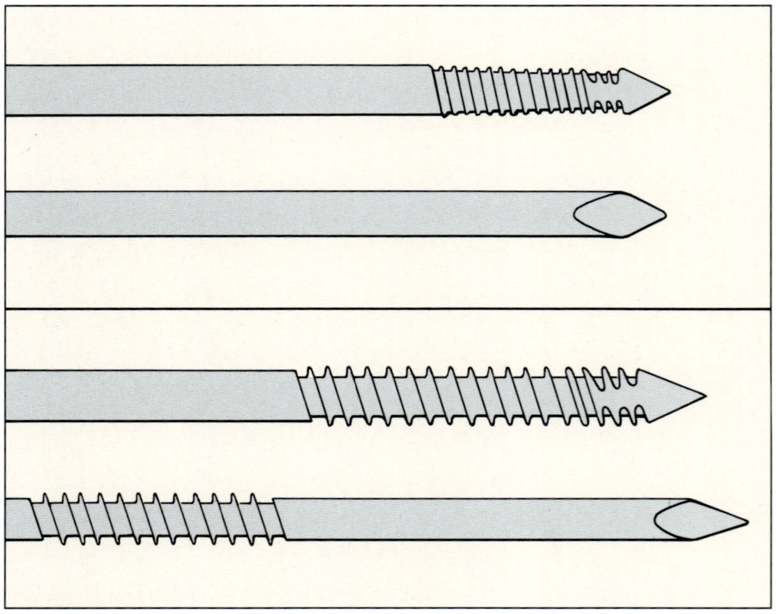

FIGURE 2.42 A copy of a brochure showing modern IM and external fixation pins.

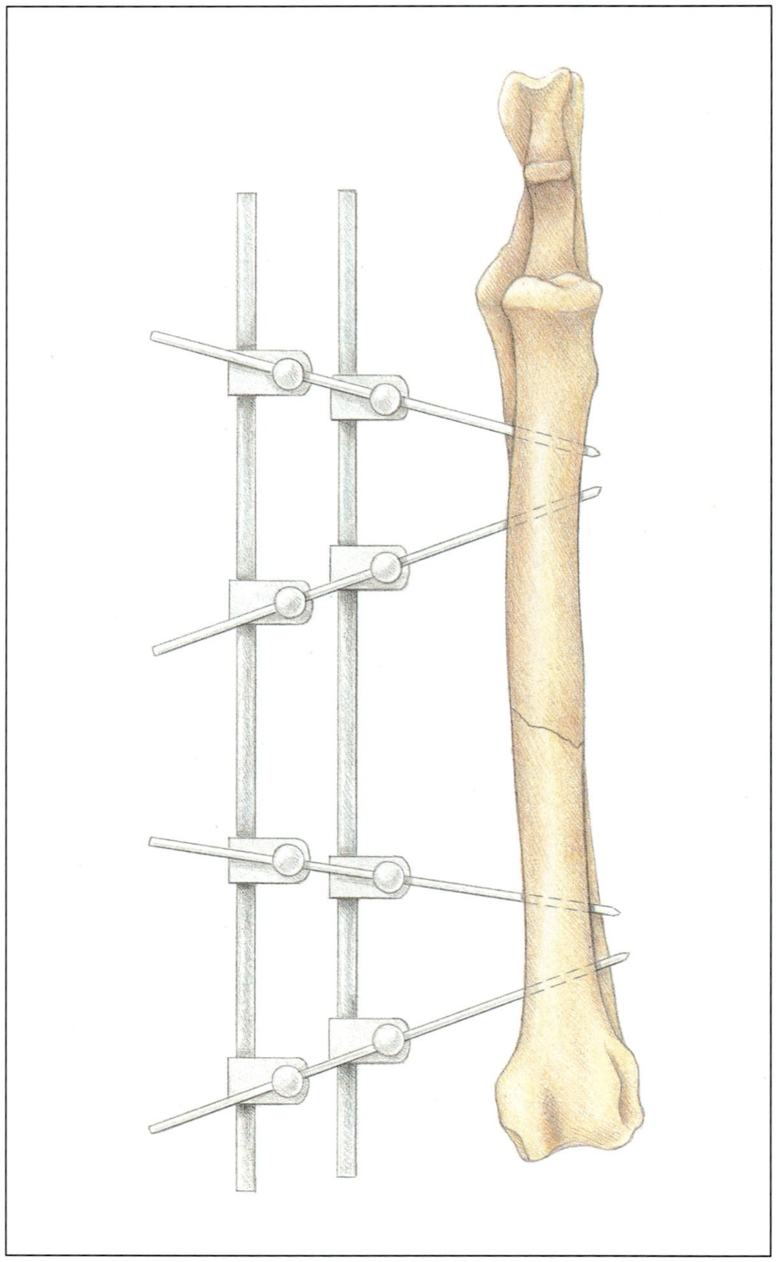

FIGURE 2.43 The two connecting bars used in a Kirschner/Ehmer external fixation splint.

made and the cast is held in this position until it hardens further. The stockinette at the elbow is reflected onto the splint and covered with additional strips. At the foot, the tapes are reflected onto the cast along with the stockinette, which is secured with a strip of plaster of Paris or plastic. The two central toes should extend from the splint. Hardening of the cast usually takes only a short time. A cast cutter will be required for removal.[1,2]

External Fixation

External fixation devices are particularly useful in fractures of the radius and ulna that cannot be readily plated or pinned because of infection, severe tissue damage, comminution, or short proximal or distal fragments. They are relatively easy to apply, can be used as an adjunct to intramedullary pinning, are well tolerated and, except for the pins, can be reused and are therefore less expensive than plating. They also require less equipment for application.

Pins are inserted through the tissues into the bone fragments, usually at a 70° angle to the long axis of the bone. They are attached to the rigid supporting device—the connecting bar—with metal clamps tightened with bolts. The connecting bar may also be formed with methylmethacrylate plastic.

When first developed, the pins were inserted and used to control the fragments in a closed reduction. The clamps were then tightened to maintain the fixation. The original configuration had two pins at converging angles in each fragment, which were attached to a small bar. A connecting bar was applied to the short bars. Stability was often difficult to maintain, since the clamps had a tendency to loosen. A number of variations have been developed to provide increased immobility. Open reduction is done to ensure proper bone alignment. The pins are never inserted through the surgical incision. Partially or completely threaded pins are available (Fig. 2.42) that have increased holding power. These are threaded into the bone or, preferably, inserted into previously tapped holes. The pins can be inserted by hand or with a power drill at slow speed. Where practical, pins of larger diameter bend less and are less likely to loosen. They should not exceed one third the diameter of the bone. All pins must penetrate both cortices.

A craniomedial location over the radius is recommended, since it minimizes the distance between the clamp and the bone. The clamps must not contact the skin surface. A distance of about 1 cm is allowed. Postoperative swelling may press the skin against the clamp, causing tissue necrosis. Readjustment of the clamps is done to prevent this. Some amount of seepage can be expected where the pins penetrate the skin. The skin must not be tensed against the pins. A more rigid configuration can be obtained when the inserted pins are attached directly to the connecting bar. In large dogs, two connecting bars are used (Fig. 2.43).

Additional pins can be inserted to give greater strength and to control fragments. In some cases, better control and rigidity are obtained by a bilateral configuration with the pins transfixing the bone and being attached to connecting bars on both sides of the fractured bones (Fig. 2.44). Many variations can be developed by the surgeon to meet the demands of the situation at hand to provide the required fixation.

The device is covered with some roll cotton, bandaged, and covered with adhesive tape. Gauze pads are placed around the pins.

SURGICAL TECHNIQUE

Fractures of the diaphysis of the radius are exposed by a craniomedial approach. The skin and subcutaneous tissue are incised over the craniomedial border of the radius, taking care to avoid the cephalic vein and, distally, the radial artery and vein. The extensor carpi radialis is retracted cranially and the pronator teres and flexor carpi radialis are retracted caudally. The fracture is reduced. It can be held with bone forceps, or a small K-wire can be inserted across the fracture to hold it in place. In large dogs an interfragmentary lag screw can be used.

Because of its attachment to the radius, the corresponding fracture of the ulna is usually brought into proper position simultaneously.

A single connecting bar with four clamps is prepared and the proximal and distal pins are inserted in the same plane. A small nick is made in the skin and the pin is driven into the bone to penetrate both cortices. For threaded pins, a small skin incision is made and the tissues are separated down to the bone. A drill guide is used to protect the tissues while the hole is drilled and tapped. The pin is threaded into the bone. After placement of the distal pin, the bar is attached and tightened. The two central pins are placed through the clamps into the proximal and distal fragments. They should be at least 5 mm from the fracture site. The pins are tested for solid seating and the clamps are tightened. The pins are cut off about 1 cm above the clamps. Cancellous bone graft material is placed at the fracture site. Closure is done in the usual manner. Sterile sponges are split halfway and placed between the pins and the clamps. The device is wrapped in roll cotton, bandage, and adhesive tape. This covers the sharp ends of the cut pins and prevents damage to the patient's surroundings. It also provides a more finished appearance.

Dressings for treatment of gunshot wounds, infections, and loss of tissue at the fracture site are easily applied. The device is removed after healing has been confirmed by examination and radiography. The pins can often be removed without anesthesia. After the device is removed some support to the leg is provided for a week with a coaptation splint or Robert Jones splint.[3]

INTRAMEDULLARY FIXATION Intramedullary pinning is not the internal fixation of choice for most radial and ulnar fractures. It is used effectively in the ulna to align that bone and, in larger dogs, to provide additional support when the radius is plated.

The radius is slightly curved cranially and has a flattened ovoid intramedullary cavity, with articular surfaces at each end. These features require a pin of smaller diameter to be introduced close to the distal radial articulation through the distal fragment, then driven up the medullary cavity of the proximal fragment. Rotation may not be adequately controlled. A second intramedullary pin is introduced at the top of the olecranon to stabilize the ulnar fracture and to help control the rotation and motion of the radius. A coaptation splint is always used to provide additional support.

A small intramedullary pin or K-wire is used in distal fractures of the ulna, often in conjunction with a distal fracture involving the articular surfaces. There is little or no medullary cavity at this location.

Fractures of the styloid process of the ulna are similarly repaired with a K-wire and a figure-8 tension band wire similar to

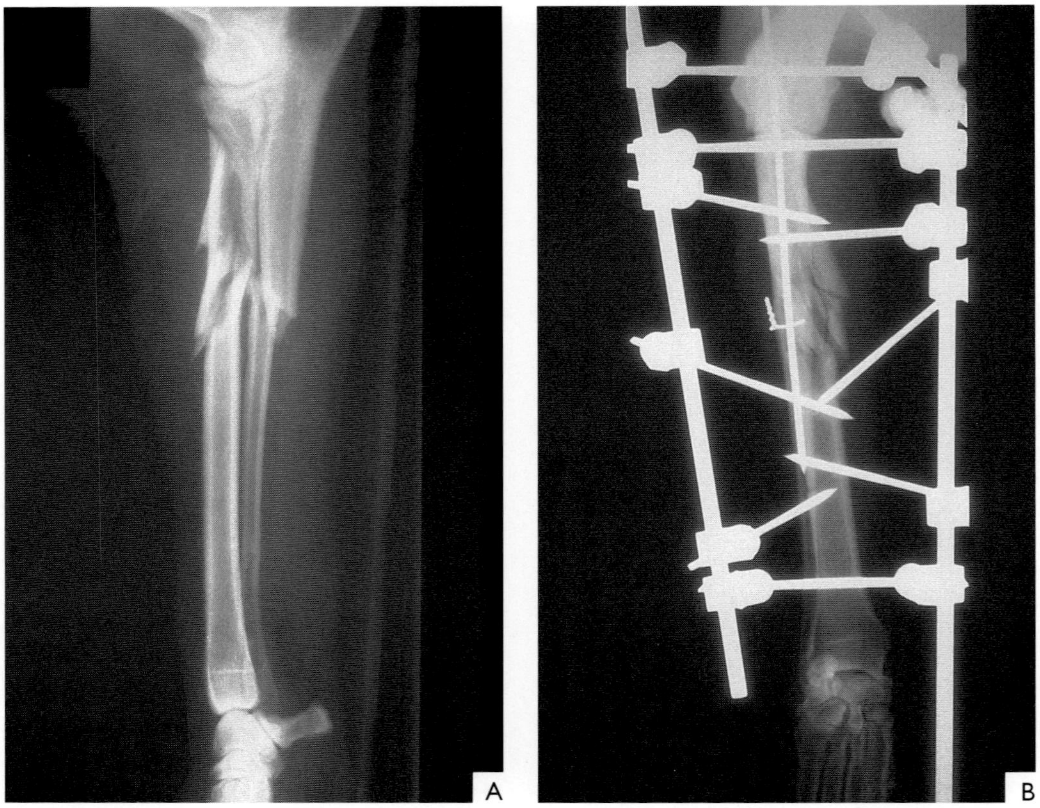

FIGURE 2.44 (A) Comminuted fracture of the proximal radius and ulna. (B) Comminuted fracture of the proximal radius and ulna treated with a bilateral configuration external fixation splint, with additional pins for fragment control. A K/E apparatus was selected because of the extremely short proximal radial fragment.

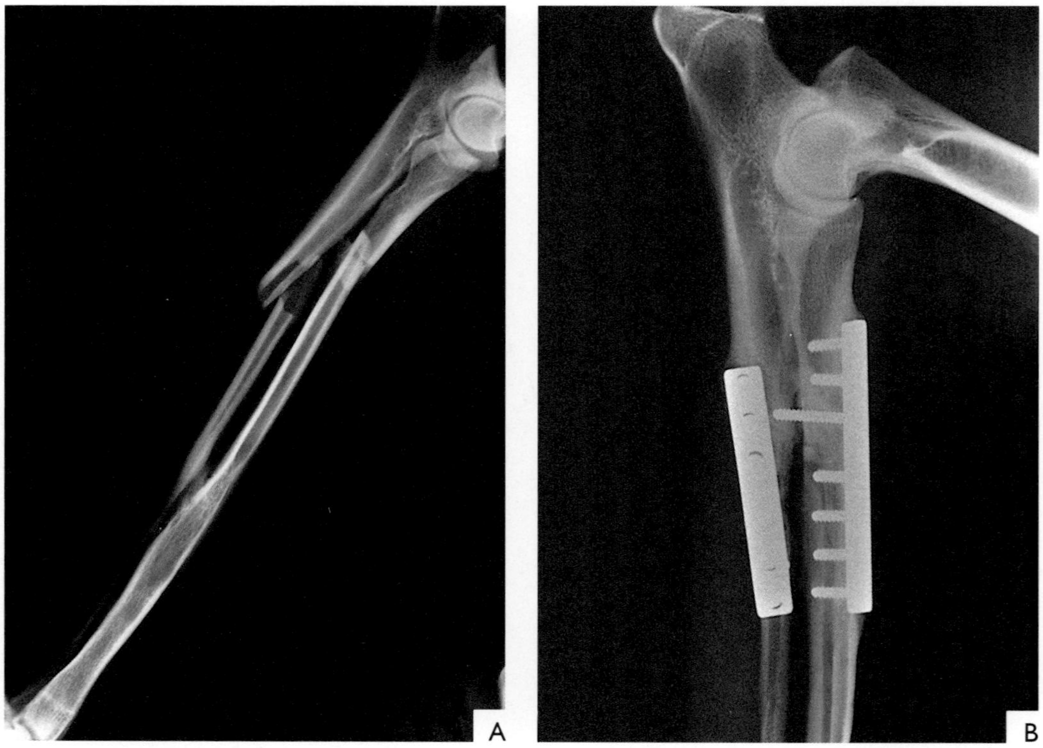

FIGURE 2.45 (A) Proximal fracture of the radius and ulna. The atrophy of the distal ulna and its fusion to the radius were from a previous fracture. (B) Proximal radial and ulnar fracture treated with bone plates.

that used in a malleolar fracture. A coaptation splint is applied. Rapid healing can be expected.

Fractures of the styloid process of the radius involving the distal radial articulation require open reduction through an incision directly over the fractured fragment to obtain joint congruency. The fragment is re-placed and held by a small K-wire, after which a lag screw is inserted. Smaller fragments are held by K-wires and a figure-8 tension band wire.

A single intramedullary pin is used in young dogs with epiphyseal fractures. The growth plate is less likely to fuse than it would be if compressed by a plate, crossed pins, or a screw.

SURGICAL TECHNIQUE

The fracture site is exposed by a craniomedial incision through the skin and subcutaneous tissues over the craniomedial border of the radius.

An intramedullary pin is selected of a diameter that will fit the intramedullary cavity of the radius. The pin will be slightly flexible. It is introduced at a slight angle into the cranial aspect of the distal radius so that the point of the pin enters the medullary cavity of the distal fragment. The fracture is reduced and the pin is driven up the medullary cavity of the proximal fragment to be seated firmly like a Rush pin. The pin is bent at a right angle where it emerges from the bone distally and is cut off, leaving a small, angled end. This will provide something to grip when the pin is to be removed after healing.

The pin can be introduced from the medullary cavity of the distal fragment to exit on the cranial surface of the distal fragment just cranial to the articular surface. The pin is drawn distally, introduced into the proximal medullary cavity at reduction, and well seated. Its end is cut off after being bent at a right angle.

The leg is placed in a coaptation splint. It takes from 3 to 6 weeks for the fractures to heal, after which the pin is removed.[4]

BONE PLATING Where applicable, bone plates provide an elegant and effective means of treating most radial and ulnar fractures. They are particularly useful in more proximal fractures (Fig. 2.45) and in corrective surgery for malunions, nonunions, highly comminuted fractures, and in radial fractures in the toy breeds for which very small plates and screws are available (Fig. 2.46).

Plates are applied to the flat cranial surface of the radius. Occasionally, as in the case of very large dogs, both the radius and the ulna are plated (Fig. 2.47). Additional support can also be

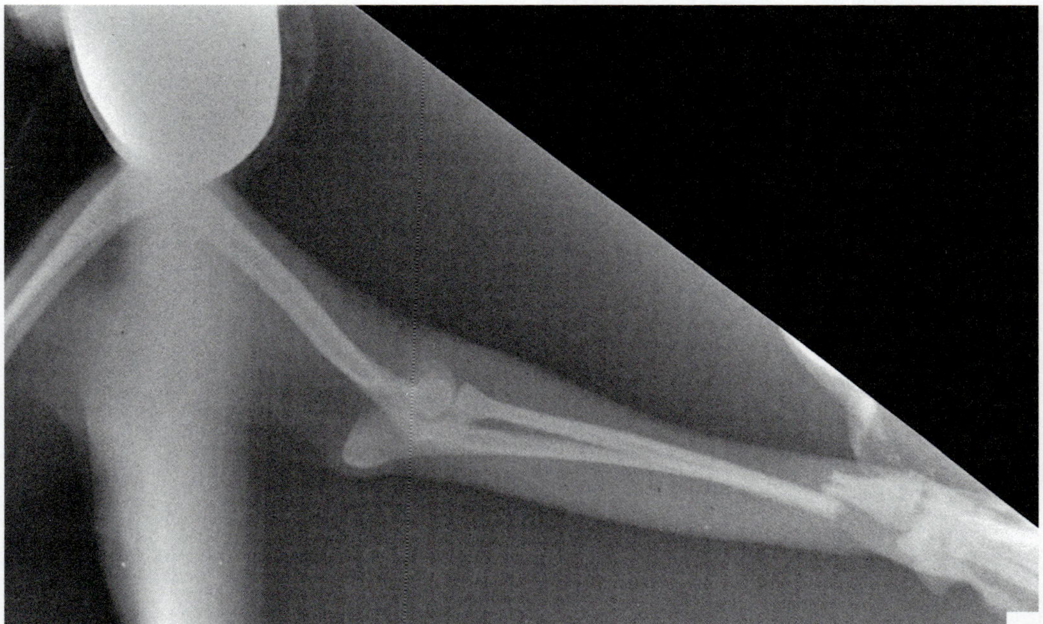

A

FIGURE 2.46 (A) Radiograph of bilateral radial and ulnar fractures in a Pomeranian. (B) Radiograph of bilateral radial and ulnar fractures in a Pomeranian treated with miniplates.

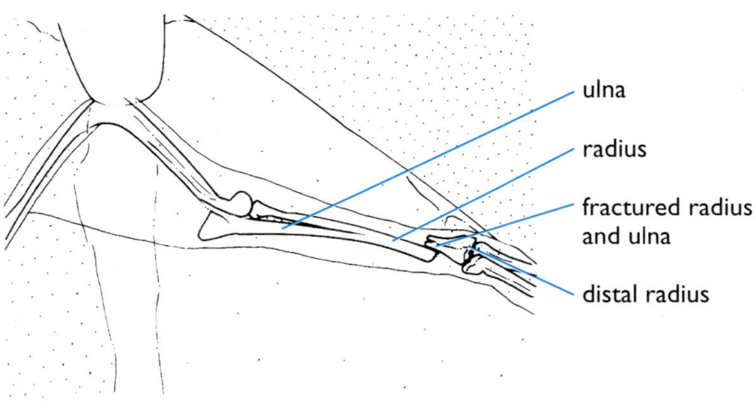

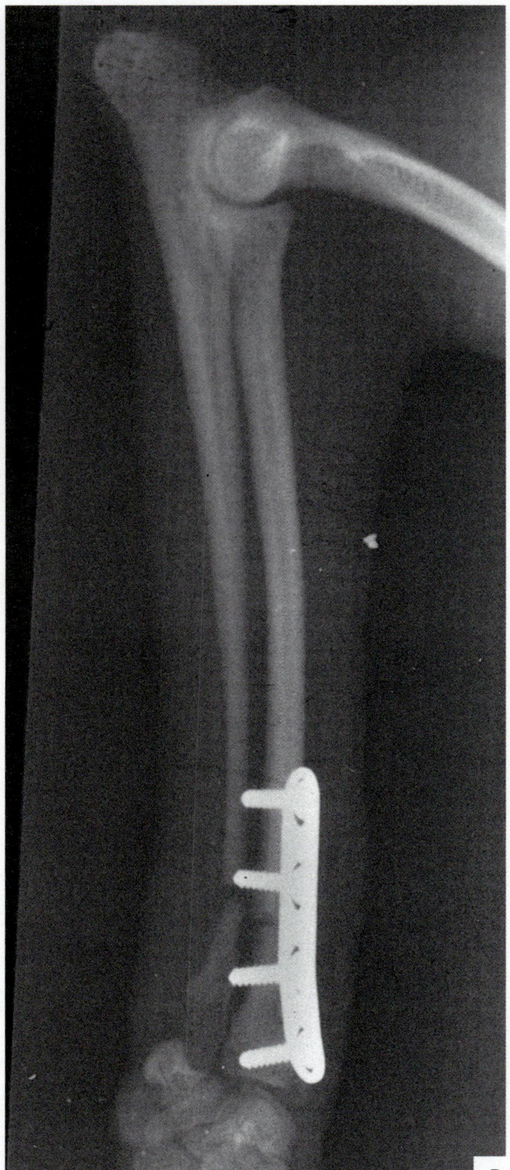

B

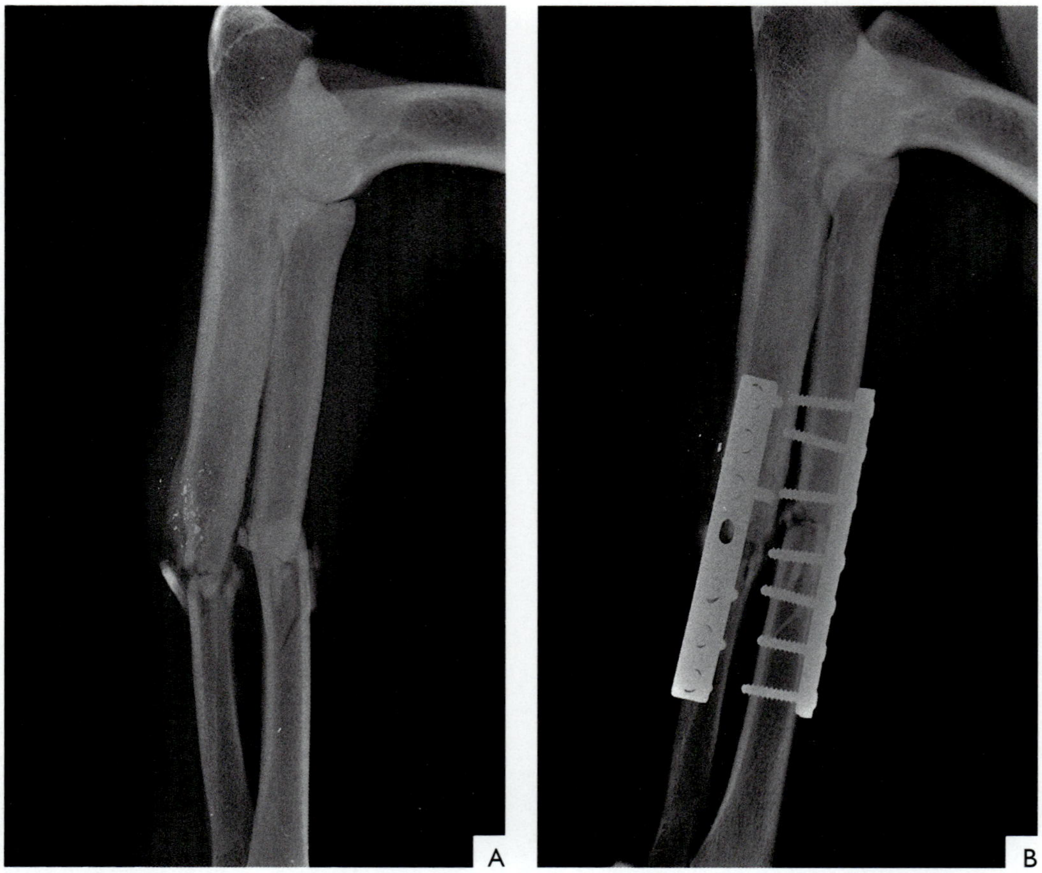

FIGURE 2.47 (A) Midshaft gunshot fracture of the radius and ulna in a German shepherd. (B) Midshaft gunshot fracture of the radius and ulna treated with a bone plate.

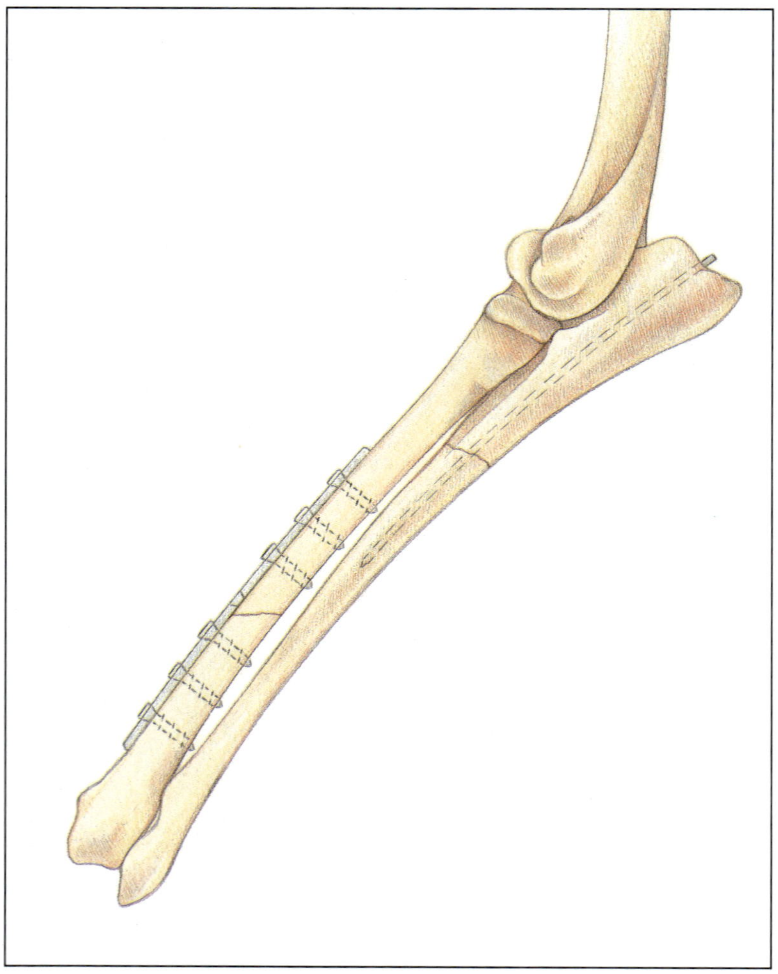

FIGURE 2.48 A fracture of the radius and ulna treated with an IM pin in the ulna and a plate on the radius.

obtained by placing an intramedullary pin in the ulna (Fig. 2.48). This is most effective in proximal third fractures of the radius and ulna.

Transverse fractures can be impacted by use of a dynamic compression (DC) plate. Long oblique and comminuted fractures are stabilized with lag screws or small K-wires. A neutralization plate is applied. Bone plates are very effective in proximal third fractures. Distal fractures are plated on the medial aspect of the radius, away from the cranially located extensor tendons.

Plates provide essential support when normal position must be maintained and when there is loss of bone substance and a cancellous graft has been performed. A minimum of two screws per dorsal or distal fragment is required. Screws should not be closer than 4–5mm to the fracture line. DC plates are pre-bent slightly upwards to provide 1 mm of space between the plate and the bone underneath at the fracture site.

Tubular plates are used in lighter weight dogs and in cats. They are not as easily contoured. The choice of plate size is dependent on the weight and size of the patient. Too firm a plate may result in stress protection with diminution of bone substance. Plated fractures of the radius and ulna are given additional support with a coaptation splint for 1 to 3 weeks. Although less callus is seen on radiographs and healing time may be somewhat prolonged, the coaptation splint provides continuous support. Plates may remain as long as they cause no problems, but eventually should be removed. Loosening of the screws and plate breakage can cause pain, and the plate and screws must be removed, reset, or replaced.

SURGICAL TECHNIQUE

The shaft of the radius is approached from the medial aspect of the limb. An incision is made through the skin and subcutaneous tissues along the medial border and is extended as needed from the head of the radius to its styloid process. Bone plates require a more extensive exposure.

The deep and superficial digital flexors are retracted caudally and the extensor carpi radialis is retracted cranially. For proximal fractures the antebrachial fascia is incised along with the muscle insertions of the supinator and pronator teres. These muscles are retracted to expose the dorsal surface of the radius. For distal fractures, the incision is curved towards the dorsal surface, taking care not to damage the large cephalic vein located cranially and the smaller radial artery and vein located caudally.

A single transverse fracture is reduced by angulation and with a bone clamp. A suitable DC plate is bent slightly upward about 1mm over the fracture site. The plate is contoured to fit the cranial curvature of the flat surface of the radius. Screws should not be inserted closer than 5 mm to the fracture site. Holes are drilled, measured with a depth gauge to aid in proper screw length selection, and tapped. Two holes are drilled at locations nearest the fracture site, one in load and the other in neutral mode.

The neutral screw is seated. As the load screw is tightened, it will impact the fracture. The load screw is always in the fragment with the greater part of the bone against the plate at the fracture site (Fig. 2.49). The rest of the screws are inserted in neutral mode.

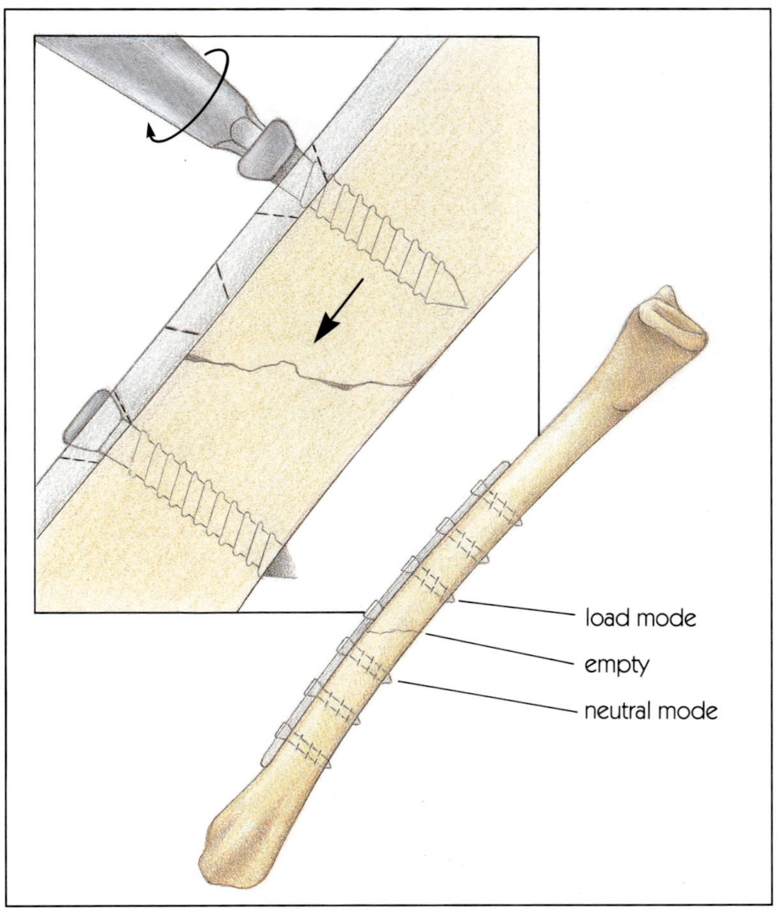

FIGURE 2.49
The placement of a bone plate on a radial fracture using a dynamic compression (DC) plate.

Larger oblique fractures are reduced and held with short K-wires, while the lag screws are inserted. A neutralization plate is applied.

The major fragments of comminuted fractures are re-placed, to be held with short K-wires and, if possible, subsequently held with lag screws. Sometimes a lag screw is inserted through one of the screw holes in the plate. Cancellous bone grafts are performed and a neutralization plate is applied.

Plates that are too short must be avoided. A minimum of two screws in a major fragment is required. At least three or four screws should be applied above and below a fracture if at all possible. A long plate increases the number of screws, therefore the holding power (Fig. 2.50).

Closure is performed by resuturing any muscle attachments that have been incised, such as the supinator or pronator teres, to their fascial insertions or if the plate interferes with adjacent muscles. Skin closure is routine.

The leg is placed in a coaptation splint, which is removed in 2 weeks. Check radiographs are made weekly, and activity is restricted for a month. Healing may take 2 or 3 months. Although plates should be removed at 6 to 8 months, it is often difficult to convince owners of the necessity. Chronically loose bone plates have been shown to cause bone tumors.[5]

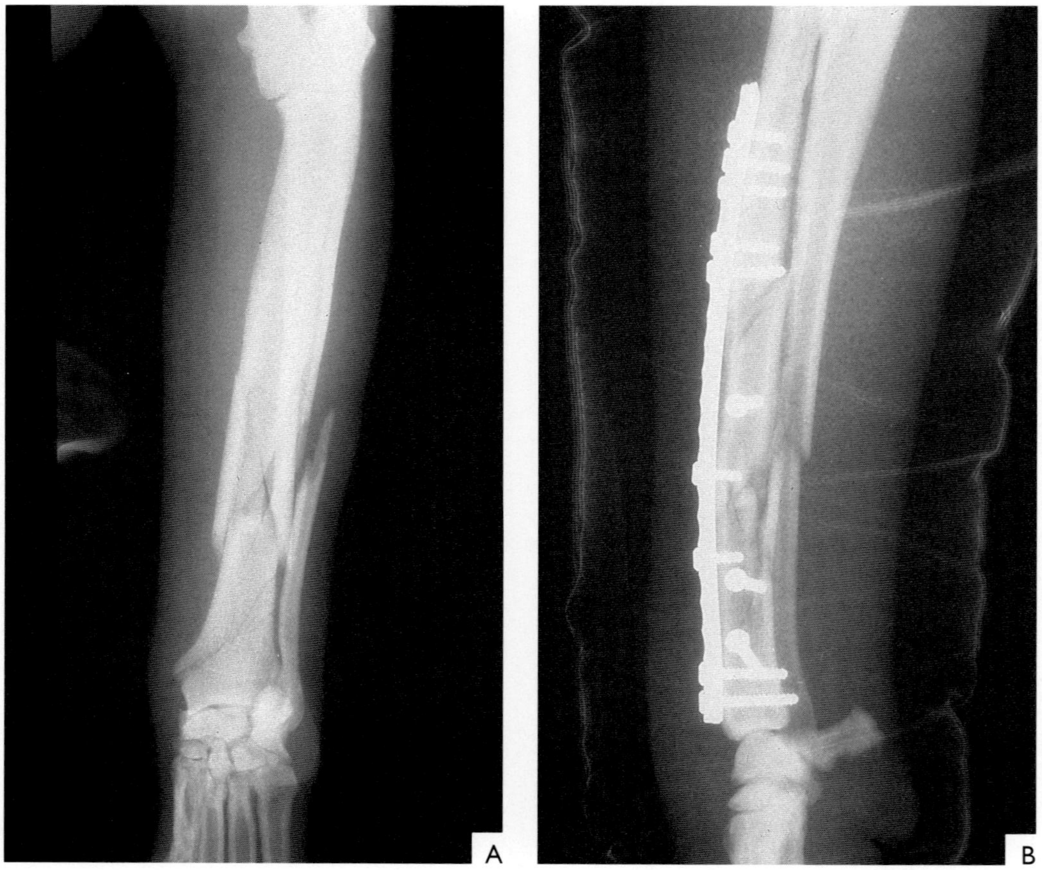

FIGURE 2.50 (A) Comminuted fracture of the radius and ulna. (B) Comminuted fracture of the radius and ulna showing the use of a long plate and interfragmentary lag screws.

REFERENCES

1. Knecht CD, et al. *Fundamental Techniques in Veterinary Surgery*, 3rd ed. Philadelphia: WB Saunders; 1987.
2. Leighton RL. Principles of conservative fracture management: splints and casts. *Semin Vet Med Surg (Small Anim)*. Fracture Management 1, Philadelphia: WB Saunders; 1991; 6(1):39–51.
3. Toombs JP. Principles of external skeletal fixation using the Kirschner-Ehmer splint. In Murtagh RJ, ed. *Semin Vet Med (Small Animal)*. Fracture Management 1, Philadelphia: WB Saunders; 1991; 6(1):68–74.
4. Howard PE. Principles of intramedullary pin and wire fixation. *Semin Vet Med Surg (Small Animal)*. Fracture Management 1, Philadelphia: WB Saunders; 1991; 6(1):52-67.
5. Boudrieau RJ. Principles of screw and plate fixation. *Semin Vet Med (Small Animal)*. Fracture Management 1, Philadelphia: WB Saunders; 1991; 6(1):75–89.

CHAPTER 3 HIND LIMB

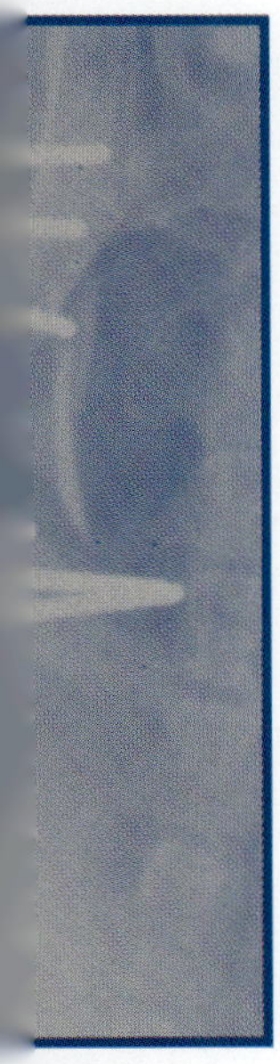
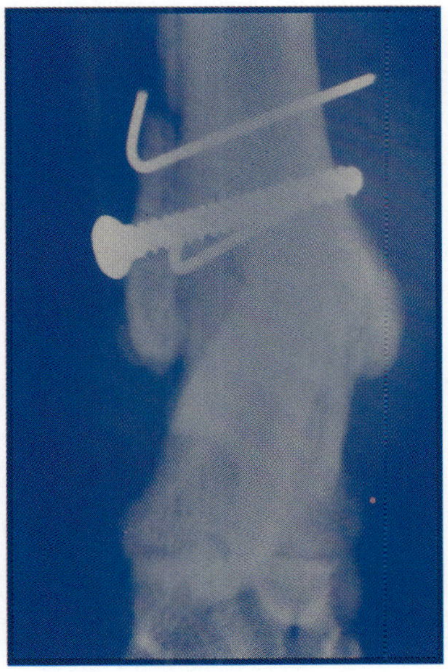
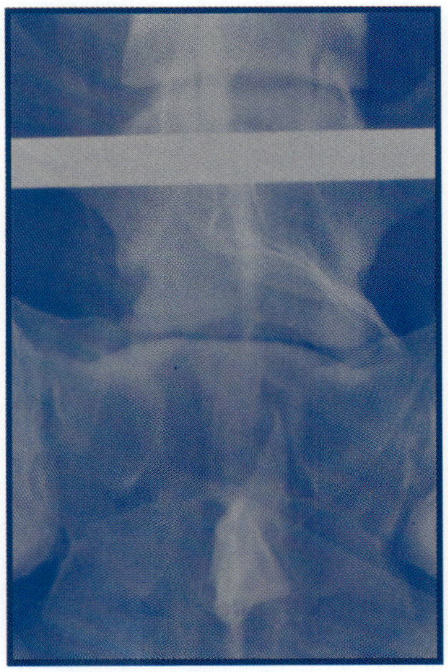
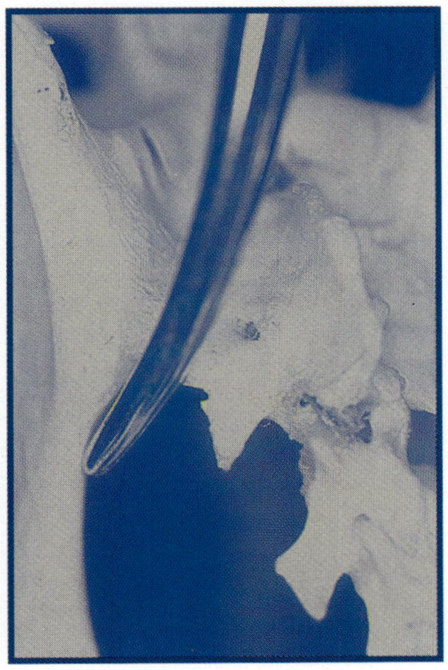
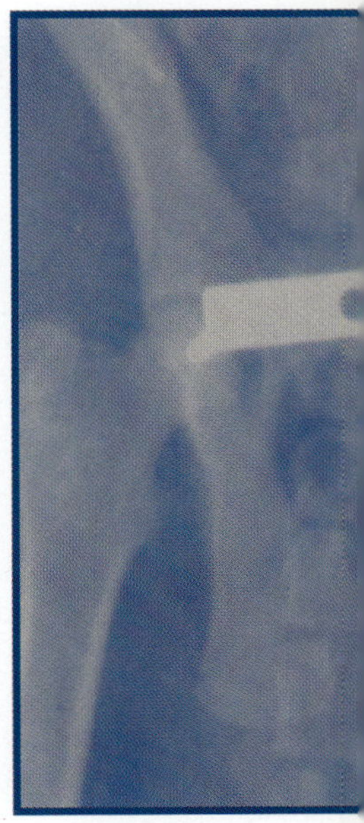

FRACTURES OF THE PELVIS

The pelvis is one of the most commonly broken bones in the dog. Almost all pelvic injuries are the result of automobile accidents. An examination must be conducted for soft-tissue damage such as rupture of the bladder, severed urethra, bowel rupture, fractured vertebrae, diaphragmatic hernia, traumatic lung lesions and tail paralysis from avulsion or fracture of the coccygeal vertebrae. Injury to the ischiatic nerve may cause temporary or permanent hind limb paralysis. Similarly, perineal and pudendal nerve injuries can result in urinary and fecal incontinence. These paralyses are usually unacceptable to the owner, who then requests that the patient be euthanatized.

In many cases, pelvic injuries without severe displacement or involvement of the acetabular articular surfaces can heal without surgical intervention (Fig. 3.1). The heavy musculature surrounding the pelvis aids in controling the fragments. All that is needed is nursing care for the animal's comfort. Many patients are ambulatory in a few days.

Pelvic injuries that heal in malalignment can obstruct the pelvic birth canal. If this condition cannot be rectified, the female should be spayed (Fig. 3.2).

Nutritional hyperparathyroidism with multiple fractures and collapse of the pelvis is rarely seen nowadays (Fig. 3.3).

Surgically repairing sacroiliac luxations, fractures of the wing and body of the ilium, acetabular fractures, ischial fractures, and symphyseal separations provides anatomic realignment, shortened healing time, and reduction of pain.

Acetabular fractures require anatomic reduction to maintain joint congruency and to avoid posttraumatic arthrosis.

Surgical intervention should be done as soon as the patient's condition permits. It becomes increasingly difficult to maneuver the fragments more than four or five days after the accident.

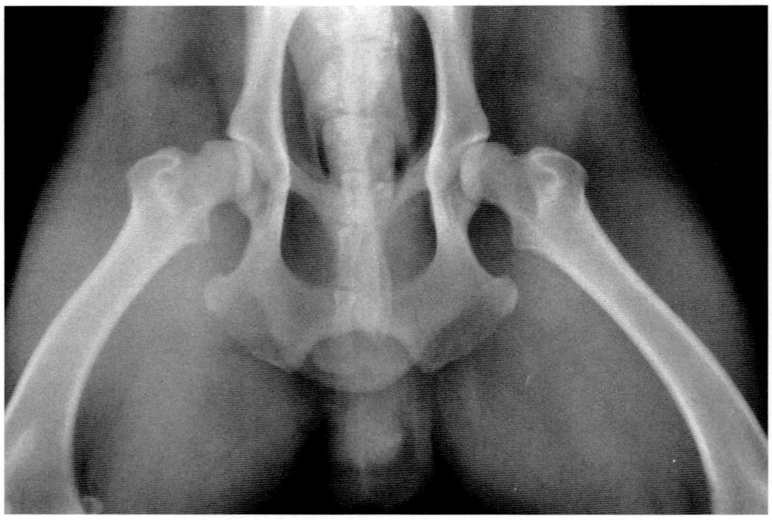

FIG. 3.1 V-D radiograph of a pelvic injury in a dog. No surgical intervention was required.

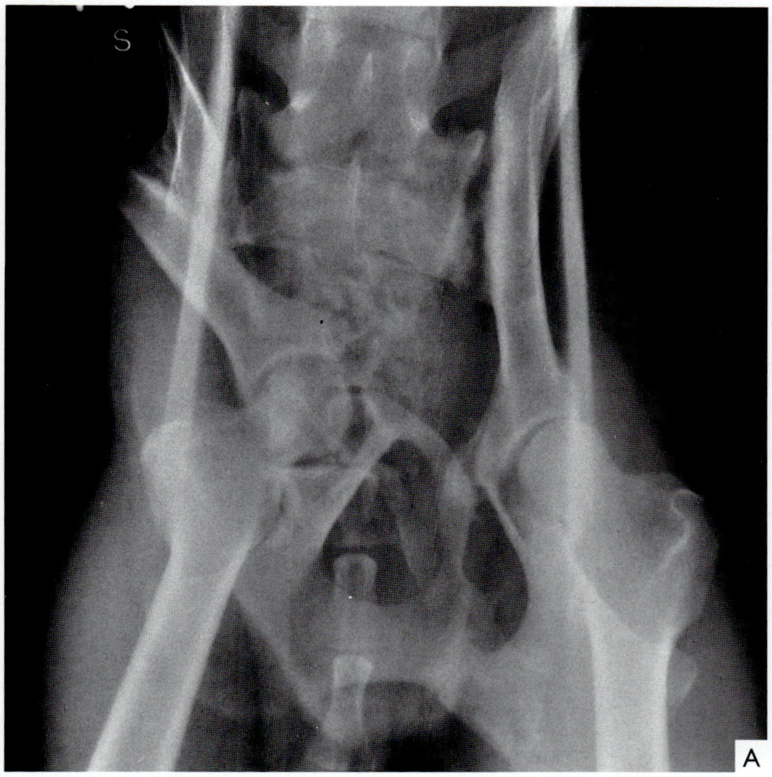

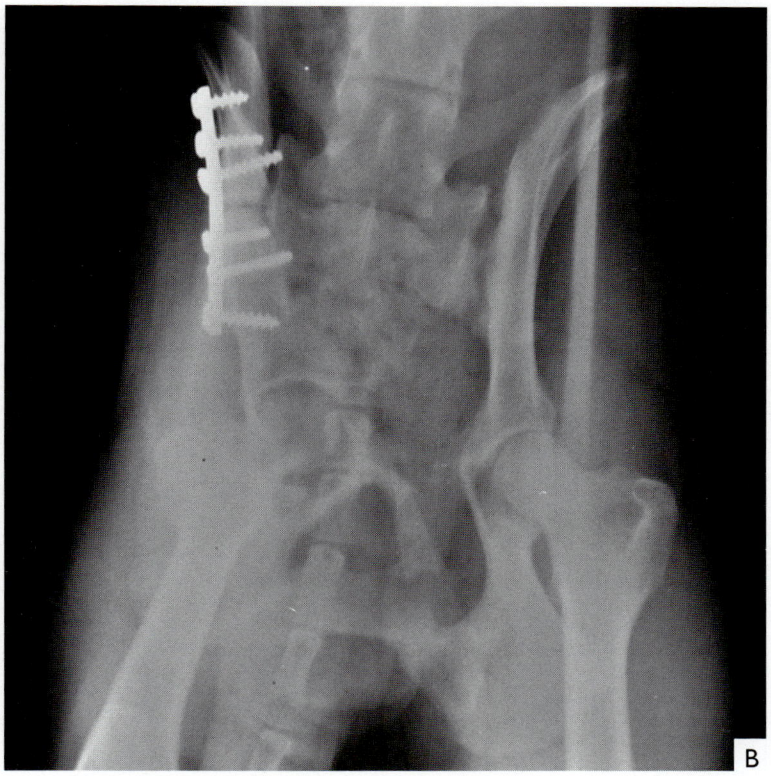

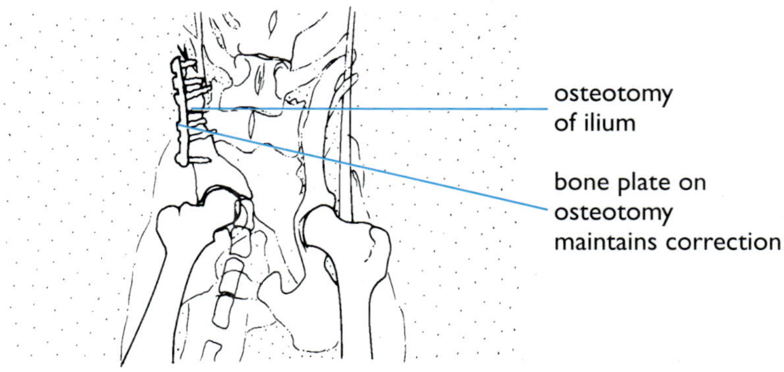

FIG. 3.2 (A) V-D radiograph of severe pelvic fractures that require surgical intervention, which was not done. (B) V-D radiograph of severe pelvic fractures that were not surgically corrected early, resulting in narrowing of the pelvic canal. Surgical repair was done by osteotomy of the ilium, which was secured with a bone plate. Some partial improvement was obtained.

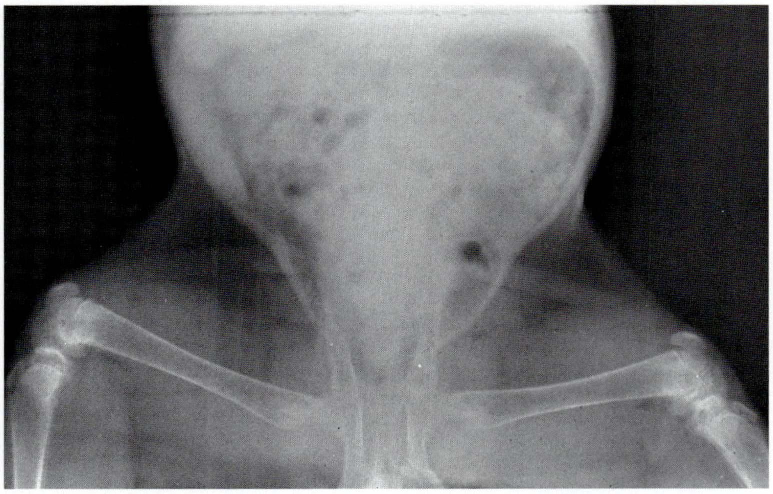

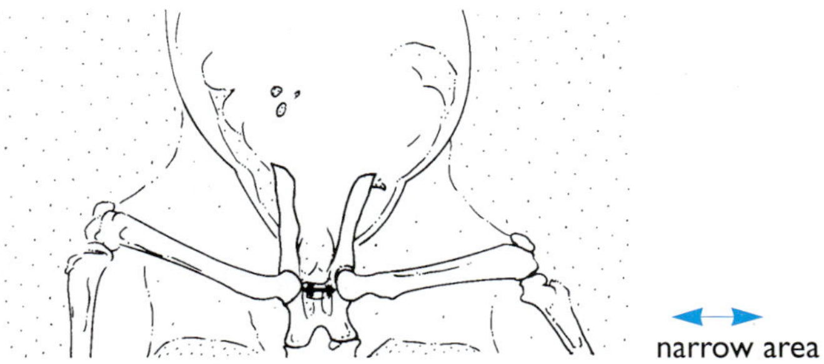

FIG. 3.3 Radiograph of a cat's pelvis with narrowing of the pelvic canal from nutritional hyperparathyroidism.

Ilium

Small bone fragments from injury to the wing of the ilium that cause pain are removed surgically. Epiphyseal fractures of the wing of the ilium are replaced and secured with K-wires (Fig. 3.4).

Ilial fractures, which are usually oblique, involve the body and the wing. They may be bilateral. The ischium and pubis are also often fractured at the same time. Reduction and fixation of the ilial fracture is usually all that is needed except when the acetabular or ischial fragment is severely displaced.

Although intramedullary pins, wires, lag screws, and external fixation devices can be used, bone plating is the most successful method of treatment.

SURGICAL TECHNIQUE

The wing and body of the ilium are approached through an incision extending from the iliac crest to just cranial to the trochanter major. The subcutaneous tissues and fat are cleared, exposing the separation between the middle gluteus dorsally and the tensor fascia lata ventrally. Subperiosteal reflection of the middle gluteus exposes the wing and body of the ilium. As the acetabulum is approached, the deep gluteus is elevated to expose the underlying bone. Centrally, the cranial gluteal nerve, artery, and vein cross the body of the ilium. Ventrally, the iliolumbar artery and vein lie close to the bone. The lateral circumflex artery and vein are located just cranial to the acetabulum in the tissues around the femoral neck. If necessary, both the cranial gluteal and the iliolumbar vessels are incised and

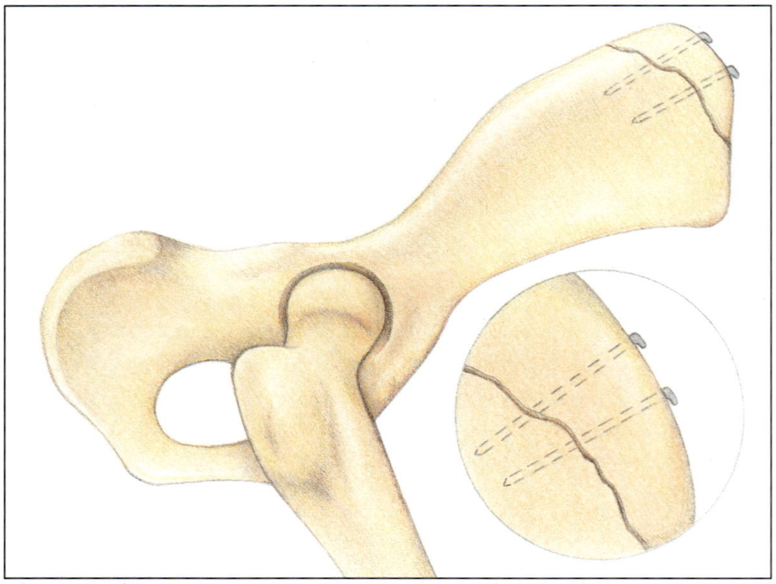

FIG. 3.4 Repair of epiphyseal fracture of the wing of the ilium repaired with two K-wires.

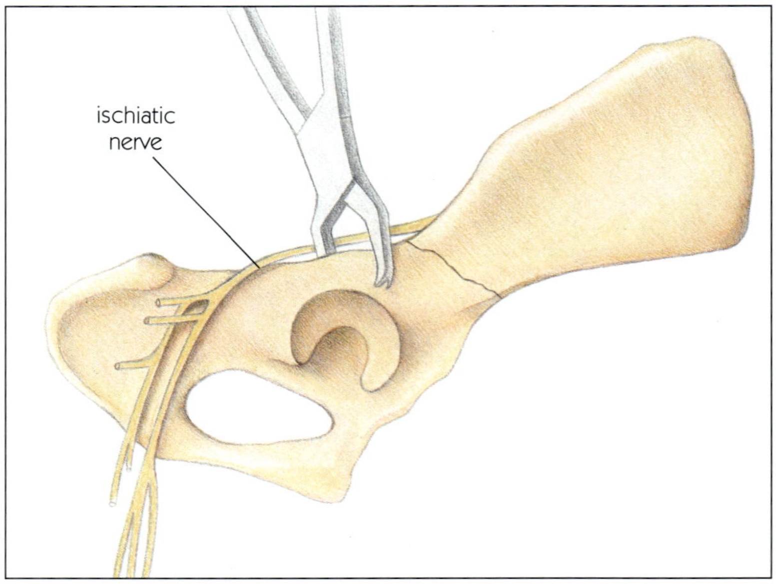

FIG. 3.5 Bone clamp on the body of the ilium.

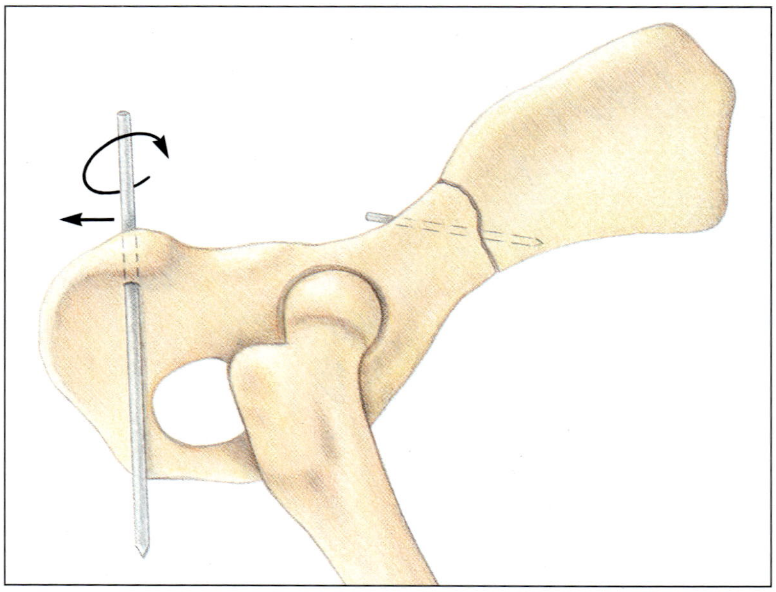

FIG. 3.6 An intramedullary (IM) pin placed ventrodorsally in the ischium to provide a handle with which to move the caudal fragment of a pelvic fracture.

ligated. When applying bone clamps, care must be taken not to injure the ischiatic nerve, which lies just medial to the ilial body (Fig. 3.5).

The caudal fragment usually lies medially under the cranial portion of the fractured ilium. The caudal fragment may be controlled by transfixing the tuber ischii ventrodorsally with an intramedullary pin (Fig. 3.6) or by making a small incision over the tuber ischii, exposing the bone dorsally and ventrally so that it can be grasped with a bone forceps.

The caudal fragment is lifted with a blunt bone hook, while traction is applied to the bone forceps or pin in the ischial tuberosity. An assistant may elevate the hip area by lifting the hind limb, holding it parallel to the table. Once the fracture is reduced, it is held with a bone forceps. If possible, a K-wire is driven across the fracture site to maintain the reduction.

A suitable bone plate is selected and contoured to fix the concavity of the bone. If possible, one of the screws in the cranial fragment should penetrate the body of the sacrum. This provides excellent holding power, which is needed because the rest of the screws will seat in rather thin bone (Figs. 3.7, 3.8).

The contoured plate is secured to the distal fragment. Each screw is placed in a hole that has been drilled, measured with a depth gauge, and tapped. The cranial screws are inserted. The surgical area is flushed with saline or Ringer's solution and suctioned dry.

Closure is done by suturing the fascial separation between the middle gluteus and the tensor fascia lata. The deep gluteus is sutured in place. Closure of the skin and subcutaneous tissue is routine.

The dog is confined for three weeks in a nicely padded cage. These patients at first require support when walking. Healing is usually rapid. The plate remains in place unless the screws loosen or pain develops.

Dislocation of the Sacroiliac Joint

With a severe blow from behind, the pelvis is pushed forward with such force that the ilium breaks away from the sacrum cranially. The

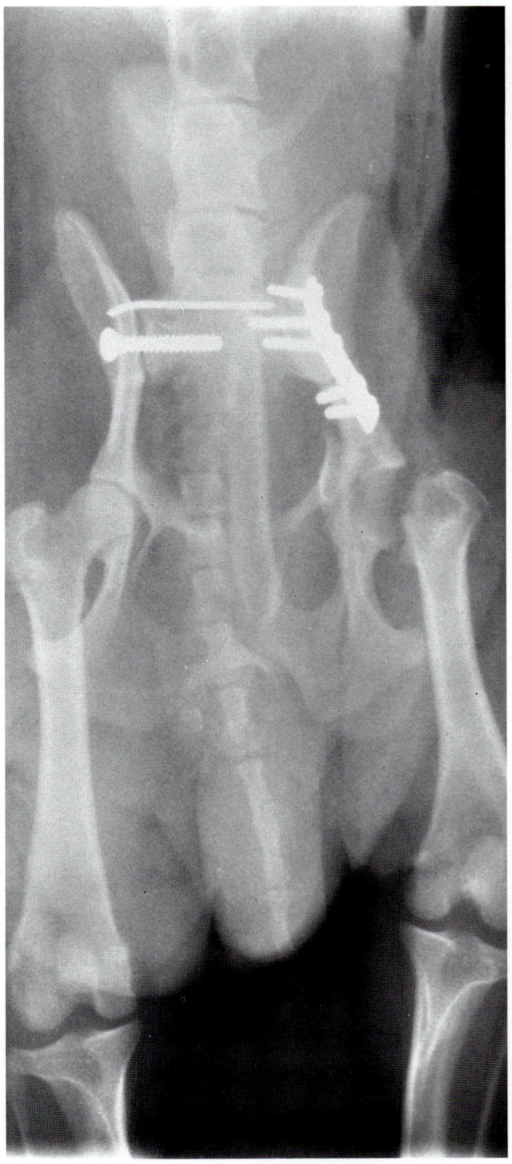

FIG. 3.7 Fractured ilium treated with bone plate. Second screw is placed nicely into body of the sacrum. The sacroiliac luxation is held in place with well-placed bone screw and K-wire.

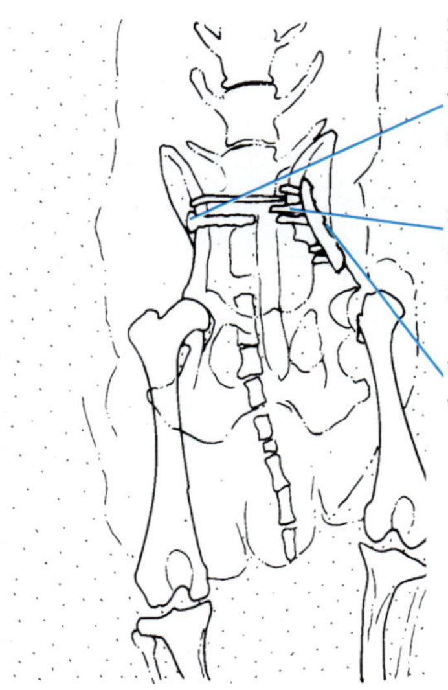

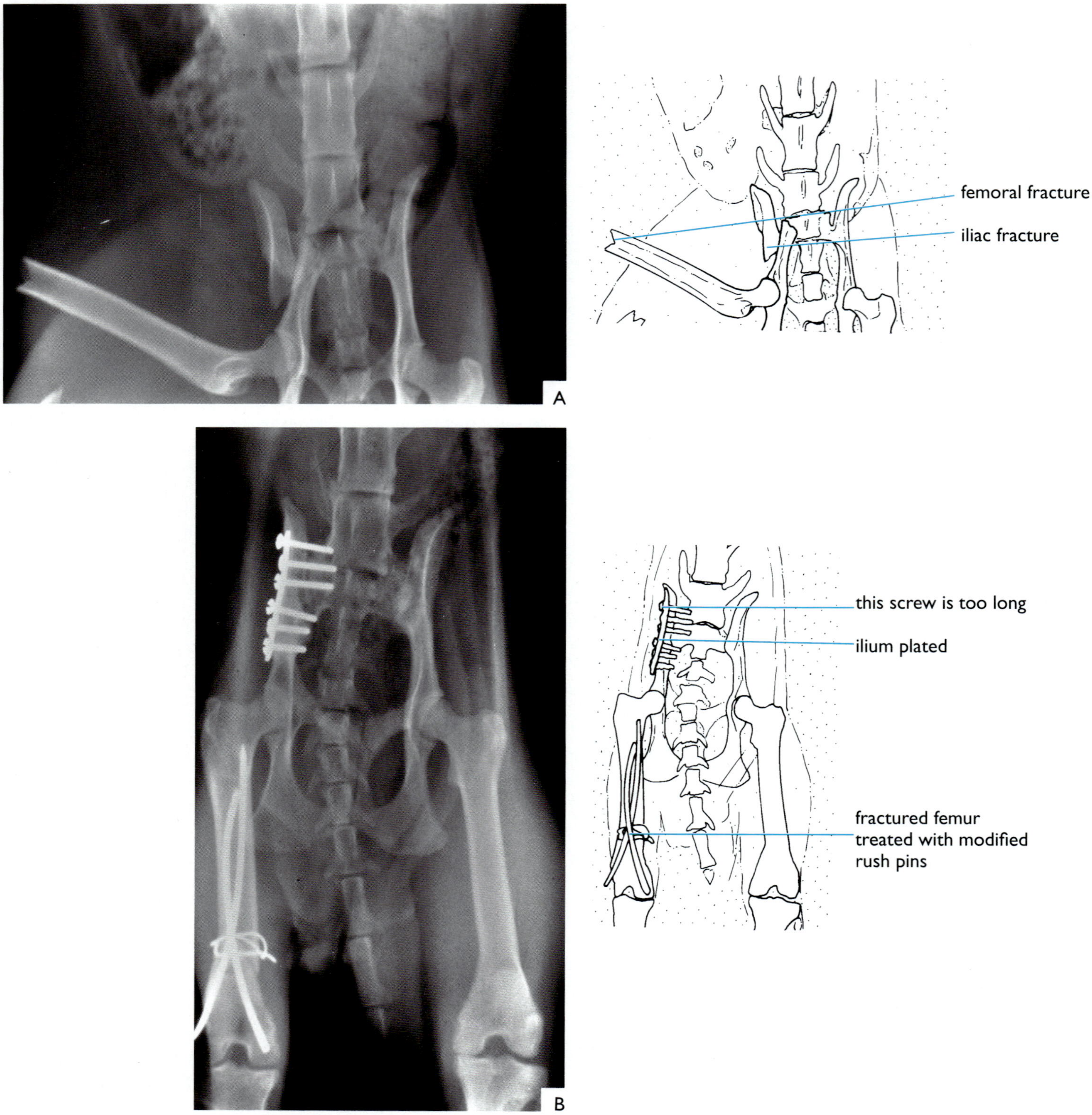

FIG. 3.8 (A) Radiograph of a fracture of the body of the ilium and a distal femoral fracture. (B) Fractured body of the ilium treated with a bone plate. Note that first screw is too long and penetrates the seventh lumbar vertebra. The femoral fracture was treated with modified Rush pin technique; this will be taken up in treatment of femoral fractures.

ischium and pubis are also fractured. The condition is often bilateral or associated with ilial fractures or hip dislocations. Severe fractures of the acetabulum may be present (Fig. 3.9).

Treatment of the iliosacral luxation consists of moving the ilium back to its proper position and securing it with a bone screw. Only a limited area in the body of the sacrum can receive the screw. A K-wire or another screw, if feasible, helps maintain the reduction (Fig. 3.10).

Additional support is provided by inserting an intramedullary pin from one ilial wing to the other, passing on top of L-7 (Fig. 3.11). In small dogs and cats, a threaded screw is used (Fig. 3.12).

SURGICAL TECHNIQUE

The ilium's wing is approached either dorsally, with the incision along the dorsal crest of the ilium and the dorsal iliac spine, or ventrally as described for an approach to the body of the ilium. This approach is used if there is an additional injury to the ilium.

For the dorsal approach the dog is placed in ventral recumbency and an incision is made through the skin and subcutaneous tissues over the crest of the ilium extending caudally over the dorsal iliac spine. The thin cutaneous trunci muscle is incised to expose the cranial border of the ilium's wing. The fascial origin of the middle gluteus is incised, then reflected subperiosteally to expose the underlying bone.

The cranial gluteal nerve, artery, and vein pass over the iliac spine at the level of the caudal articular surface of the sacrum. These structures are protected and the caudal border of the sacrum is located with a large, curved hemostat (Fig. 3.13).

The tissues between the iliac crest and the sacrum are reflected to expose the iliosacral joint surfaces. A bone-holding forceps is

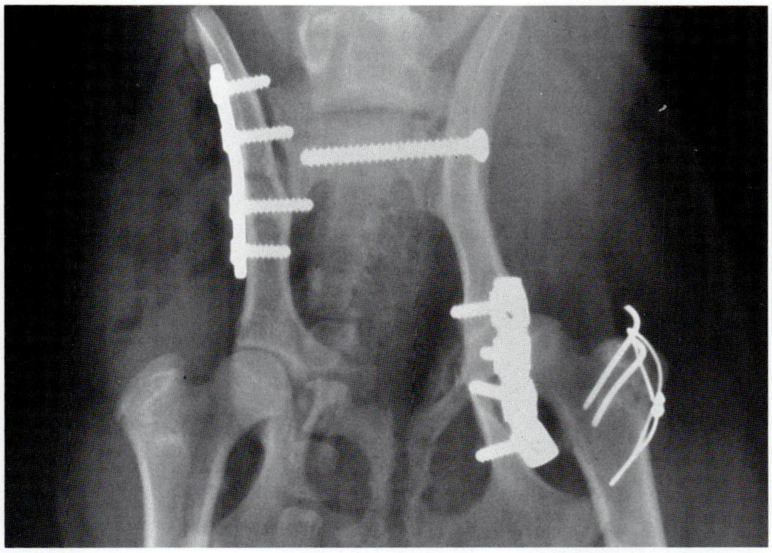

FIG. 3.9 Radiograph of a fractured body of the ilium treated with a bone plate, a luxation of the sacroiliac articulation treated with a well-placed bone screw and an acetabular fracture treated with a reconstruction bone plate.

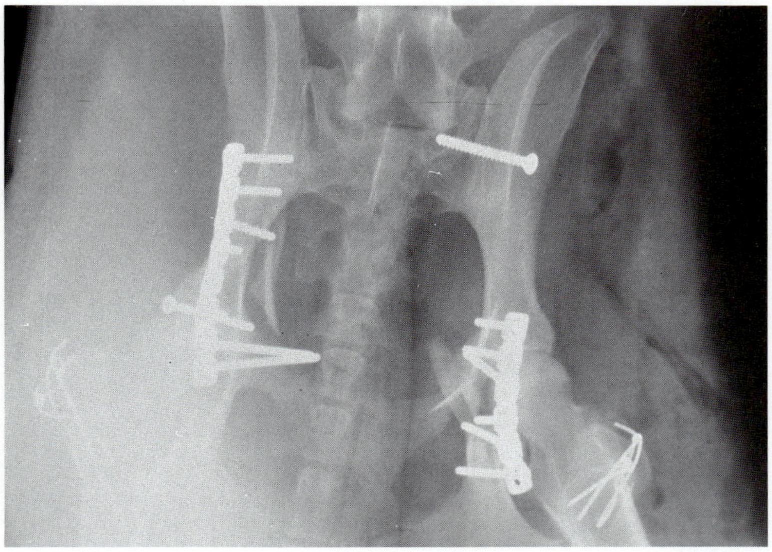

FIG. 3.10 Radiograph of a left sacroiliac luxation treated with a bone screw and bilateral acetabular fractures treated with reconstruction bone plates. Note the sacroiliac screw should be more caudal. The right acetabular plate has a loosened screw and the two caudal screws are much too long.

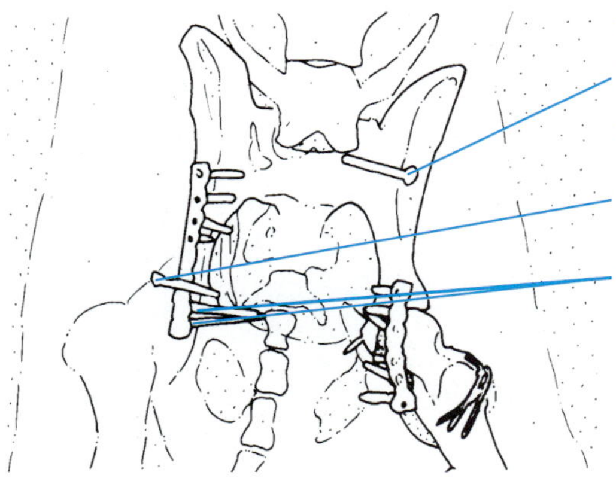

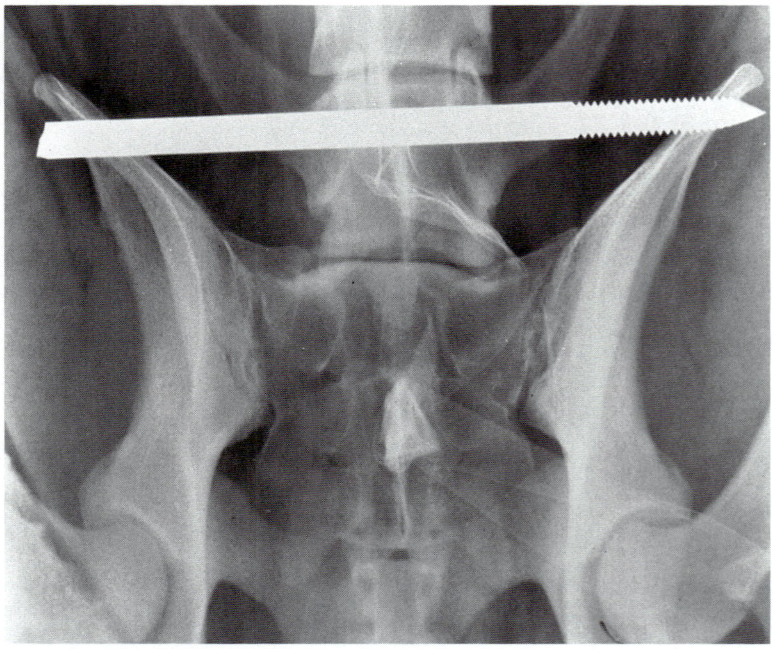

FIG. 3.11 Radiograph of a transilial pin used in a bilateral sacro-iliac luxation.

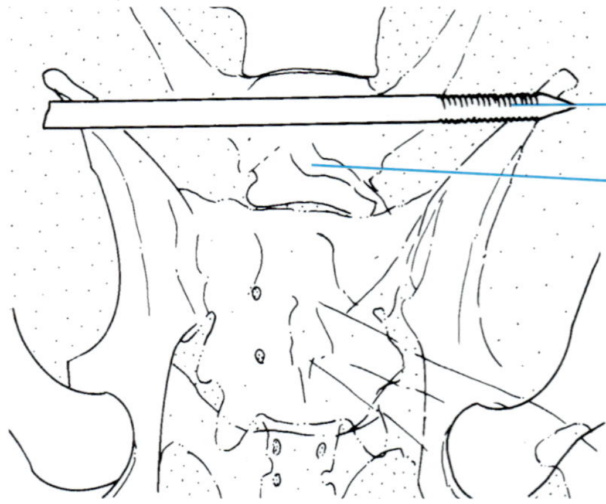

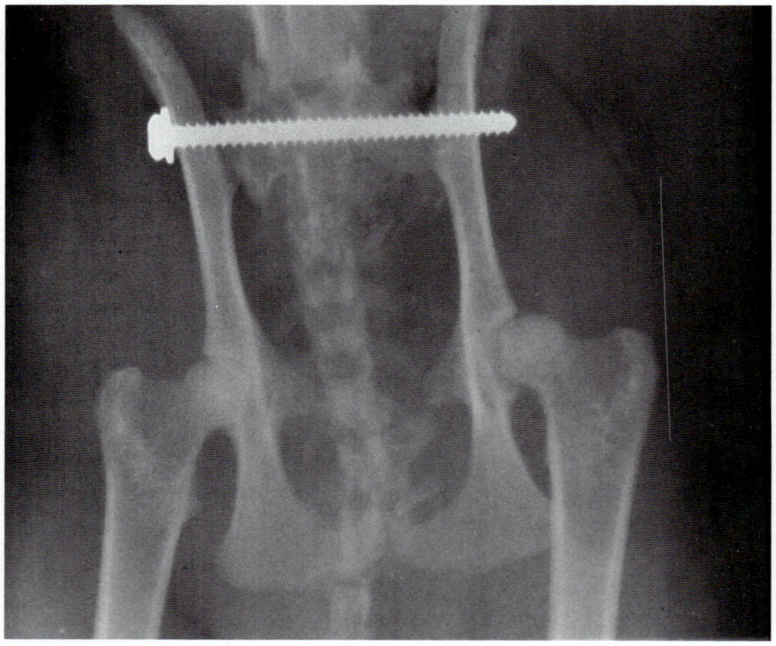

FIG. 3.12 Radiograph of a transilial screw used in a bilateral sacroiliac luxation.

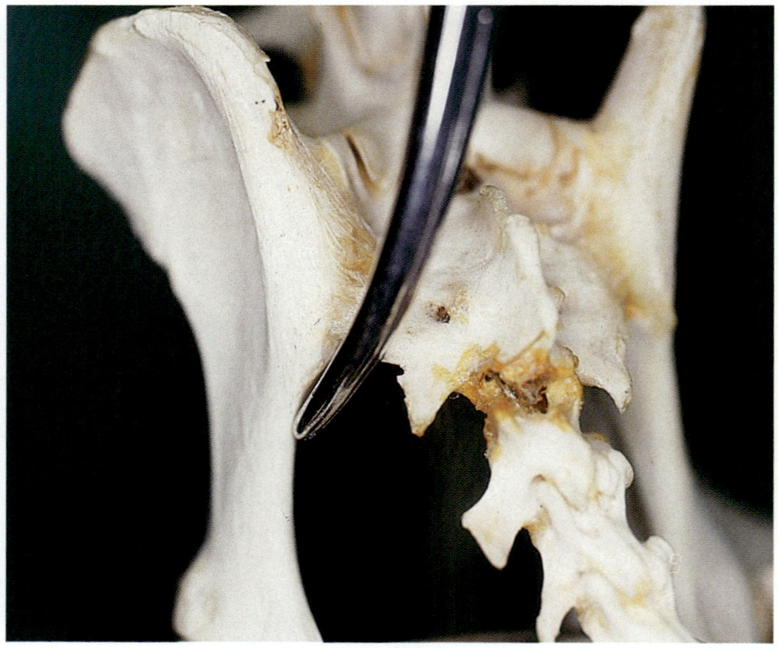

FIG. 3.13 Sacroiliac junction with curved hemostat identifying caudal aspect and retracting ischiatic nerve. Nerve would be caudal and medial to the hemostat.

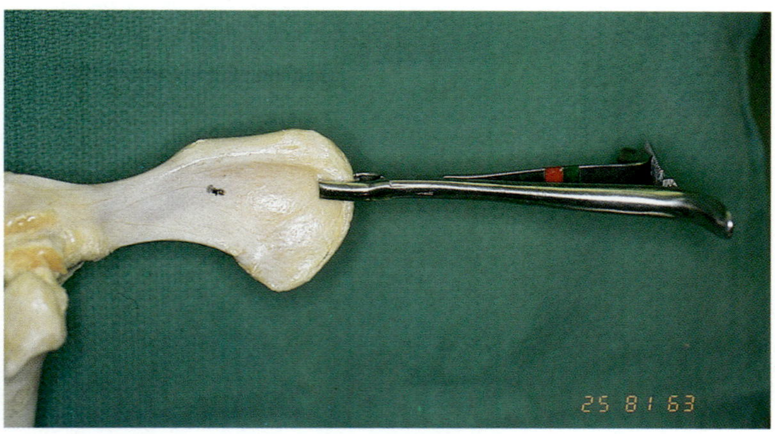

FIG. 3.14 Kern forceps on wing of ilium.

secured to the wing of the ilium and traction is applied to force the ilium caudally (Fig. 3.14). An assistant applies traction on the hind leg at the same time.

There is a small, limited area where a lag screw may be inserted to seat into the body of the sacrum. Misdirected screws have little holding power and can damage nerves.

The location for inserting the screw is obtained by drawing an imaginary line from the cranial dorsal iliac spine parallel to the iliac crest. Another line is drawn parallel to this line from the caudal dorsal iliac spine. Vertical and horizontal midlines are drawn. The site for the screw is midway on the caudal half of the horizontal line (Fig. 3.15).

When the reduction is obtained, it is held in place by a K-wire. The hole for the bone screw is drilled into the body of the first sacral vertebra. The hole is measured and tapped; the screw is inserted and tightened. The K-wire can be left in place or, if space permits, a second screw can be inserted to obtain a more rigid control.

Closure is done by replacing the middle gluteus and suturing the fascia at its origin. The rest of the tissues are replaced. Closure of the panniculus, subcutaneous tissues, and the skin is routine.

If a ventral approach is taken, the location of the luxation is obtained by inserting the index finger from the ventral border of the ilium up along the medial surface. A separation large enough to permit entry of the finger is made by separating the iliacus muscle from the ventral border of the ilium's wing.

Additional control can be provided by inserting an intramedullary pin from one dorsal area of the wing of the ilium to the other, passing it just above the seventh lumbar vertebra.

Acetabulum

Fractures of the acetabulum vary from a single dorsal split to severe fragmentation accompanied by hip luxation. The ischium and pubis are also often fractured. Frequently, reducing the acetabular fracture restores the ischium and pubis. Acetabular fractures require anatomic reduction to reestablish the joint's congruity so as to avoid posttraumatic joint disease.

In minor fractures in small dogs, K-wires are inserted cranio-caudally and caudo-cranially through the fracture with a figure-8 tension band wire applied to compress the fracture (Fig. 3.16). Similarly, a bone screw is placed in each fragment and a figure-8 tension band wire is placed on them (Fig. 3.17). External fixation devices are cumbersome, difficult to apply and tend to loosen. The best and most consistent results are achieved with bone plates.

Several types of bone plates are available. They must be contoured to the arched, rounded, and sloping surface of the dorsal acetabulum. At least two screws need to be inserted in the ischial portion of the fracture.

Reconstruction plates are rather difficult to contour. Acetabular plates, although specifically designed for this area, are unsatisfactory. Cuttable plates are also very stiff and resist contouring.

For dogs over 50 pounds, a 2.7 five- or six-hole dynamic compression plate is satisfactory. The surgeon should precontour the plate to a skeletal acetabulum similar to the patient's. This will save time and surgical exposure. For smaller dogs, 2.0 miniplates in "T" and "L" formations (Fig. 3.18) are used.

An oscillating bit attachment to the power drill is useful, since it does not pick up tissue and is very safe to use near the ischiatic nerve. An additional advantage is that it is easy to guide, since it will not slip off the selected area, as happens with a rotary bit.

SURGICAL TECHNIQUE

The acetabulum is exposed through a dorsal approach. An incision through the skin and subcutaneous tissue is begun midway between the trochanter major and the dorsal spine, extending just cranial to the trochanter, parallel to the shaft of and extending to the proximal third of the femur. The fascia lata is incised along the cranial edge of the biceps femoris. These two structures are retracted. The superficial gluteus is transected near its insertion on the femur and retracted dorsally. The insertion of the middle gluteus on the

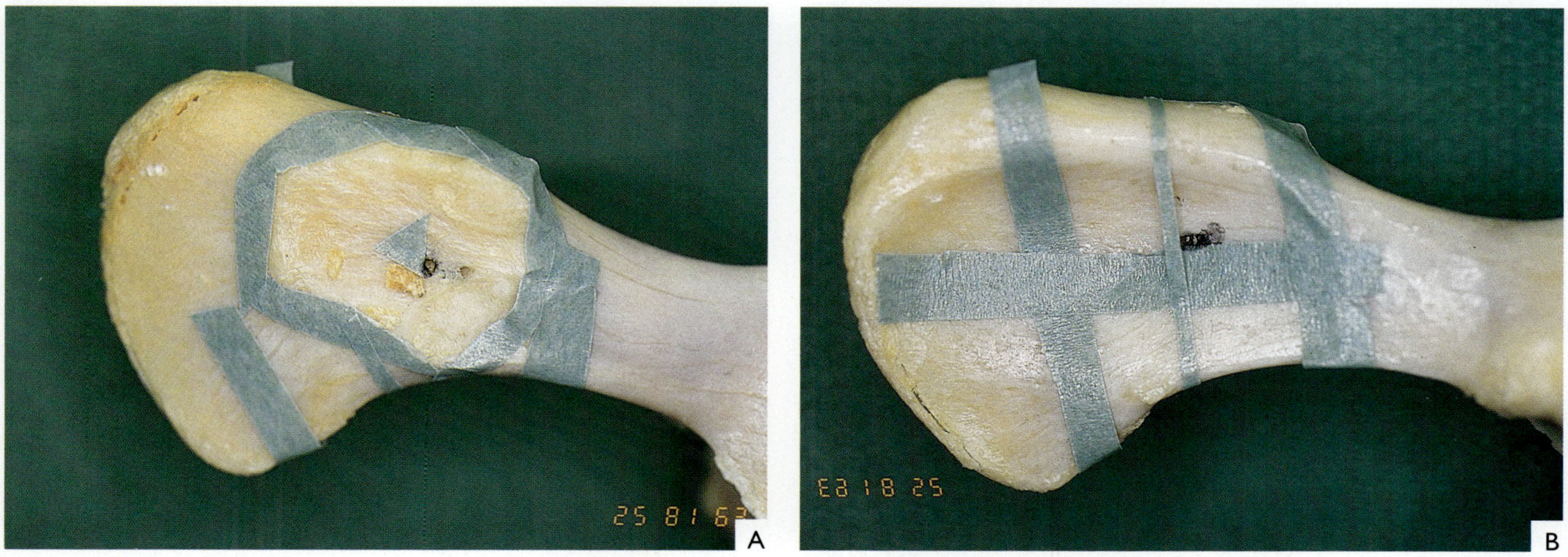

FIG. 3.15 (A) Location of best site for insertion of screw for stabilizing sacroiliac luxation. Tapes identify the imaginary lines. (B) Medial view showing central location of the screw in the sacroiliac articulation.

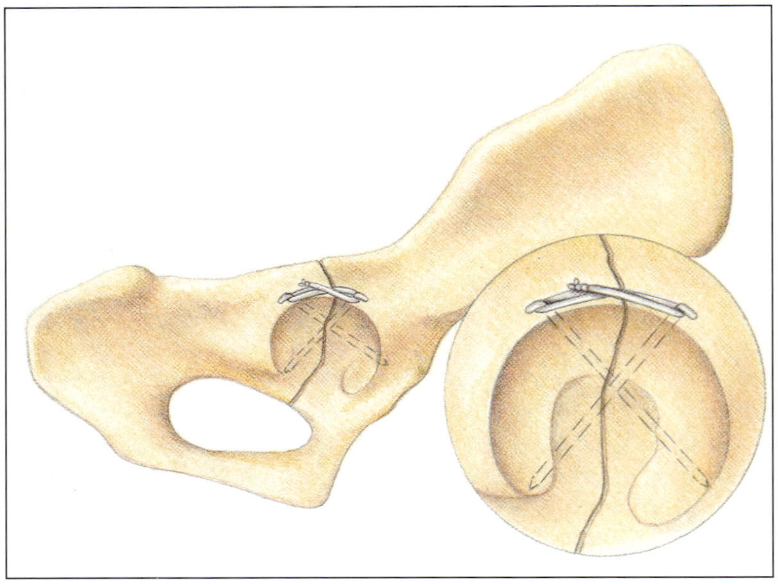

FIG. 3.16 An acetabular fracture secured with K-wires inserted across the fracture. Tension is applied with figure-8 wire.

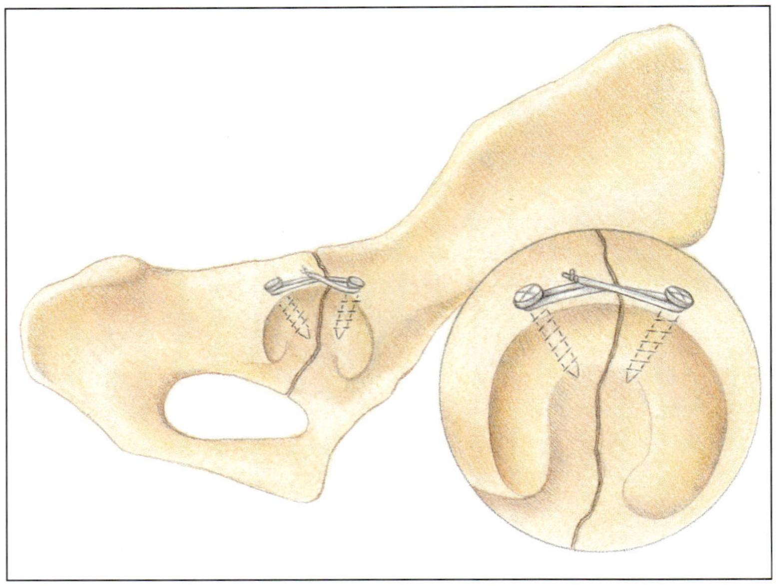

FIG. 3.17 An acetabular fracture secured with two bone screws and a tension band figure-8 wire.

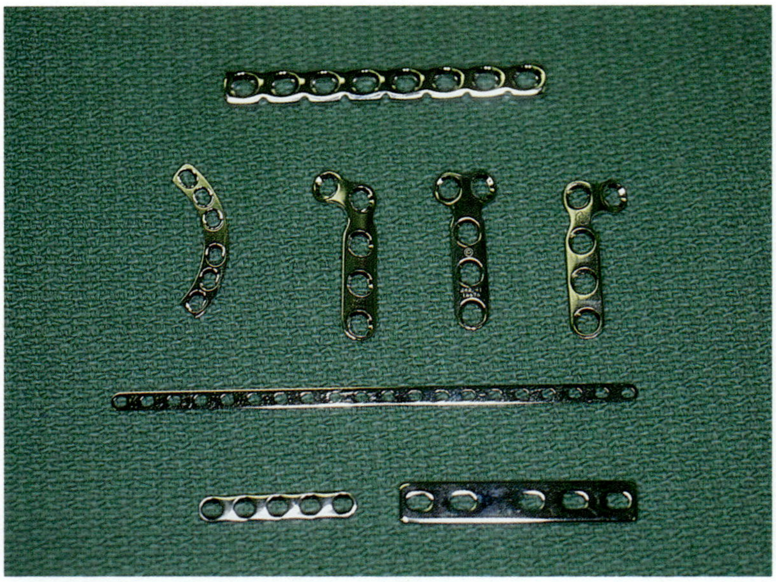

FIG. 3.18 Varieties of plates used in treatment of acetabular fractures.

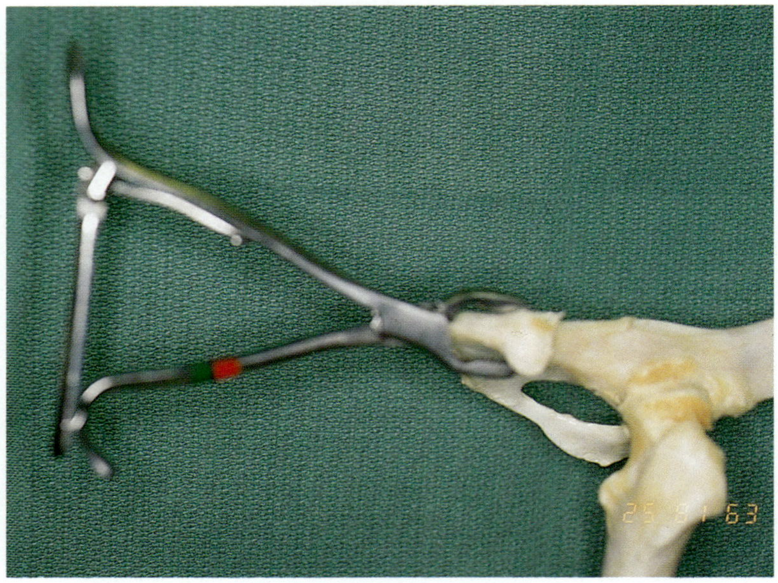

FIG. 3.19 Slide of Kern forceps on ischium.

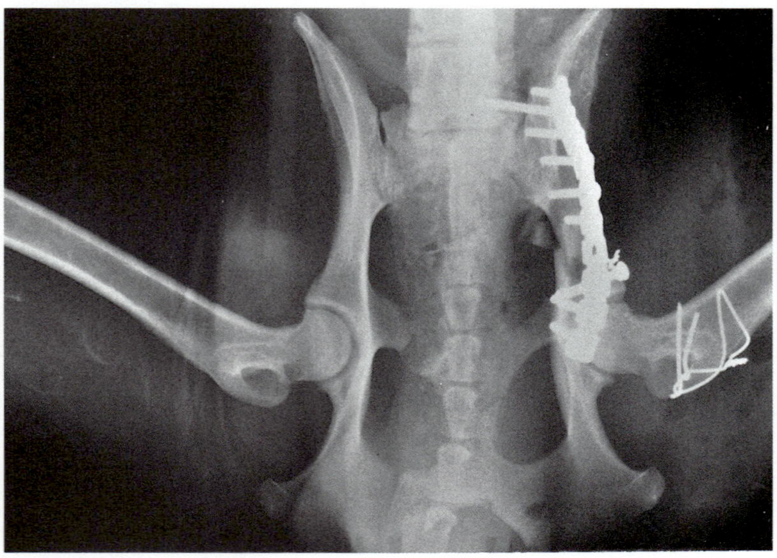

FIG. 3.20 Radiograph of a caudal ilial fracture treated with a bone plate.

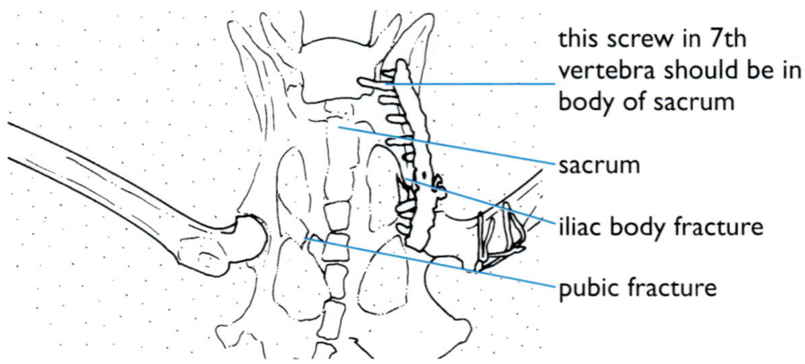

trochanter is outlined by mostly blunt dissection. A Gigli bone saw wire is used to osteotomize the trochanter so that the middle gluteus can be retracted cranially. The deep gluteus is freed from its attachment to the dorsal rim of the acetabulum and the ilial body.

The area of fracture is exposed. Further caudal exposure is obtained by transecting the insertion of the gemelli and the obturator internus near the trochanteric fossa. Identifying sutures are placed in the cut ends. The ischiatic nerve is identified and protected.

Reduction of the fracture is begun. A bone forceps fastened to the ischiatic tuberosity through a small incision allows an assistant to rotate and elevate the fragments into position (Fig. 3.19). A K-wire is inserted across the fracture to provide temporary anchoring while the plate is contoured. It should have at least two screws in the ischial component and three or more in the ilial. Screws are inserted in the caudal segment first. The K-wire may be cut off and left in place or removed (Fig. 3.20).

The joint capsule is frequently torn, permiting observation of the joint surface reduction. The capsule is sutured closed. Other fractures of the ischium and pubis usually require no treatment.

Closure is done by reattaching the gemelli and internal obturator to their tendinous insertion. The osteotomy of the trochanter is reattached by inserting two K-wires and applying a figure-8 tension band wire. The K-wires are bent at a right angle and cut off. The short-angled ends are turned medially and the pins are driven in with light taps of an orthopedic hammer. The superficial gluteus is reattached. The fascial separation of the fascia lata and the biceps femoris is sutured. Closure of the subcutaneous tissues and the skin is routine.

Ischium

Most ischial fractures occur in conjunction with other more major fractures and tend to be reduced when these are repaired.

Small fractures of the ischiatic tuberosity rarely require treatment (Fig. 3.21). Larger ones are distracted by the pull of the biceps femoris, semi-tendinosus and semi-membranosus muscle, which causes pain and interrupts healing.

The loose fragment is reattached with K-wires in small dogs and lag screws in large ones (Fig. 3.22). Fractures of the ischial body are treated with a screw-tipped intramedullary pin. On occasion the ischiatic symphysis is wired together.

SURGICAL TECHNIQUE

For repair of a fracture of the ischiatic tuberosity, the surgical approach is made directly over the tuberosity, proceeding down to the bone. Dorsal and ventral muscle attachments are lifted away with a periosteal elevator to expose the fracture. The fragment is grasped with a small bone forceps and replaced. A K-wire is inserted to maintain the reduction. One, or preferably two, lag screws are placed. The K-wire may remain or be removed.

Closure is done by suturing fascia subcutaneous tissue and skin in the usual manner.

For repairing a fracture of the ischial body, exposure is gained by incising directly over the caudal third of the sacrotuberous ligament. A fracture makes the ligament more difficult than usual to identify. The pelvic fascia is incised, revealing the origin of a portion of the biceps femoris on the sacrotuberous ligament. The fascial attachment is incised and the muscle mass is retracted, exposing the gemelli and the obturator internus muscles as they cross over the ischial body. The ischiatic nerve lies cranially. It may be involved in the fracture and must be handled with care.

After placing mattress sutures on both sides of the incision, the obturator internus muscle is transected. The stitches should be placed first, because muscle retraction makes suturing difficult after a transection.

The fracture is exposed and elevated. An intramedullary pin with one threaded end is selected. The unthreaded end is introduced into the medullary portion of the ischial body and the pin is

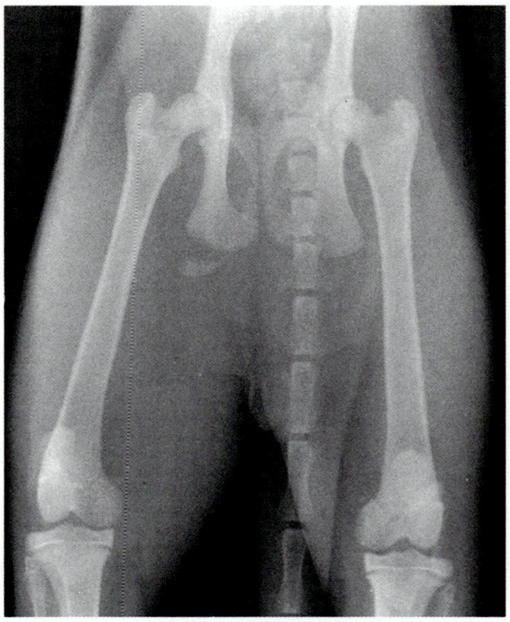

FIG. 3.21 Radiograph of a small fracture of the ischiatic tuberosity.

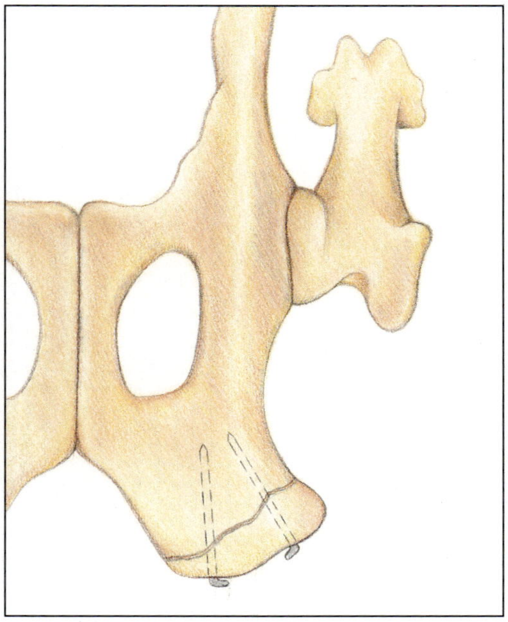

FIG. 3.22 A large caudal ischial fragment secured with K-wires.

driven retrograde to exit near the ischiatic tuberosity. The pin is withdrawn caudally until only the tip is visible at the fracture site. Using the pin as a lever, the fracture is reduced and the screw tip is threaded firmly into the bony mass, medial to the acetabulum. The pin is cut off at its exit point on the caudal ischium (Fig. 3.23).

The gemelli and obturator internus are closed by tying the mattress suture ends together. The biceps is replaced on the sacrotuberous ligament, which will be drawn tightly into position with the reduction of the fracture. The fascia and subcutaneous and skin tissues are closed. The pin is usually removed in three or four weeks.

Pubis

These fractures usually require no surgical intervention. As a component of other fractures they are aligned when the major fracture is reduced.

Fractures of the pubis (and ischiatic) symphysis may spread so far apart that the patient cannot adduct the hind limbs. This occurs more frequently in the cat. Often the hind legs need only to be placed in hobbles. The animal should be confined to a cage, and receive nursing care.

The symphysis may be wired together, providing relief from pain and speeding the recovery of use of the hind legs.

Formerly, fecal obstruction was seen in cats whose pelvises had collapsed from nutritional hyperparathyroidism. Malunited pelvic fractures also prohibit passage of feces and are a cause of dystocia. Surgical correction consists of splitting and wedging apart the symphysis or removing it. The symphysiotomy or partial symphysiectomy is prevented from collapsing by inserting a bone graft or steel prosthesis (Fig. 3.24). A sectioning of the ilial body is required with malunions. The osteotomy is plated.

SURGICAL TECHNIQUE

In the female dog and in cats, the pelvic symphysis is approached by a midline incision directly above it. In the male dog, the skin and subcutaneous tissue incision are directed away from the midline at the attachment of the penis to run parallel to this structure. A branch of the external pudendal artery and other vessels must be isolated and ligated. The penile body is undermined by blunt dissection and retracted to expose the midline. The incision on the midline is now made to expose the symphysis, which is freed of fascia and muscle insertions with a periosteal elevator.

The fractured symphysis is wired together by preplacing wire sutures through holes drilled in the pubic and ischial portions. The hind legs are elevated to bring the symphysis together. The wires are twisted, cut, and the ends laid flat to the bone (Fig. 3.25).

With a collapsed pelvis, the symphysis is cut away with a small rongeur. A metal spreader or a bone graft is placed across the ischial area to prevent collapse (Fig. 3.26).

Closure of the soft tissues is performed in the usual manner. Removal of the symphysis enables cats to defecate normally.

With malaligned pelvic fractures, the symphysis is cut and the soft tissues are closed. The body of the ilium is exposed at a separate surgery. An assistant aids the repositioning by rectal palpation. The osteotomy is plated.

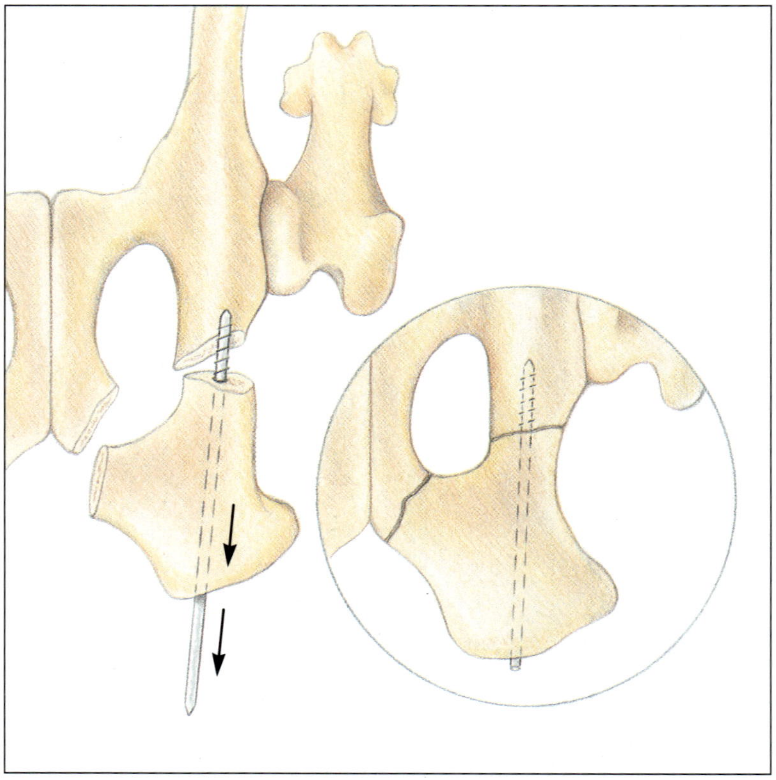

FIG. 3.23 Intramedullary fixation of a fracture of the ischial body.

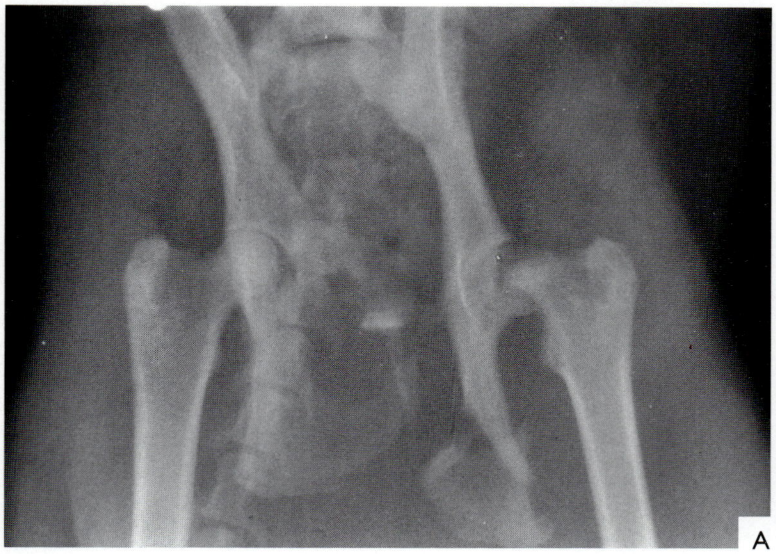

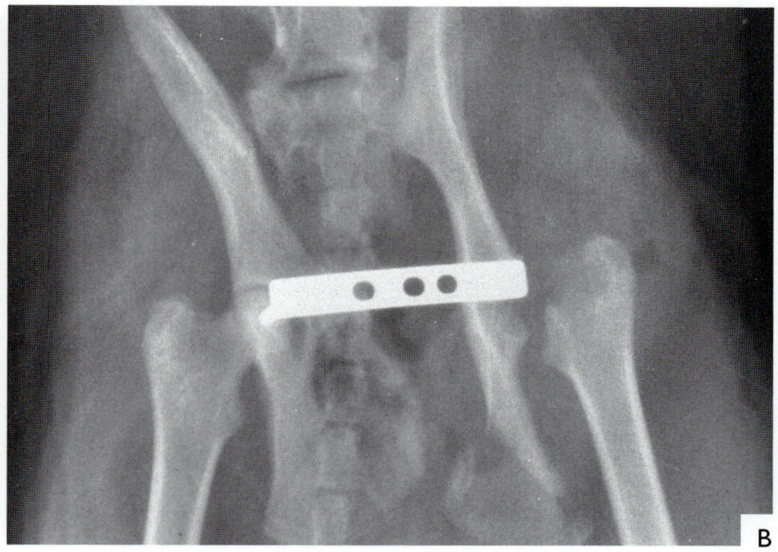

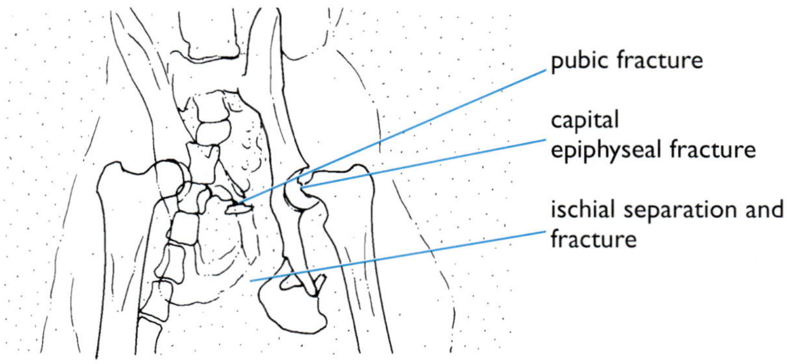

FIG. 3.24 (A) Radiograph of a severe fracture of the pubis and ischium. There is a capital epiphyseal fracture of the left femur. (B) Radiograph of a fractured pubis and ischium. The surgeon elected to plate the pubic space, since the caudal ischial fragment offered no support.

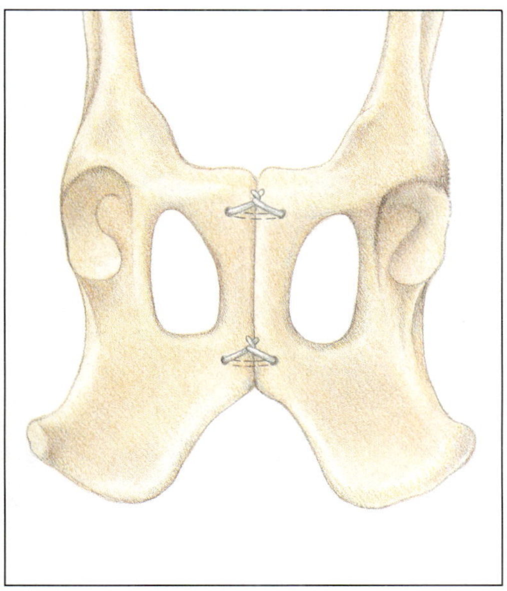

FIG. 3.25 The pelvic symphysis, secured with wire sutures.

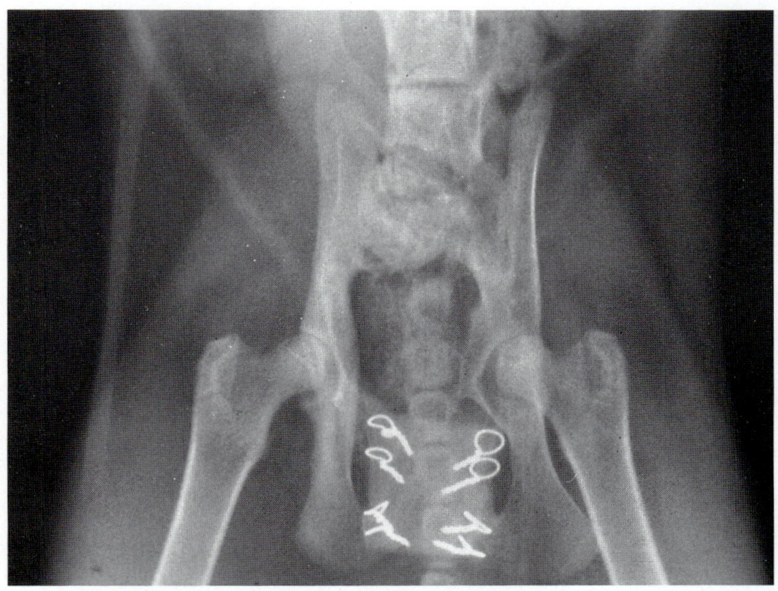

FIG. 3.26 Radiograph of a pelvic symphysiectomy with a bone graft placed to maintain the width of the pelvic canal.

Triple Osteotomy for Relief of Hip Dysplasia

Osteotomizing the pubis and ischium at the obturator foramen and transversely transecting and plating the body of the ilium with a special angled Slocum® plate (Slocum Enterprises, Eugene, OR) improves the coverage of the femoral head by outwardly rotating the acetabulum.

The degree of angulation depends on the severity of the dysplasia. Dogs between the ages of six months to a year with evidence of moderate hip dysplasia benefit most (Fig. 3.27). Very severe hip dysplasia requires a total hip replacement when mature.

Special Slocum® plates with angles of 20°, 30°, and 40° are used (Fig. 3.28). A standard DC plate can be bent to shape, but requires a lot of trial and error fitting.

SURGICAL TECHNIQUE

The dog is placed in dorsal recumbency. An incision is made through the skin and subcutaneous tissues over the origin of the pectineus muscle in the groin. The underlying fascia is incised, as is the fibrous attachment to the ileopectineal eminence. The pectineus muscle retracts. A periosteal elevator is used to expose the bone caudally to the rim of the cranial portion of the obturator foramen. A Hohmann retractor is inserted to retract and protect the tissues as the pubis is transected with an osteotome. All hemorrhage is controlled.

Closure is done by suturing the heavy fascia, the subcutaneous tissue, and skin.

With the dog in ventral recumbency, a dorsoventral incision through the skin and subcutaneous tissues is made over the caudal aspect of the ischium at a point where it is nearest to the caudal rim of the obturator foramen. The incision is retracted and the muscle attachments are elevated with a periosteal elevator. Care must be taken to stay close to the bone. A right-angled hemostat is inserted ventrally to the caudal edge of the obturator foramen, where it is turned dorsally to grasp the Gigli bone saw wire that is inserted dorsally. The ischium is transected caudally (Figs. 3.29, 3.30).

For closure, the fascia, the subctaneous tissue, and the skin are sutured. The dog is placed in lateral recumbency. The ilial body is approached by an incision extending from the center of the iliac crest to just cranial to the trochanter major. Skin, subcutaneous tissues, and the incised fascia are retracted to expose the intermuscular

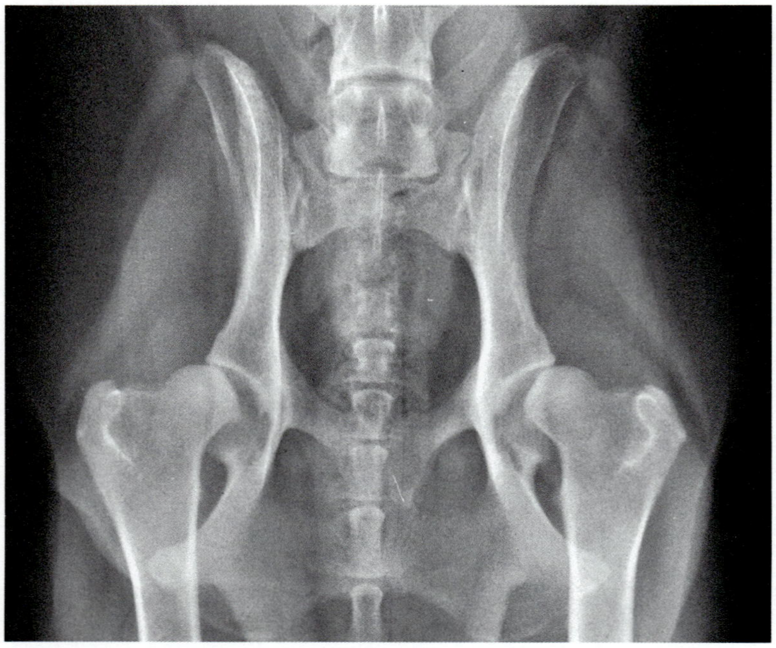

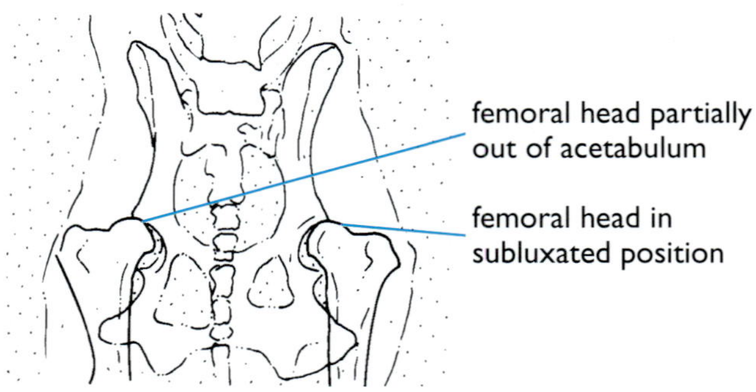

FIG. 3.27 Radiograph of a dog with a degree of hip dysplasia that would benefit from a triple pelvic osteotomy.

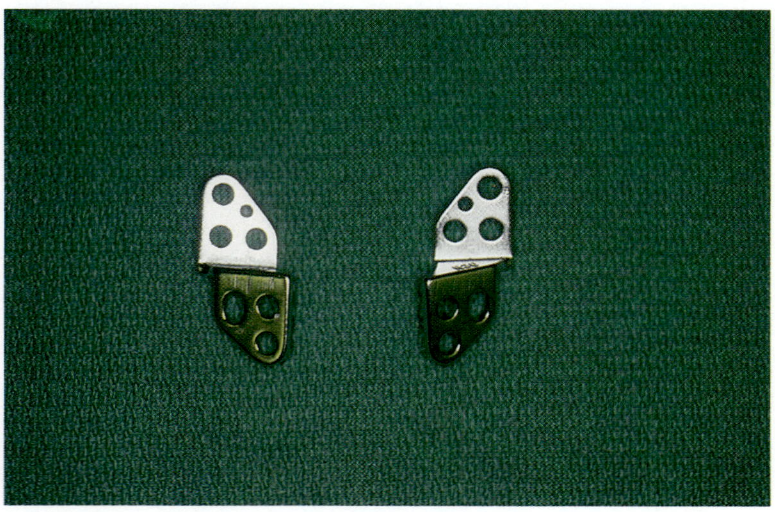

FIG. 3.28 Slides showing right and left Slocum plates used in triple pelvic osteotomies.

septum between the middle gluteus and the tensor fascia lata. A separation between these muscles is made and the middle gluteus is elevated dorsally. Sharp and blunt dissection separates the cranial portion of the middle gluteus from the wing of the ilium. The deep gluteal muscle is elevated from the ilial body. The cranial gluteal artery and vein are incised and ligated and the nerve is sectioned.

The iliacus muscle is freed of its attachment to the ventral border of the ilial body. The nutrient artery of the ilial body is located here and will require ligation. Further elevation of the deep gluteus caudally exposes the cranial portion of the acetabulum.

Where greater exposure is needed, the primary incision is continued at a right angle, parallel to the cranial third of the femur. Reflecting the skin and subcutaneous tissues exposes the superficial gluteus, which is transected at its insertion on the femur and reflected dorsally. An osteotomy of the trochanter major is done and the middle gluteus is retracted dorsocranially.

The special plate has three holes in each half, two side-by-side near the center and one away from the center. When applied, the screw in the most cranial hole should be located so that it penetrates the body of the sacrum. The index finger is inserted under the ilium to identify the caudal articular surface of the sacrum, as an aid in placing the screw.

A malleable retractor is inserted medially to protect the soft tissues, especially the ischiatic nerve. A perpendicular transection of the ilium is made with a power saw just caudal to the dorsal iliac spine. This should permit the cranial screw, and sometimes an additional screw, to be placed into the sacral body.

Slocum® plates in 20° and 30° angulations are usually sufficient. Too much outward rotation will impinge the brim of the acetabulum onto the femoral neck. The surgeon must use judgment in this regard.

The caudal portion of the ilium is held with a bone forceps to maintain the outward rotation until all the screws are in place. The osteotomized trochanteric fragment is reset caudally onto a pre-

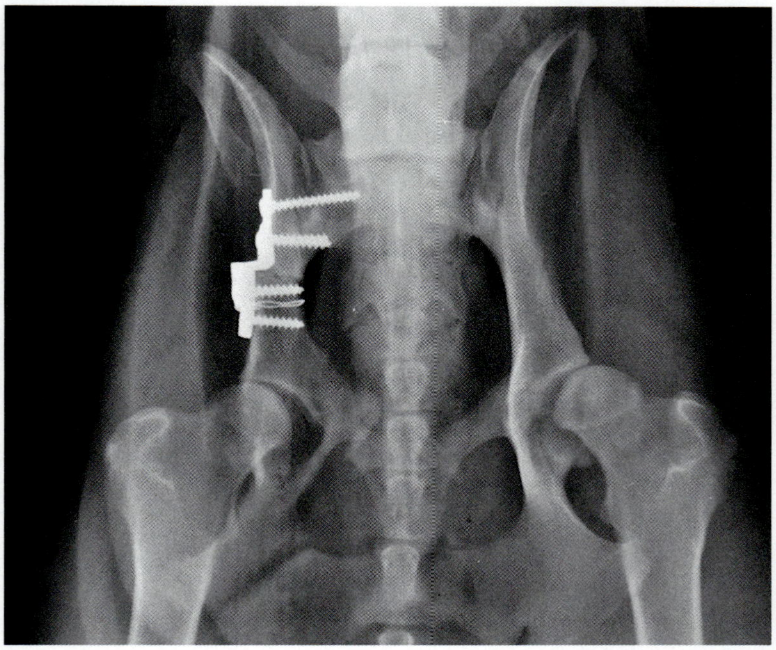

FIG. 3.29 Radiograph of a triple pelvic osteotomy with a Slocum® plate in the ilium for improvement of acetabular coverage of the femoral head. Lines of osteotomy cuts are indicated.

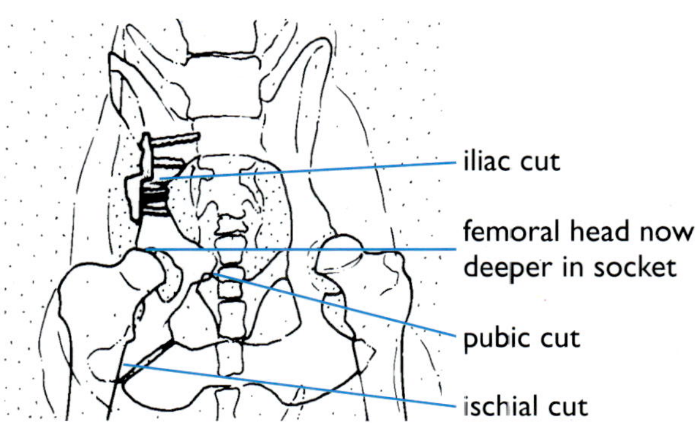

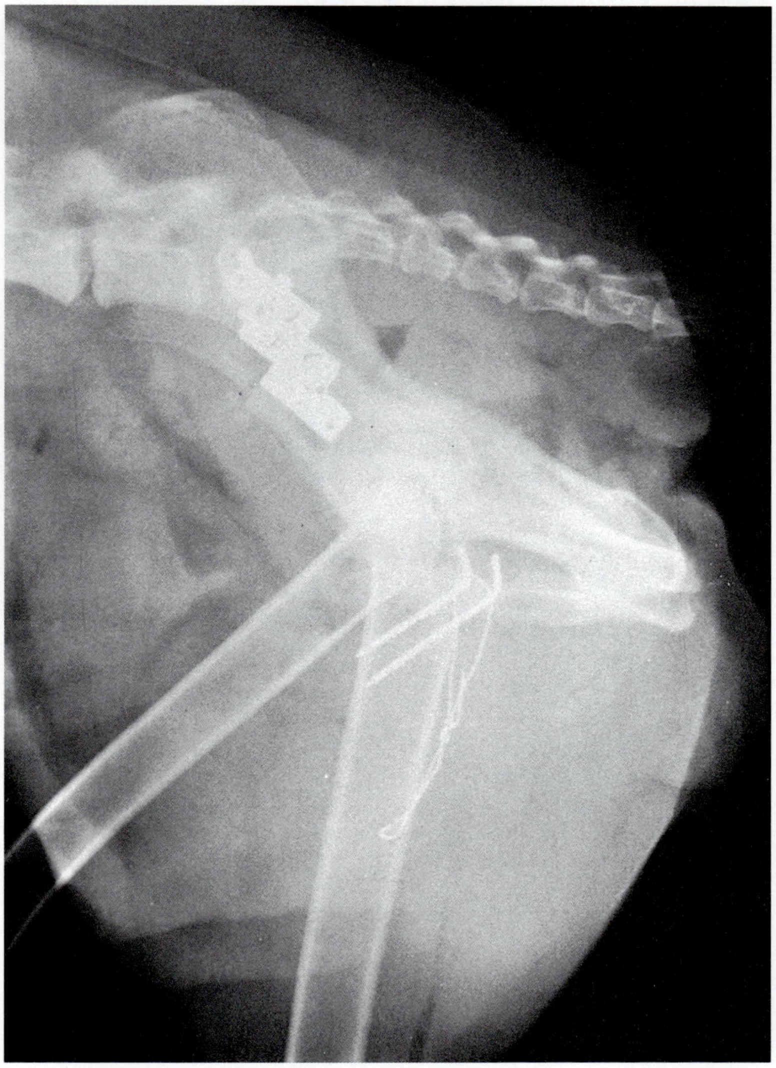

FIG. 3.30 A lateral radiograph of the ilium in a triple pelvic osteotomy. The line of incision for the osteotomy is indicated.

pared surface on the femur to tighten the hip into the acetabulum. It is secured with K-wires and a figure-8 tension band (Fig. 3.31). The redundant joint capsule is plicated with mattress sutures.

Closure is done by reattaching the superficial gluteus, suturing the tensor fascia lata and middle gluteus in place, and suturing the fascia, subcutaneous tissue, and the skin in the usual manner.

The opposite limb may be done in three or four months (Fig. 3.32).

Postoperative care is critical because so much weight will be borne by the plate. Close confinement is provided for three weeks. This is followed by exercise on a leash for another three weeks.

FRACTURES OF THE FEMUR

The femur is the most commonly fractured long bone of the dog and cat. In almost every instance, except for greenstick fractures in puppies, surgical intervention is required. Open reduction provides optimal fragment apposition and fixation. Failures in the form of non- and malunions, osteomyelitis, sequestrum formation, pseudoarthroses, delayed union, osteoporosis, and muscle contracture, alert the surgeon to the need for accurate diagnosis, early intervention and aseptic surgery, as well as adequate reduction and fixation.

The earliest form of therapy was a cast or splint. In most cases

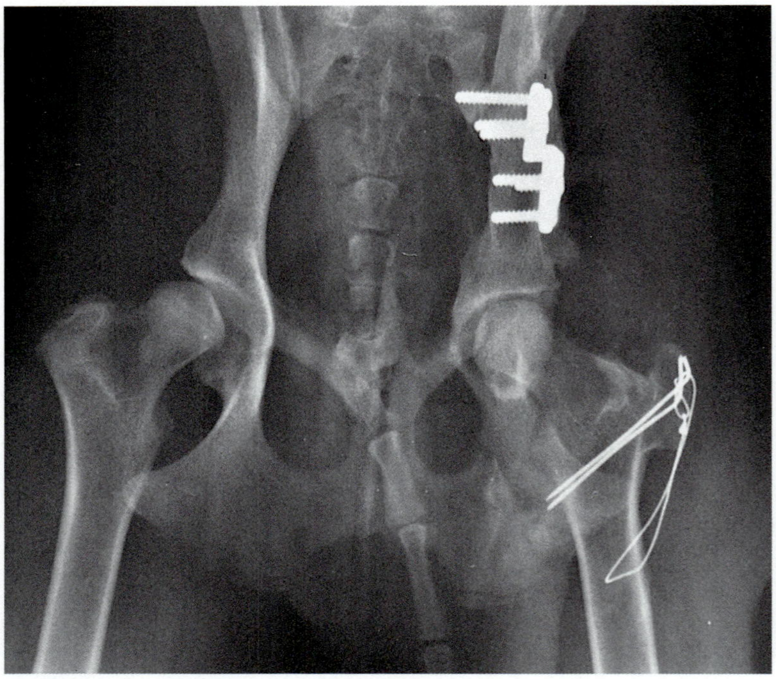

FIG. 3.31 Radiograph of a triple pelvic osteotomy showing transposition of the trochanteric osteotomized fragment to tighten the head into the acetabulum. The screw placements are excellent.

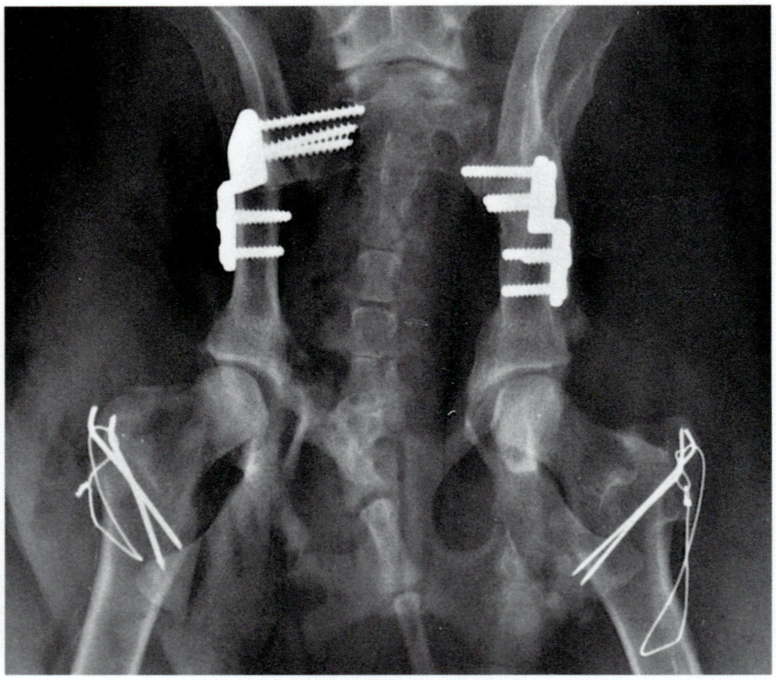

FIG. 3.32 Radiograph of a bilateral triple pelvic osteotomy. A period of about three months is allowed before the second surgery.

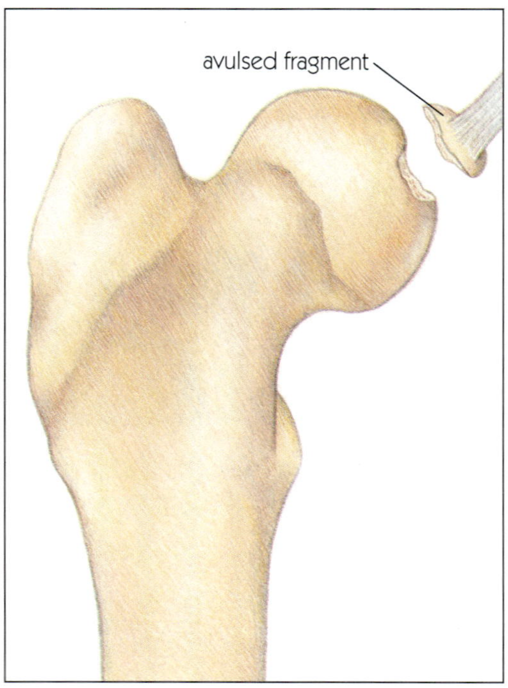

FIG.3.33 An avulsed fragment of the femoral head.

they are inadequate or, when misused, harmful. The Ehmer sling and the Robinson sling are useful in preventing weight-bearing and maintaining hip reductions. The Schroeder-Thomas splint was an improvement over splints and casts because it provided traction, especially when used with bone tongs inserted in the femoral condyles. Its use was limited to these distal fractures and required constant supervision to maintain any benefit. It can be used as a supplemental device to rest a limb after surgery, but the modified Robert Jones splint is better.

The first major advance in the treatment of femoral fractures was the external fixation splint, which was shortly overshadowed by the advent of the intramedullary pin. A combination of these techniques was soon established, offering a very satisfactory procedure. The use of bone plates, cerclage and hemi-cerclage wires, K-wires and interfragmentary compression with lag screws has become the method of choice. Specialized plates permit dynamic compression. There are plates designed specifically for subtrochanteric fractures.

One of the great advantages of internal fixation and external fixation is early ambulation, which helps prevent osteoporosis, joint stiffness, and muscle atrophy. Another is the capability for anatomic reduction with primary healing and more rapid return to normal function.

Femoral Head

Occasionally a portion of the femoral head is avulsed at the insertion of the round ligament, or small fractures occur when a hip is luxated (Fig. 3.33). Fragments over one third the area of the femoral head cause the hip to luxate, and therefore should be replaced. In immature dogs, separation of the proximal femoral physis is common. It is usually a smooth separation, but minor fractures may be present. The joint capsule may be intact or partially or wholly torn away. Repair is initiated as soon as possible, because of the damage to nutrient vessels and rapid demineralization of the femoral neck.

Severely damaged femoral heads can be treated by excision arthroplasty (Fig. 3.34) or replacement with a total hip prosthesis.

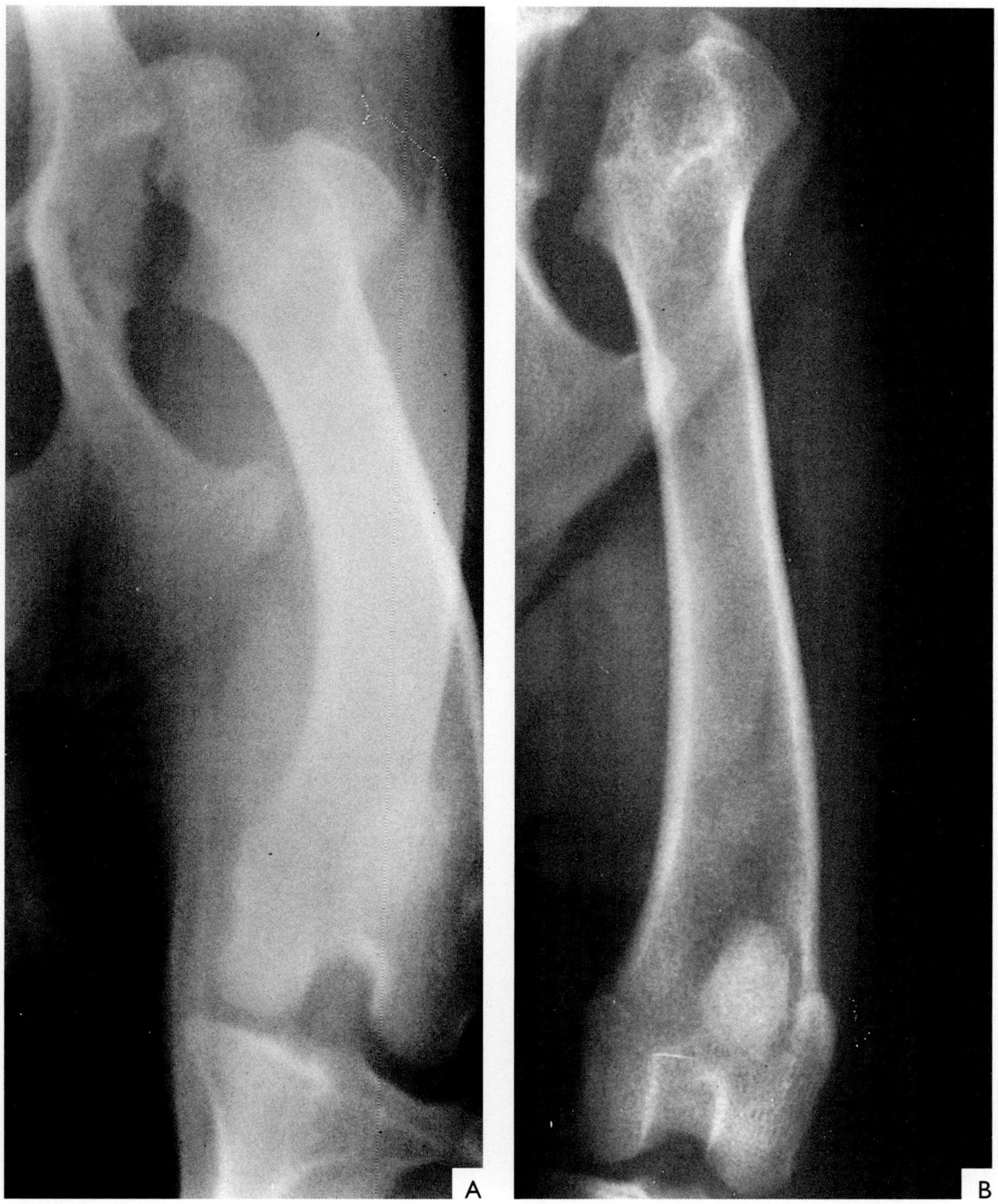

FIG. 3.34 (A) In this fractured femoral head, the fragment is undergoing resorption. (B) Excision arthroplasty was necessitated by severe damage to the acetabulum.

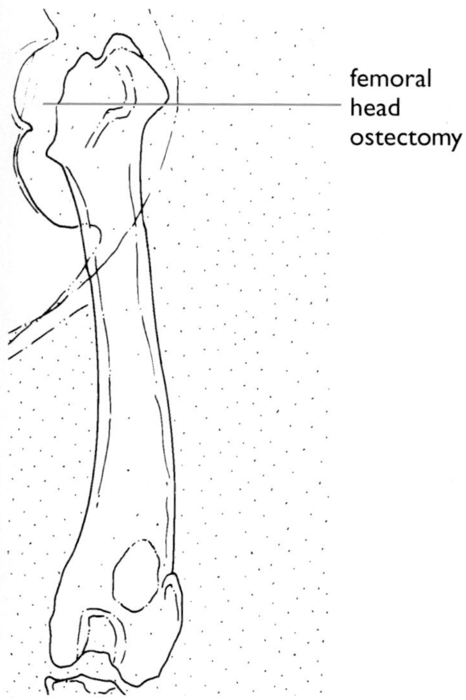

SURGICAL TECHNIQUE

For removal or replacement of femoral head fragments, a dorsal approach is used. This is done either by osteotomy of the greater trochanter or by tenotomy of the gluteal muscles.

An incision through the skin and subcutaneous tissues should be made midway between the trochanter major and the dorsal spine, extending slightly cranial and parallel to the proximal third of the shaft of the femur. The fascia lata is incised along the edge of the biceps femoris. These structures are reflected cranially and caudally. The tensor fascia lata and the superficial gluteus muscles are incised at their insertions and are reflected. The ischiatic nerve is located under the biceps femoris. It is identified and protected. The insertion of the middle gluteus is exposed by blunt dissection. In mature and larger dogs, an osteotomy of the trochanter is done with a Gigli wire saw or osteotome. A tenotomy of the middle gluteus is performed in immature dogs and in cats. A short section of fibrous insertion is left to provide an area to suture to when the muscle is replaced. In either case, the deep gluteus is incised, separated from the underlying joint capsule, and reflected. The joint capsule and some of the surrounding tissues may be already torn and damaged. A capsular incision is made or enlarged by cutting midway between the acetabular brim and the femoral insertion. The femoral head, which is usually somewhat luxated, is retracted to permit observation of the acetabulum. Small fragments of bone attached to the round ligament are excised. Where a larger fragment is present, it is replaced and secured with a threaded pin or K-wires. A small diameter intramedullary pin threaded at one end is used. The unthreaded end is introduced into the center of the fractured area and driven until it exits at the base of the trochanter major. The driving chuck is now placed on the opposite end and the threaded end is withdrawn until its tip is at the fracture surface. The chuck is adjusted on the pin until it is the same distance from the bone as the thickness of the bone fragment. The fracture is reduced by moving the limb so that the distal fragment is pressed into the proximal fragment, which must be seated firmly; the pin must not penetrate it. The pin is cut off near the bone, at the base of the trochanter (Fig. 3.35). Alternatively, the fragment may be cut free of the round ligament, placed in position, and secured with two K-wires driven through it (Fig. 3.36). These are countersunk just below the joint cartilage surface. The round ligament does not supply very much nutrition to the femoral head.

A very large fragment in a large dog can be secured with a lag screw. The fragment is first anchored in place with a K-wire. The screw hole is drilled; the gliding portion is over-drilled. The fragment hole is tapped and the screw is inserted from the base of the femoral head at the neck into the fragment (Fig. 3.37). Alternatively, the screws can be inserted from the articular surface (Fig. 3.38).

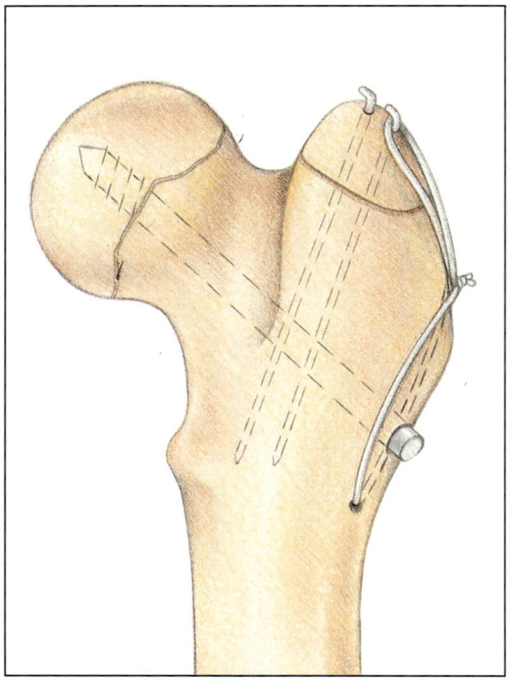

FIG. 3.35 A single threaded pin is inserted into the epiphysis for fixation of a proximal femoral epiphyseal fracture. The osteotomized trochanter has been re-placed and secured with two K-wires and a figure-8 tension band wire.

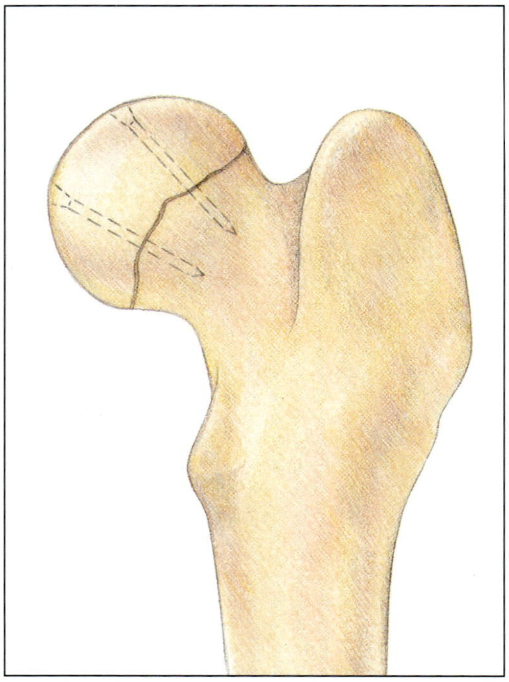

FIG. 3.36 Two K-wires inserted from the articular surface and countersunk beneath the articular surface for fixation of a fragment of the femoral head.

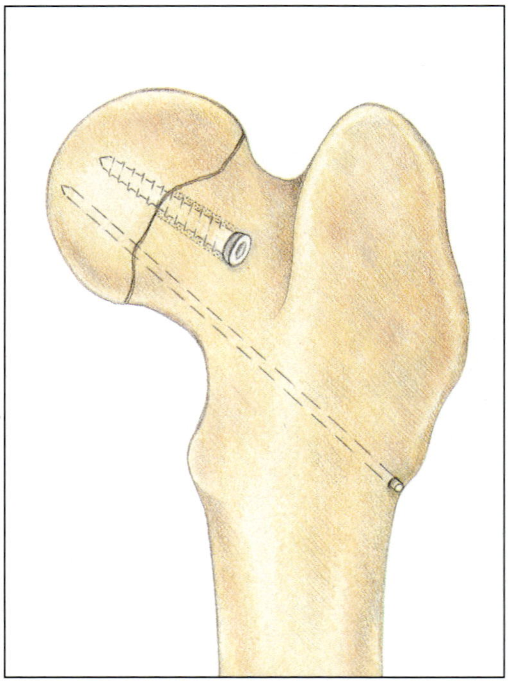

FIG. 3.37 A single lag screw is used to immobilize a femoral neck fracture. The epiphysis is stabilized with a K-wire and the screw is introduced at the neck, across the fracture site.

Either a dorsal or craniolateral approach may be taken with a proximal epiphyseal fracture. The craniolateral is preferable, but the dorsal approach by gluteal tenotomy may be needed.

Converging K-wires hold the epiphysis in place. These could be inserted from the fracture surface to exit beneath the trochanter, but this requires considerable exposure. Three converging K-wires can be inserted from the base of the trochanter to exit at the fracture site. It takes considerable maneuvering to reduce the fracture. The epiphyseal fragment is freely mobile. Its particular shape will fit perfectly in its original position. Once reduced, the hip is pressed firmly into the acetabulum by an assistant. The K-wires are driven into the epiphyseal fragment to a position just under the joint cartilage. The pins are cut off near the bone surface (Fig. 3.39). The epiphyseal fragment can be stabilized with a small pry or retractor tip in-serted through a cut in the joint capsule into the acetabulum.

In these procedures, closure is done by suturing rents or incisions in the joint capsule and replacing as much of the deep gluteus as possible. The tenotomy of the middle gluteus is secured with mattress sutures of nonabsorbable material. An osteotomy of the trochanter is replaced with two K-wires and a figure-8 tension band wire. The superficial gluteus and the tensor fascia lata are reattached to their insertions. The incisions in the fascia lata subcutaneous tissues and skin are sutured in the usual manner.

The leg is placed in an Ehmer sling for five days. Limited exercise is permitted for three weeks. Thinning of the femoral neck will almost invariably be apparent on a radiograph (Fig. 3.40). Healing or failure depends upon the blood supply, completeness of the reduction, and the stability of the fixation.

Femoral Neck

Femoral neck fractures may occur in several locations and are sometimes associated with fracture of the trochanteric physis. It is essential to treat neck fractures as soon possible with accurate reduction and fixation. There is always an element of risk when there is interference with the blood supply.

In small and immature dogs and cats, three K-wires are inserted retrograde from the fracture site to exit at the base of the trochanter. They are driven back into the fragment while the reduction is held with bone forceps. The pins are cut off at the bone sur-

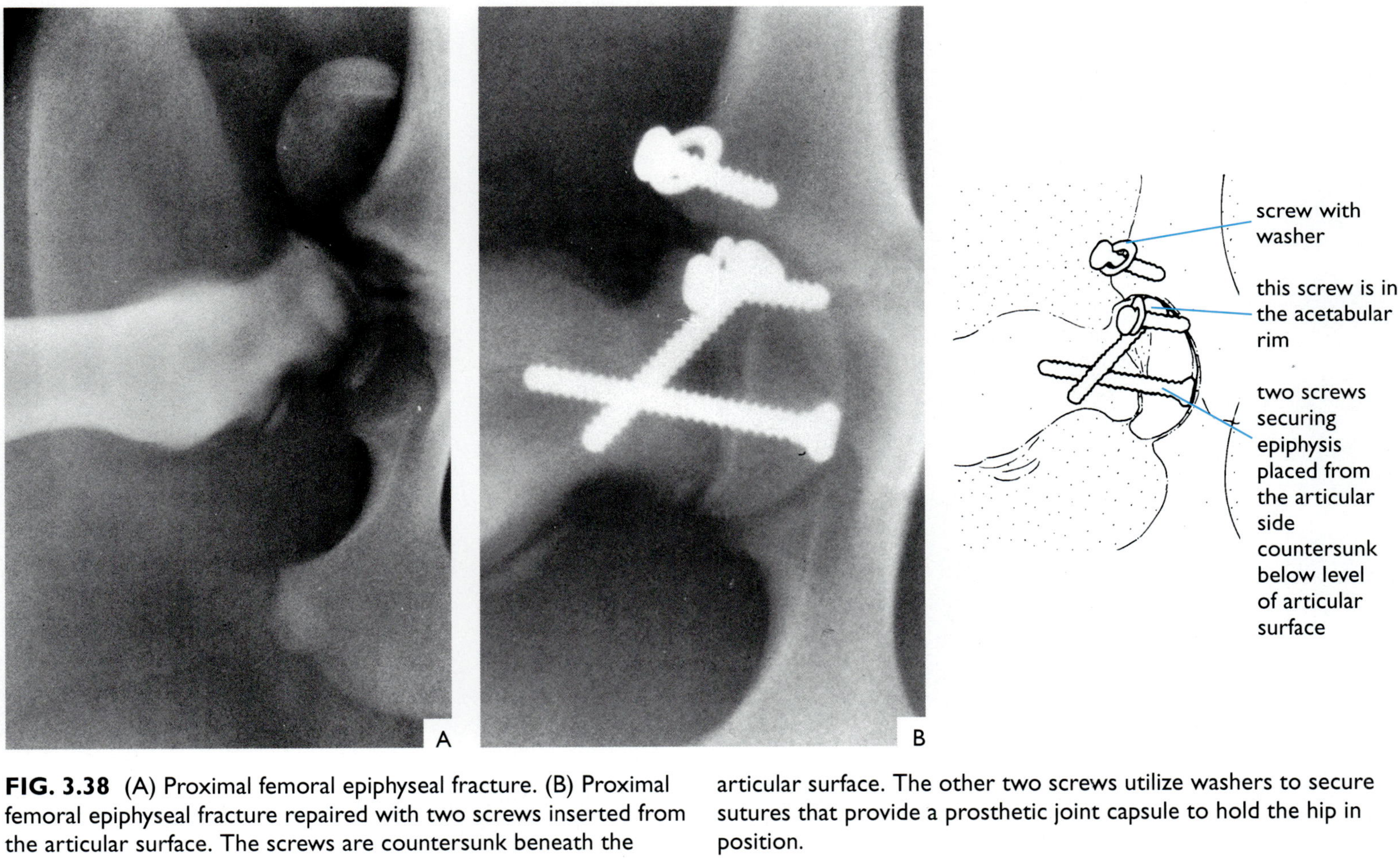

FIG. 3.38 (A) Proximal femoral epiphyseal fracture. (B) Proximal femoral epiphyseal fracture repaired with two screws inserted from the articular surface. The screws are countersunk beneath the articular surface. The other two screws utilize washers to secure sutures that provide a prosthetic joint capsule to hold the hip in position.

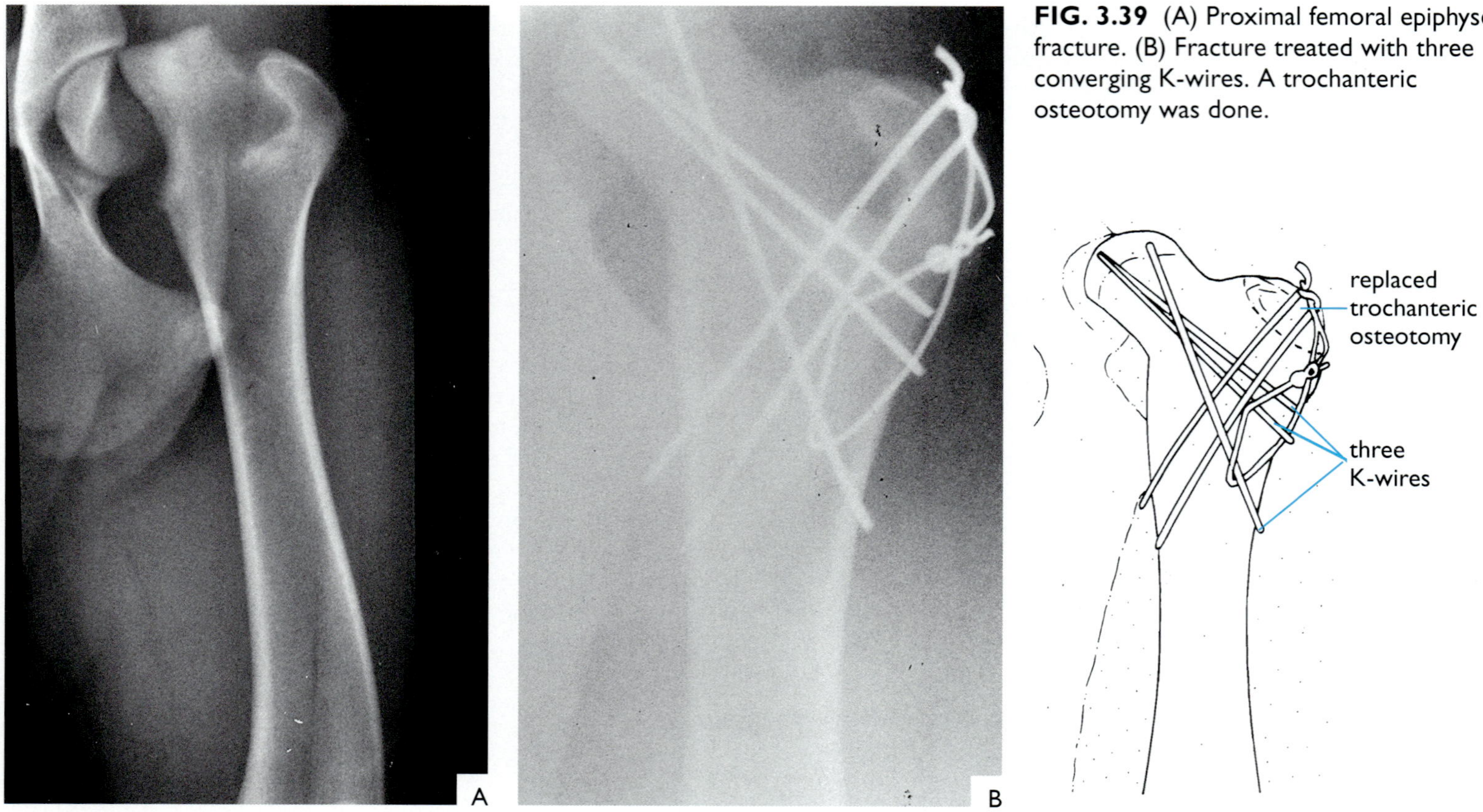

FIG. 3.39 (A) Proximal femoral epiphyseal fracture. (B) Fracture treated with three converging K-wires. A trochanteric osteotomy was done.

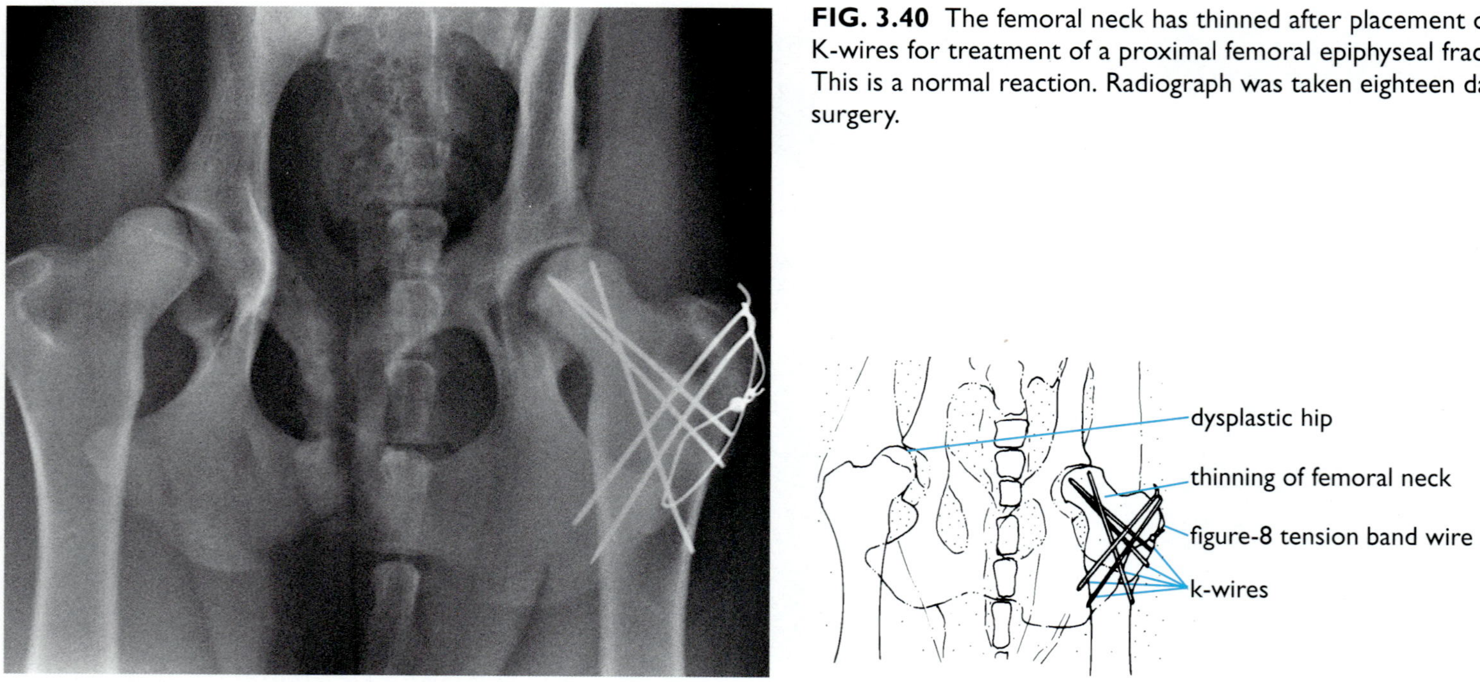

FIG. 3.40 The femoral neck has thinned after placement of three K-wires for treatment of a proximal femoral epiphyseal fracture. This is a normal reaction. Radiograph was taken eighteen days after surgery.

face (Fig. 3.41). The fracture site is not compressed. The leg is placed in an Ehmer sling for a week, followed by restricted activity for a month. In larger mature animals a combination of a K-wire and a lag screw is used (Fig. 3.42).

SURGICAL TECHNIQUE

A craniolateral approach is used and the area of the fracture is exposed by blunt dissection. A test reduction is made to see if the fracture can be reduced or if further exposure is needed. If the reduction can be made, the fracture site is exposed and a drill guide is used to drill a hole slightly larger in diameter than the screw, which will be inserted from the lateral surface of the femur to the center of the fracture, parallel to the angle of the neck. The reduction is made and a K-wire is introduced proximal to the screw hole penetrating the trochanter and the trochanteric ridge to seat into the fragment, thus stabilizing the fracture. A drill sleeve is introduced in the screw hole and a hole is drilled into the neck and head. It is measured with a depth gauge and tapped. The sleeve is removed and the cortical screw is inserted and tightened. Care is taken not to strip the threads. The K-wire is cut off close to the bone surface. It is essential that the reduction be complete, especially distally.

If there has been a fracture separation of the trochanter, it is secured with two K-wires, which are placed so as to avoid the bone screw. A figure-8 tension band wire is applied (Fig. 3.43). Muscle spasm may make it difficult to obtain the reduction.

Closure of the craniolateral approach is routine. The leg is placed in an Ehmer sling for a week and activity is restricted for a month. Even though a radiograph may show thinning of the bone at the fracture site, firm healing ordinarily follows.

Fractures involving the trochanter, the femoral neck, and the very proximal femur are treated with a bone plate. The origin of the vastus lateralis is incised and the proximal portion of the muscle is retracted to expose the subtrochanteric fractures. The plate may be a hooked plate or a dynamic compression plate. The hooked plate has hooks on its proximal end that are set into the top of the trochanter for a firm hold. Dynamic compression plates are contoured to fit. It helps to smooth away some of the lateral trochanteric surface to get a good seating. The ovoid holes in these plates allow a lag screw to be placed at an angle to hold the femoral neck fracture. The

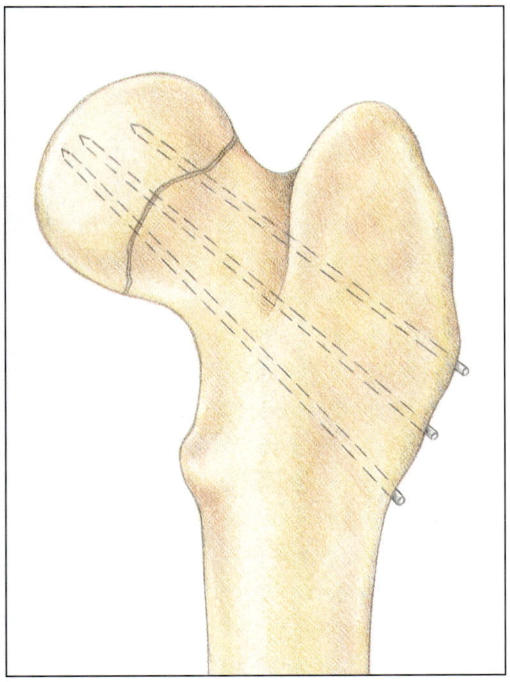

FIG. 3.41 Femoral neck fracture with three K-wires used in treatment.

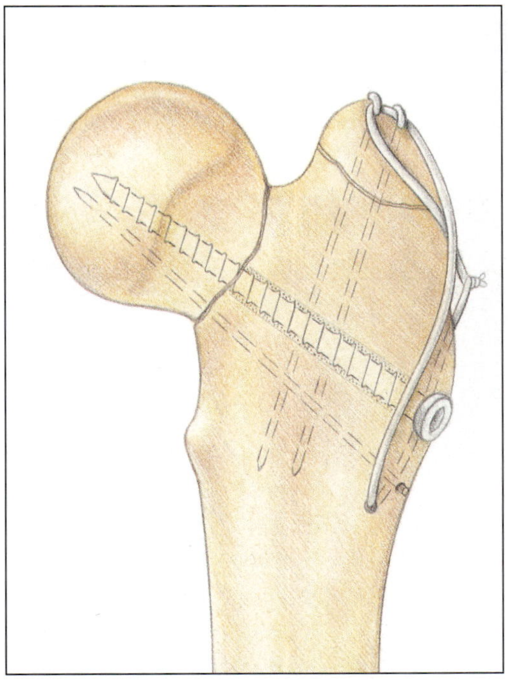

FIG. 3.42 Femoral neck fracture treated by a lag screw. The fragment was first fixed with a K-wire for control while drilling for the screw. A trochanteric osteotomy was performed.

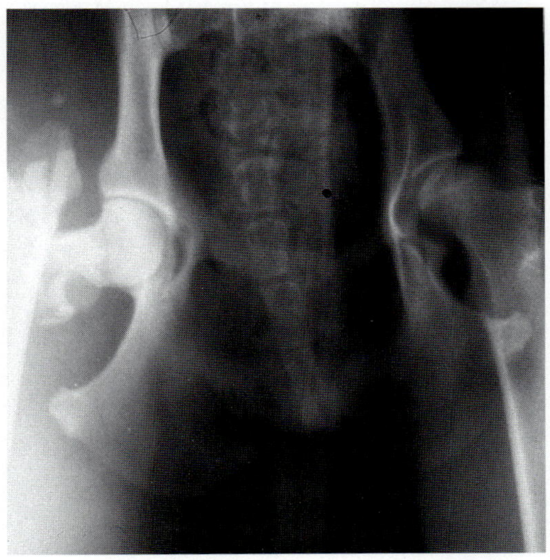

FIG. 3.43 Fractured femoral neck and fractured trochanter.

trochanteric fragment is replaced and held with a short screw. The fragment itself may be lagged in place if it is large. The femoral fracture is reduced and the plate applied. The hole nearest the fracture distally is drilled in the eccentric mode, providing compression of the fracture. The rest of the screws are inserted (Fig. 3.44).

Closure is done by resuturing the origin of the vastus lateralis, reattaching the tensor fascia lata and superficial gluteus, and closing the incisions in the fascia lata, subcutaneous tissues, and skin in the usual manner. Femoral neck fractures that fail will require either excision arthroplasty or a total hip replacement as salvage procedures.

Femoral Shaft

This is the most commonly injured area. Except for most minor injuries, good fixation is required. Splints and casts are inadequate. Currently, three modes of repair are used: intramedullary pinning, external fixation, and bone plating. A combination of intramedullary pinning and external fixation offers benefits beyond any one alone. Bone plates are frequently used in conjunction with interfragmentary screws, K-wires, and cerclage wires.

Femoral shaft fractures vary from simple transverse or short oblique to long oblique splits, multiple fractures, severely comminuted, and gunshot. They may be fresh or old, nonunions, pseudarthroses, infected, contain sequestra or foreign bodies, or be spontaneous from a tumor. Some considerable thought should be given to the manner of treatment. A stable, uncomplicated fracture may do well with an intramedullary pin. A more severe fracture with a tendency to rotate or collapse on a pin might need an external fixator. Severely infected fractures that require drainage as well as frequent dressings and care may be best treated with external fixation. Severe multiple and badly comminuted fractures are more successfully treated with bone plates. In proximal and midshaft fractures, the proximal fragment tends to rotate outwardly, a tendency that must be taken into consideration when the fracture is reduced.

Diaphyseal Femoral Fractures

Intramedullary Pin Fixation

The use of an intramedullary pin as the sole means of fixation should be confined to stable fractures, that is, a single fracture that locks together when reduced, preventing rotation, collapse, and motion. The pin should fill the medullary cavity as much as possible. This is easy in cats and small dogs with relatively straight femurs (Fig. 3.45). In larger dogs, the distal femur bows cranially and the medullary cavity is thinner centrally. Pins must be small enough to pass without splitting the bone.

Intramedullary pins come with trocar and chisel points. Each has its proponents and each functions well. Some feel that a threaded tip will hold more firmly. The holding power would be more effective if the threads were larger than the pin diameter.

Introduction of the pin may be made either from the fracture

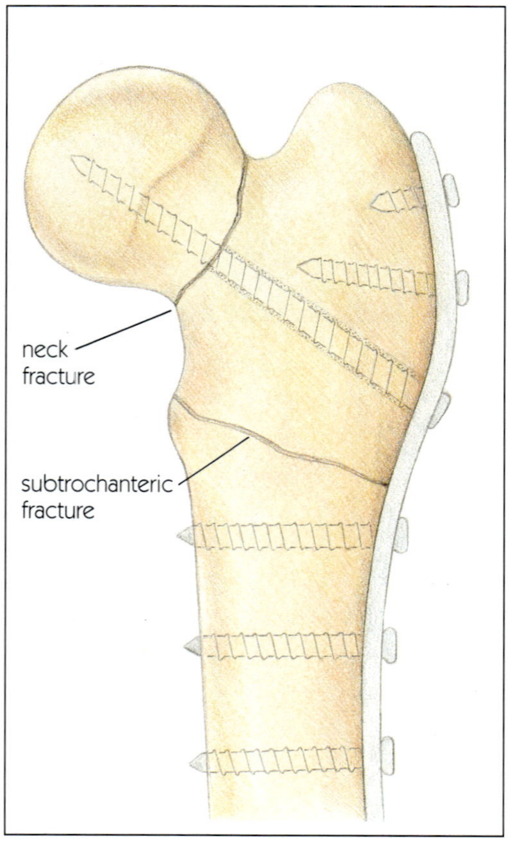

FIG. 3.44 Fractured femoral neck and subtrochanteric fracture treated with a lag screw and bone plate. The lag screw is angled through the plate.

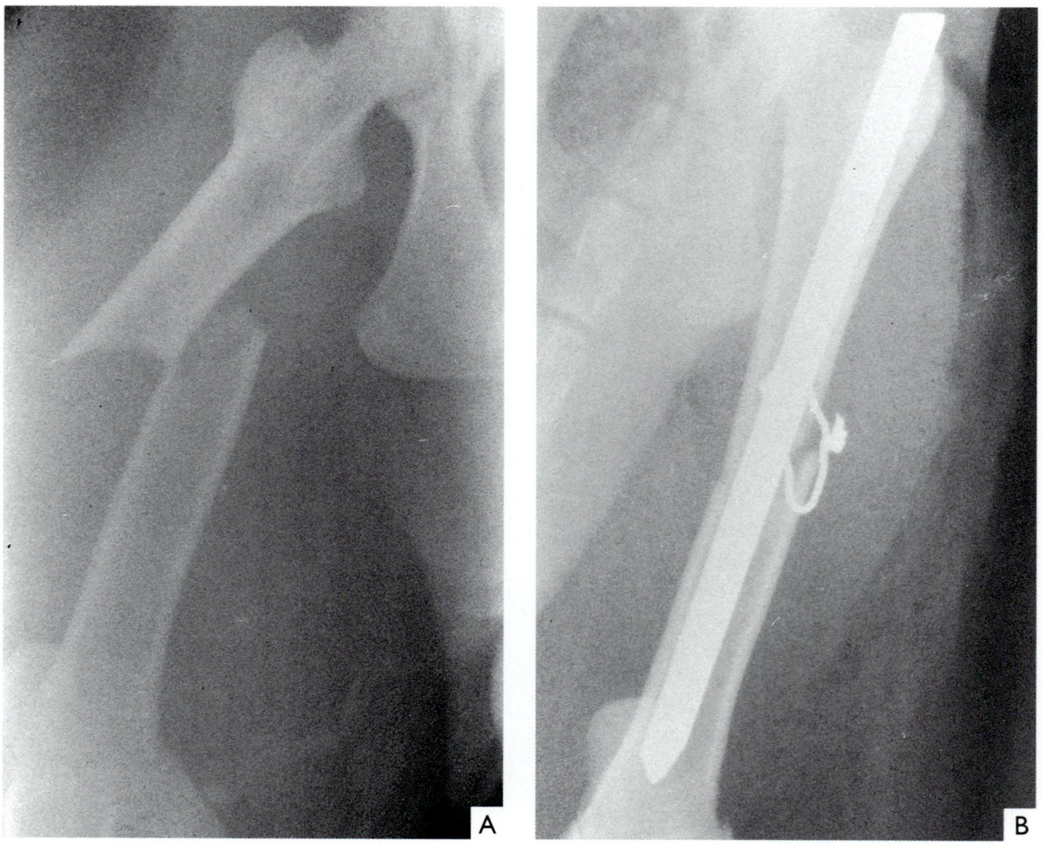

FIG. 3.45 (A) Transverse femoral fracture in a cat. (B) Radiograph of a transverse femoral fracture in a cat treated with an IM pin and cerclage wire.

site (retrograde) or from the trochanteric fossa (normograde). Many prefer the introduction through the trochanteric fossa because it offers less chance of interference with the ischiatic nerve, femoral neck, and the muscle mass at the hip.

Retrograde introduction can be satisfactory, if the femur is held in a normal standing position (parallel to the surgical table). Because of the tendency for outward rotation, it helps to turn the pin cranially when drilling it. The pin is directed along the lateral surface of the medullary cavity.

The pin is introducted into the distal fragment by angulation and traction. A pin guide is helpful (Arnold and Sons Veterinary Instruments, Reading Berks, England). The pin should follow the caudal surface of the medullary cavity of the distal fragment. The pin is seated as firmly and deeply as possible in the cancellous bone without penetrating the joint. Because the distal femur bows cranially, the exact anatomic alignment at the fracture site is exchanged for the secure seating of the pin, leaving the fracture site slightly open caudally. This causes no problem with healing (Fig. 3.46).

Intramedullary pins are cut off under the skin at the hip to avoid causing a hematoma or pain. The pins will be withdrawn after healing—usually a month to six weeks. Threaded pins must be unthreaded before they can be removed.

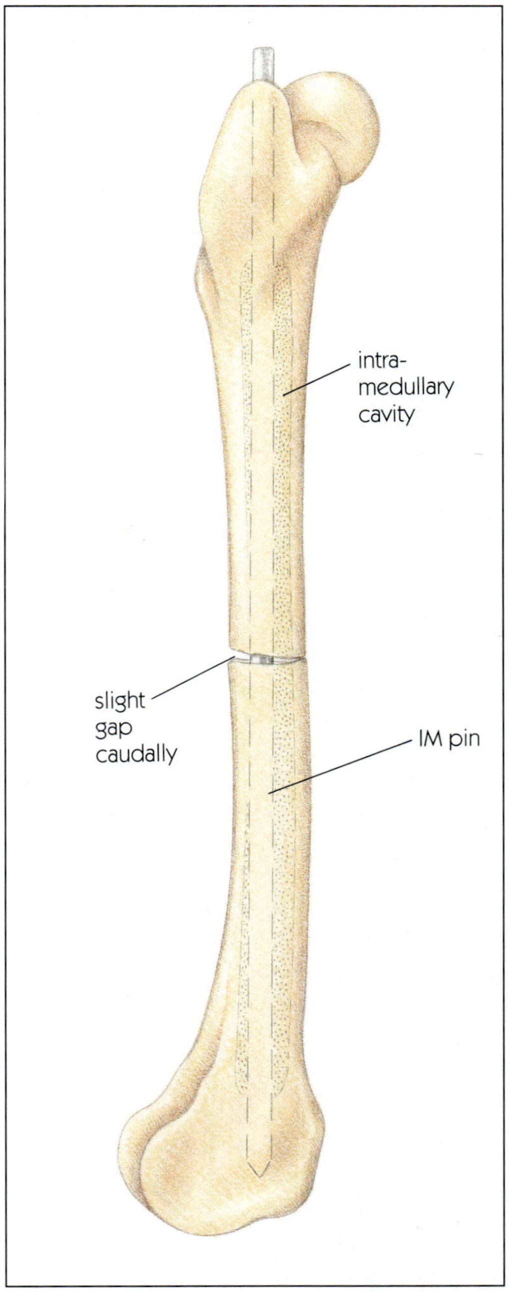

FIG. 3.46 Transverse midshaft femoral fracture. In order to insert the IM pin more securely in the distal fragment, it has been angled caudally, leaving a small caudal gap at the fracture site. With good immobility, this area will fill in with bone.

SURGICAL TECHNIQUE

The femur is approached laterally by a craniolateral incision through the skin and subcutaneous tissues directly over the area of contact between the fascia lata and the cranial edge of the biceps femoris. The exposed fascia lata is incised along this same line. Retraction of the fascia lata and the biceps femoris exposes the fracture. The proximal fragment extends cranially; the distal fragment extends caudally. The attached muscles contract in spasms and a hematoma is usually present. Caudally, the ischiatic nerve is liable to injury and must be protected. Cranially, the proximal fragment frequently embeds itself in muscle tissue. The area is suctioned dry. The fragment ends are brought into the incision area and are inspected for small fissures that might split when manipulated. Two or three cerclage wires are used to reinforce these areas. An intramedullary pin is selected that will pass into the distal fragment. A small incision is made in the skin and subcutaneous tissue just medial to the tip of the trochanter major. The pin is introduced along the medial face of the trochanter, into the trochanteric fossa. The proximal fragment is held with a bone-holding forceps to control the outward rotation and maintain it in a normal standing position. The pin is driven into the medullary canal until the tip is visible at the end of the proximal fragment. It is now introduced into the medullary canal of the distal fragment. Angulation and toggling are required to bring the fragment ends into line. An intramedullary pin guide is used as an aid. The pin is driven down the medullary canal of the distal fragment. It is placed so that it is close to the caudal edge of the medullary canal. The fracture site is angled slightly caudally to permit this. The pin is seated firmly in the cancellous bone of the distal femur. Increased resistance to drilling is a sign of reaching the proper depth. Penetration into the joint is usually caused by an overly cranial positioning of the pin and too forceful drilling (Fig. 3.47). New, sharp pins should be used. Dull ones are hard to drill and can lead to mistakes in positioning.

The leg is moved and rotated to determine the best seating of the pin and the immobility at the fracture site.

Closure is accomplished by suturing the incisions in the fascia lata, subcutaneous tissues, and skin in the usual manner. If there is seeping bleeding, a catheter is placed prior to closure and connected to a vacuum (hemovac) to prevent hematoma formation (Hemovac-Snyder Products, Wausau, Indiana). This is removed in 4 to 8 hours.

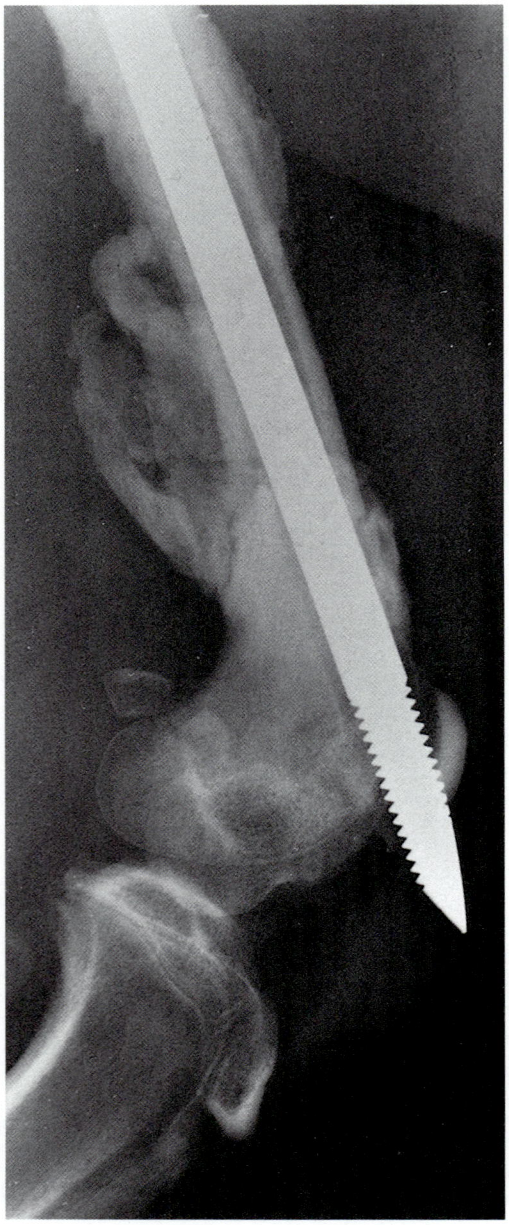

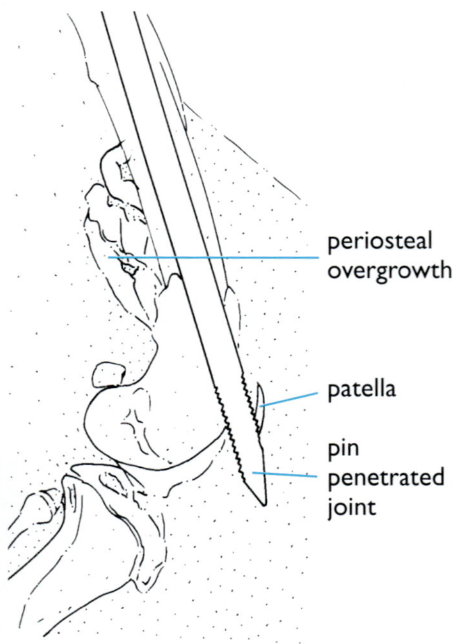

FIG. 3.47 An IM pin penetrates the knee joint in a distal femoral fracture. The fracture is unstable.

After radiographically determining the reduction and seating of the pin, it is cut off under the skin at the trochanteric area. The subcutaneous tissues and skin are sutured closed. Retrograde pinning is the same except that the pin is introduced up the medullary canal from the distal end of the proximal fragment. Bone forceps hold the bone parallel to the table in a normal standing position. The point of the pin will emerge from the trochanteric fossa and appear under the skin, which is cut with a scalpel to allow free passage. The pin driving handle (chuck) is attached proximally to withdraw the pin so that the distal tip is at the distal end of the proximal fragment.

Intramedullary Pin Fixation with External Fixation

Applying an external fixator along with an intramedullary pin helps to control rotation and maintain length.

A single bar with one pin in the proximal fragment and one in the distal is used for moderately stable fractures (Fig. 3.48). A single bar with two pins in each fragment is used where comminution and fragmentation require additional support to prevent collapse and motion at the fracture site (Fig. 3.49).

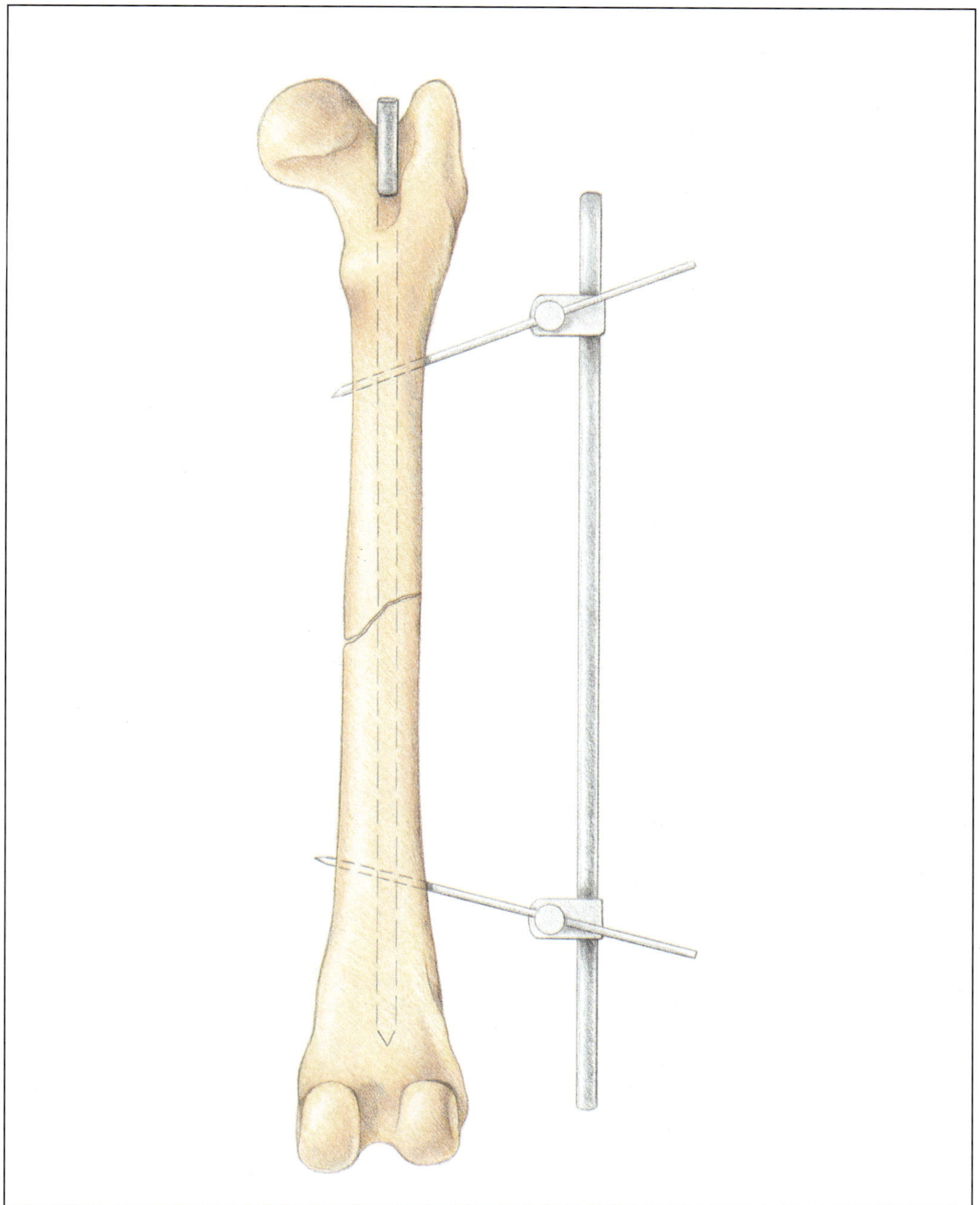

FIG. 3.48 Femur fixed with an IM pin and a single K/E (Kirschner/Ehmer) splint with two pins. The pins are inserted as far distally and proximally as feasible.

SURGICAL TECHNIQUE

A single connecting bar is selected with two pin clamps. A nick in the skin is made directly over the lateral surface of the femur. The first pin is inserted through the muscle tissue at about a 70° angle from the center. It is driven through both cortices of the proximal fragment, just below the trochanter, usually caudal to the intramedullary pin.

In using a threaded pin, the skin is incised and the muscle tissues are spread apart with a hemostat to expose the bone. A tubular drill guide is inserted and located on the proper site on the bone. A hole is drilled and tapped. The pin is threaded into place. The guide is removed.

The caudal pin is inserted laterally at the same angle, just above the condyles caudal to the intramedullary pin. Pin clamps are attached to the pins and the connecting bar is inserted. The clamps, which should be located about 1 cm above the skin, are tightened.

The pins should not be introduced through the incision. They may be inserted before closure to ascertain proper seating. When healing has progressed after three or four weeks, the external fixator is removed to permit some minor stress to the bone to encourage healing (dynamism).

Large vigorous dogs and comminuted fractures require four pins with the external fixator. The most proximal and distal pins are

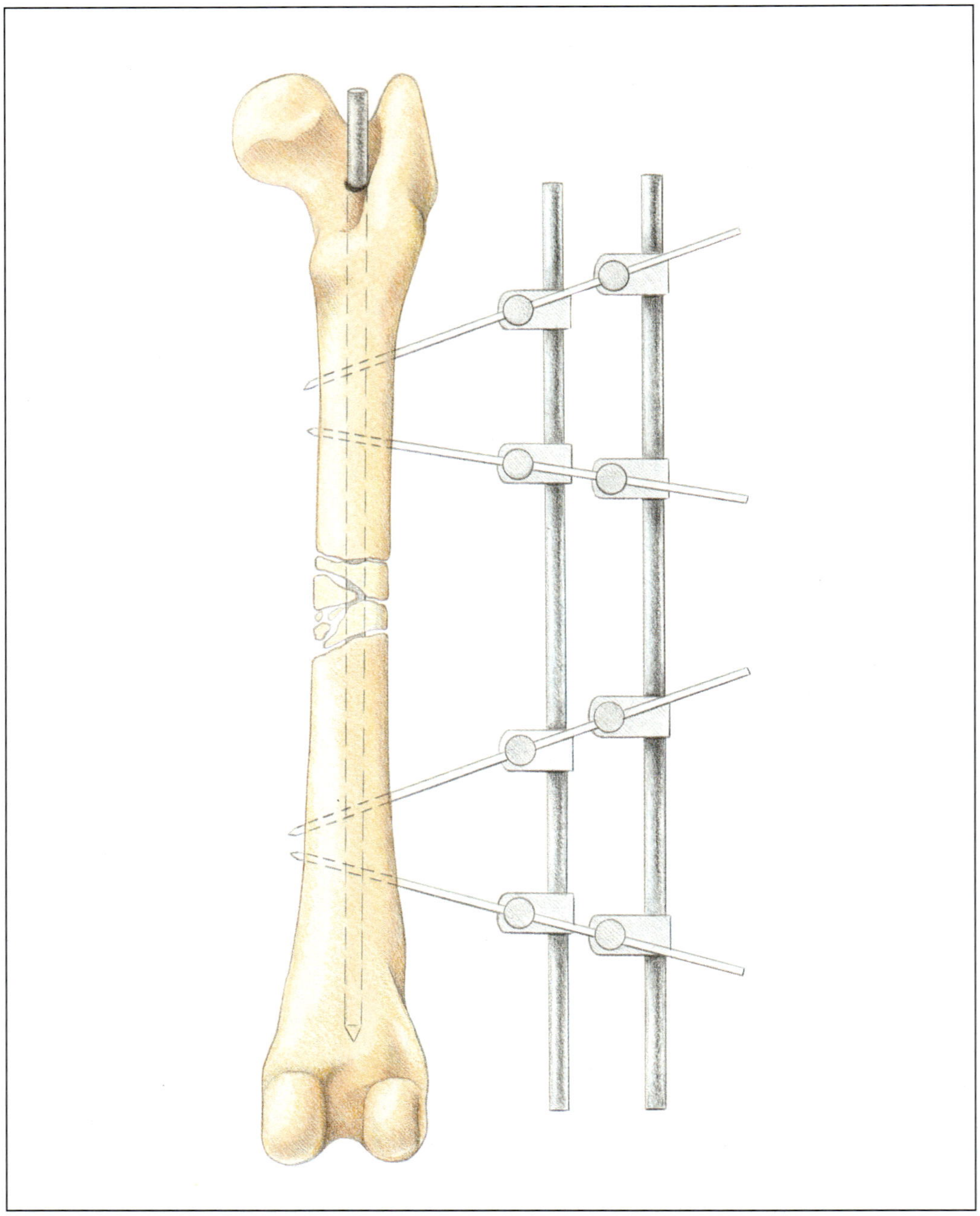

FIG. 3.49 Application of additional pins to support an IM pin, from a single bar K/E. An additional connecting bar provides reinforcement.

inserted first. The other pins are inserted through pin clamps previously placed on the connecting bar.

When the external fixator is in place, the pins are cut off about 1 cm from the clamps. A nick with a scalpel eliminates skin pressure against the pins (Fig. 3.50). Sterile sponges are placed around the point where the pins exit from the skin (Fig. 3.51). The apparatus is wrapped in cotton, bandaged and covered with adhesive tape. This prevents the device from being caught on or damaging the surroundings.

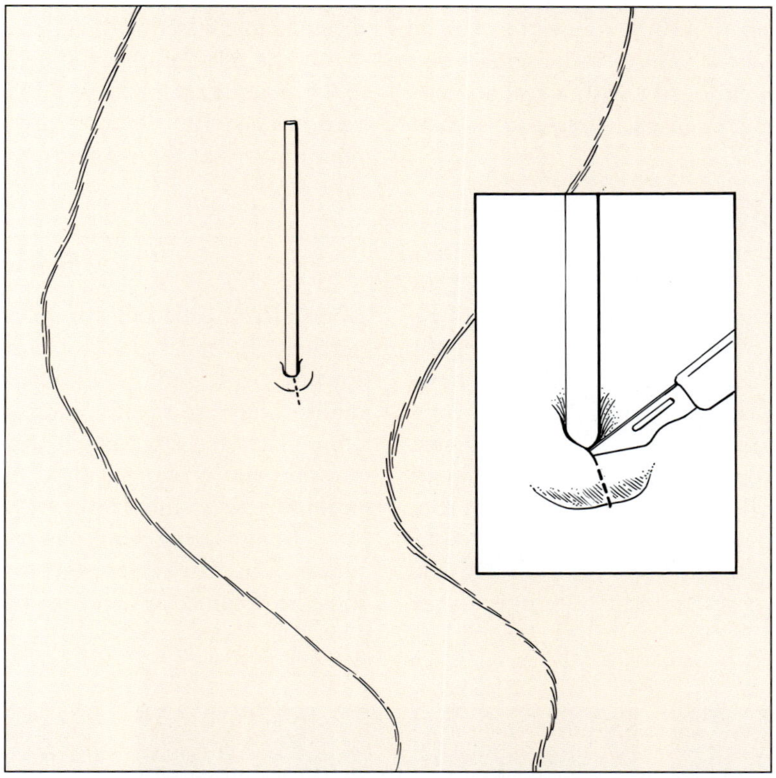

FIG. 3.50 Skin being cut with scalpel at insertion of pins for K/E external fixation.

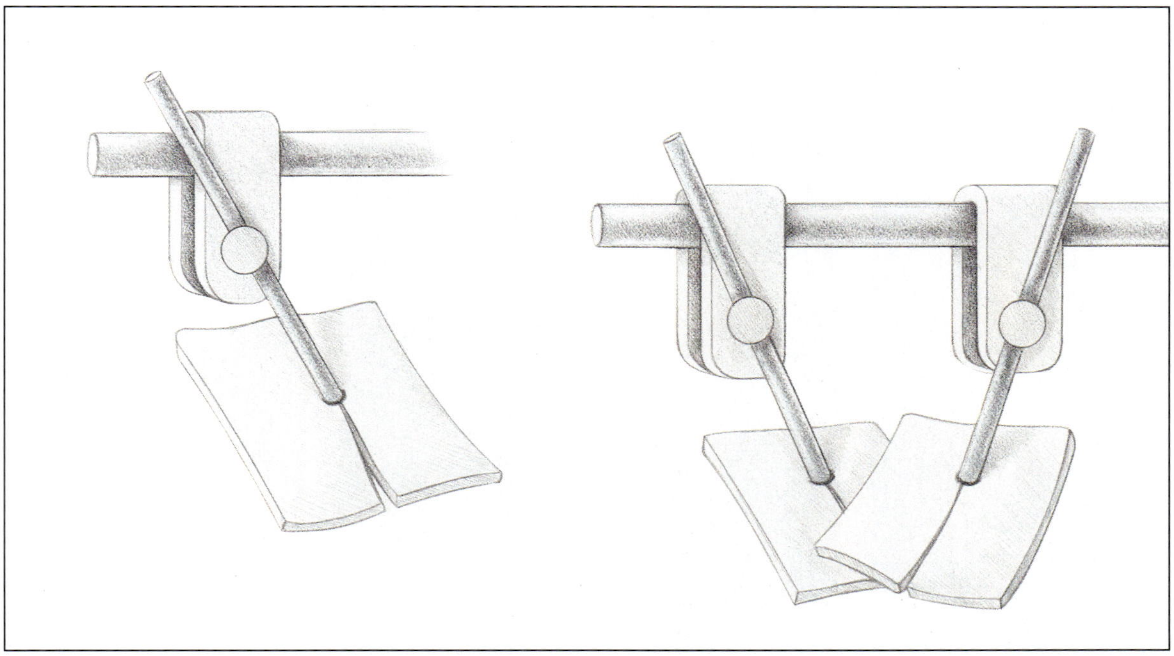

FIG. 3.51 During external fixation, a split surgical sponge protects the port of entry of the K/E pin through the skin.

External Fixation

The use of external fixation alone as the treatment for femoral fractures is indicated in small dogs, cats, and where severe infection and tissue damage will not permit the use of intramedullary pins or bone plates. The original configuration was two converging pins in the proximal and two in the distal fragments. These were connected to short bars, which were then fastened to a long connecting bar by double clamps. This arrangement was so subject to loosening that using a single connecting bar, after reinforcing with a second connecting bar and using three or four pins in each fragment is now recommended (Fig. 3.52).

SURGICAL TECHNIQUE

Although external fixation can be applied without open reduction, much better results are achieved with it. A proper assessment of the extent of bone damage can be made and fragments secured with K-wires, cerclage wires, or lag screws. The correct placement of the pins can be visualized. Threaded pins that can be inserted in holes that have been drilled and tapped to receive them are used.

One pin is placed proximally near the base of the trochanter. Another is placed distally near the condyles. Threaded pins may be inserted straight into the fragments (horizontal to the bone). A nick is made in the skin. The muscle tissue is separated down to the bone and a tubular drill guide is inserted. The hole is drilled and tapped. The guide prevents muscle tissue from being caught in the drill. With the proximal and distal pins in place, a connecting bar with four or six pin clamps is attached. Additional pins are inserted at intervals where the bone provides adequate seating. When all of the pins are placed and the clamps tightened, an additional connecting bar is attached above the first. This provides much increased rigidity. The open reduction incision is closed. Sterile sponges are placed around the pins. The apparatus is wrapped in cotton, bandaged, and covered with adhesive tape.

The pin clamps must be checked frequently for signs of loosening. Since fixators are well tolerated, they tend to encourage overly vigorous activity. The bone must be protected from stress after pin removal so that the pinholes can fill in and further calcification can take place.

Bone Plates

Bone plates, especially those providing dynamic compression, are particularly well suited for almost all kinds of diaphyseal femoral fractures. They are usually applied laterally, but can be placed cranially. They are readily contoured to the bone surface. Although bone plates require a much wider exposure, they can provide compression and prolonged rigid fixation, which enhances healing and promotes early ambulation and return to function.

Bone plating requires a considerable investment in instrumentation. The plates and screws are expensive. Training and experience must be obtained. There are great benefits to be gained.

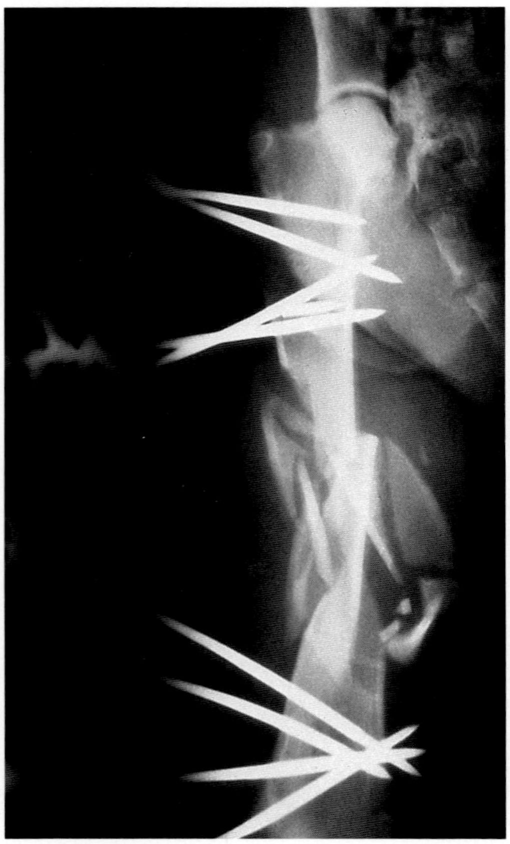

FIG. 3.52 Multiple pin placement in a single K/E bar that is treating a severely comminuted fracture (not a femur).

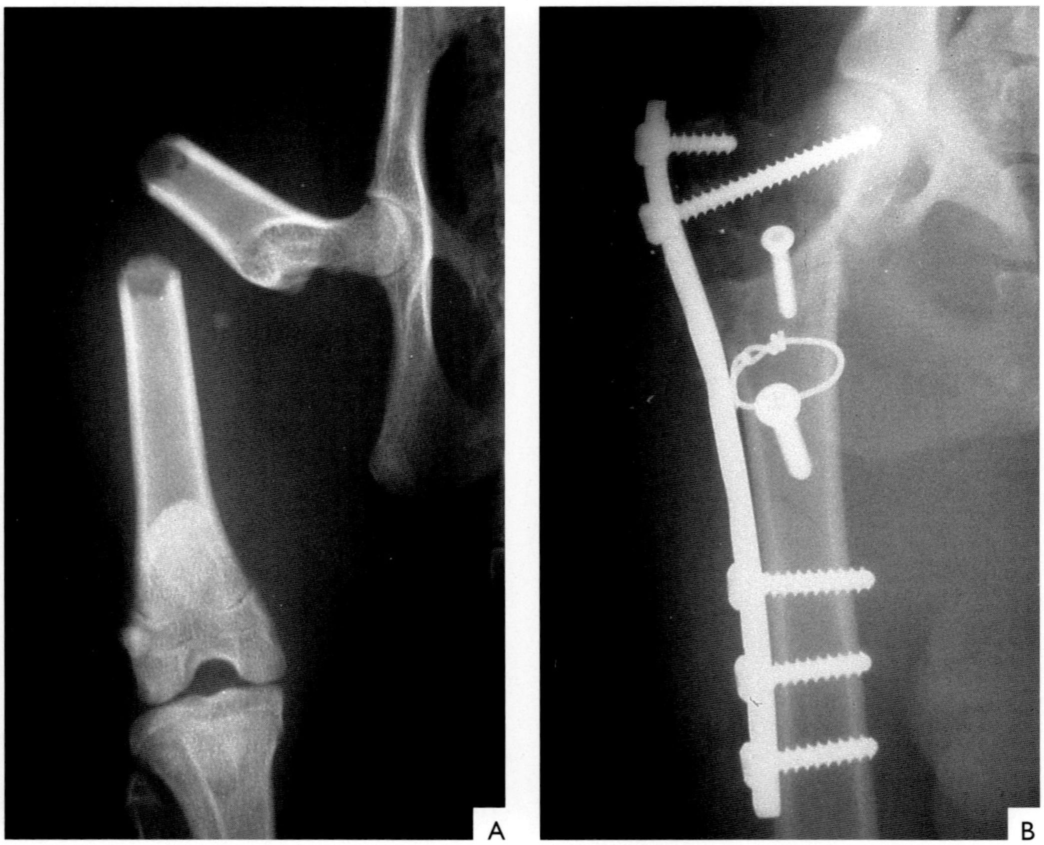

FIG. 3.53 (A) Transverse proximal femoral fracture. (B) A transverse proximal femoral fracture treated with a bone plate. Note the long screw in the femoral neck that provides greater holding power and stability.

Simple transverse or short oblique fractures are treated with dynamic compression plates (Figs. 3.53, 3.54).

Fractures with a single large fragment (butterfly fragment) or multiple fragments are treated with a neutralization plate to take the stress, while the bone fragments that have been reassembled and held with K-wires, cerclage wires, or interfragmentary screws, heal. The fracture is inherently stable but could not withstand torsional or bending stresses (Figs. 3.55–3.62).

Fractures that are reassembled but have many small or missing fragments, and are therefore inherently unstable, are treated with buttress plates to support the weak area until suitable healing takes place.

Autogenous cancellous bone grafts are placed at fracture sites to enhance healing. They are obtained from the proximal humerus, proximal tibia, wing of the ilium, and occasionally from the proximal femur. In some cases, an incurable condition is present or a portion of the diaphysis is so damaged that it cannot be put back together. A frozen allograft is then used to replace the diaphyseal segment.

Nonunions and pseudarthroses are best treated with bone plates, which provide the rigid fixation that is needed. Plates are often removed after healing is assured. Loose or broken plates must be replaced. Loose screws causing pain must be removed or replaced. Chronic irritation from a loose bone plate can cause bone tumors.

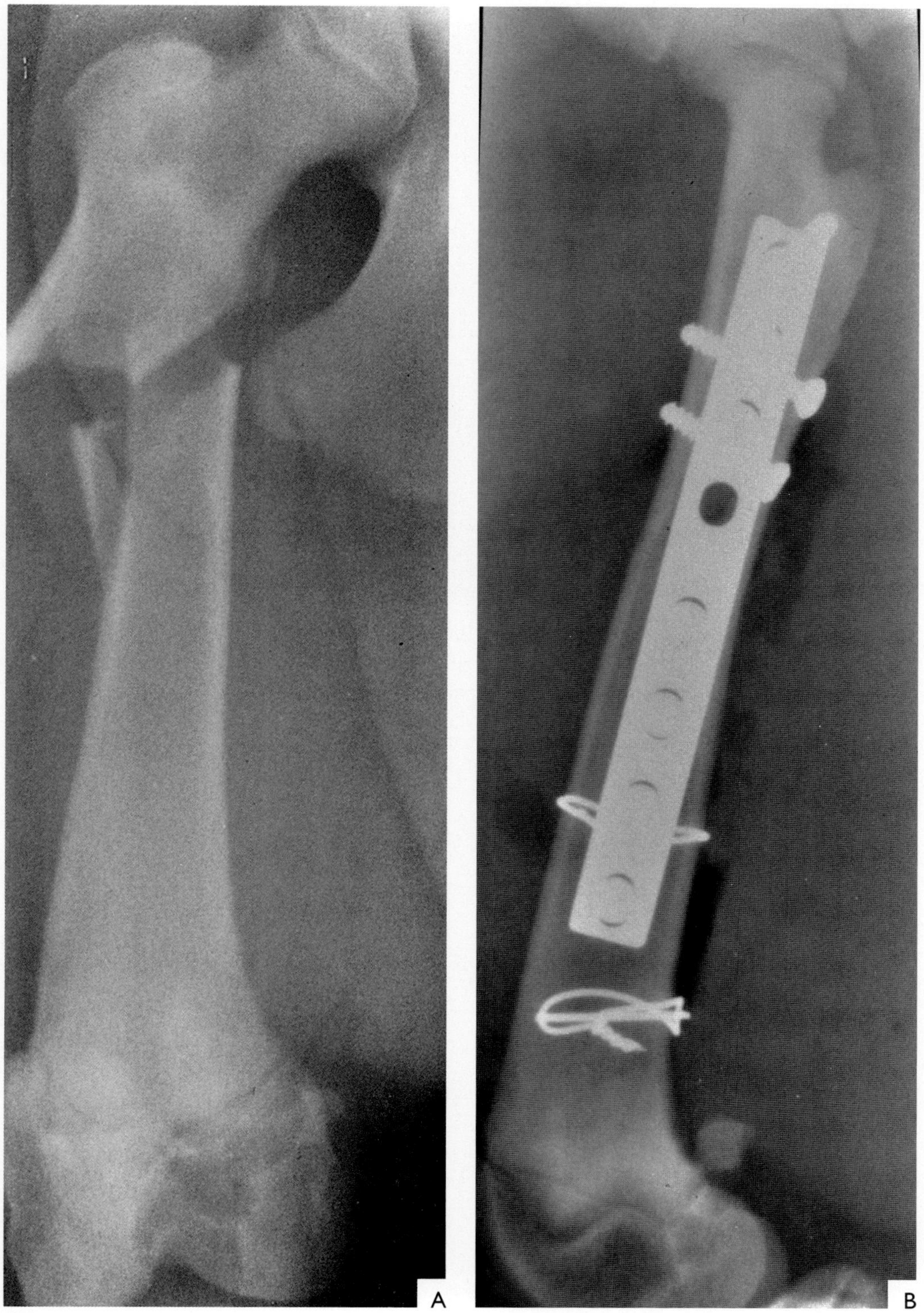

FIG. 3.54 (A) Proximal short oblique femoral fracture. (B) Lateral view of short oblique femoral fracture treated with a bone plate. Cerclage and lag screws were used. A small defect in the distal shaft was treated with a K-wire and a loop of orthopedic wire.

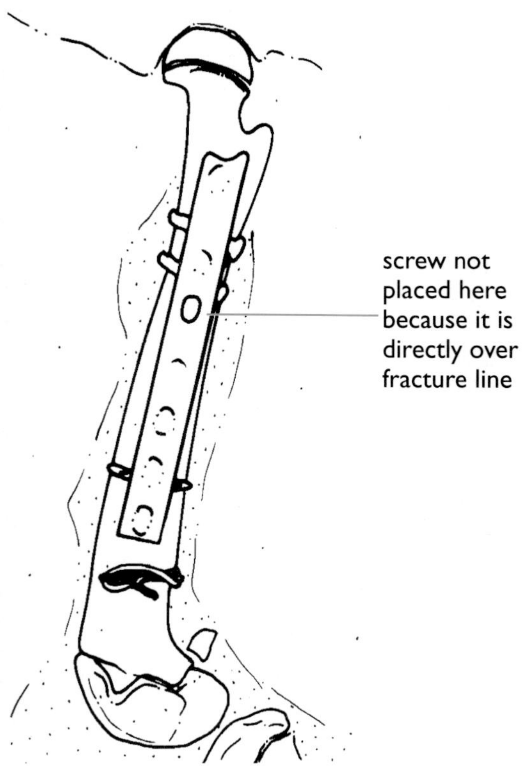

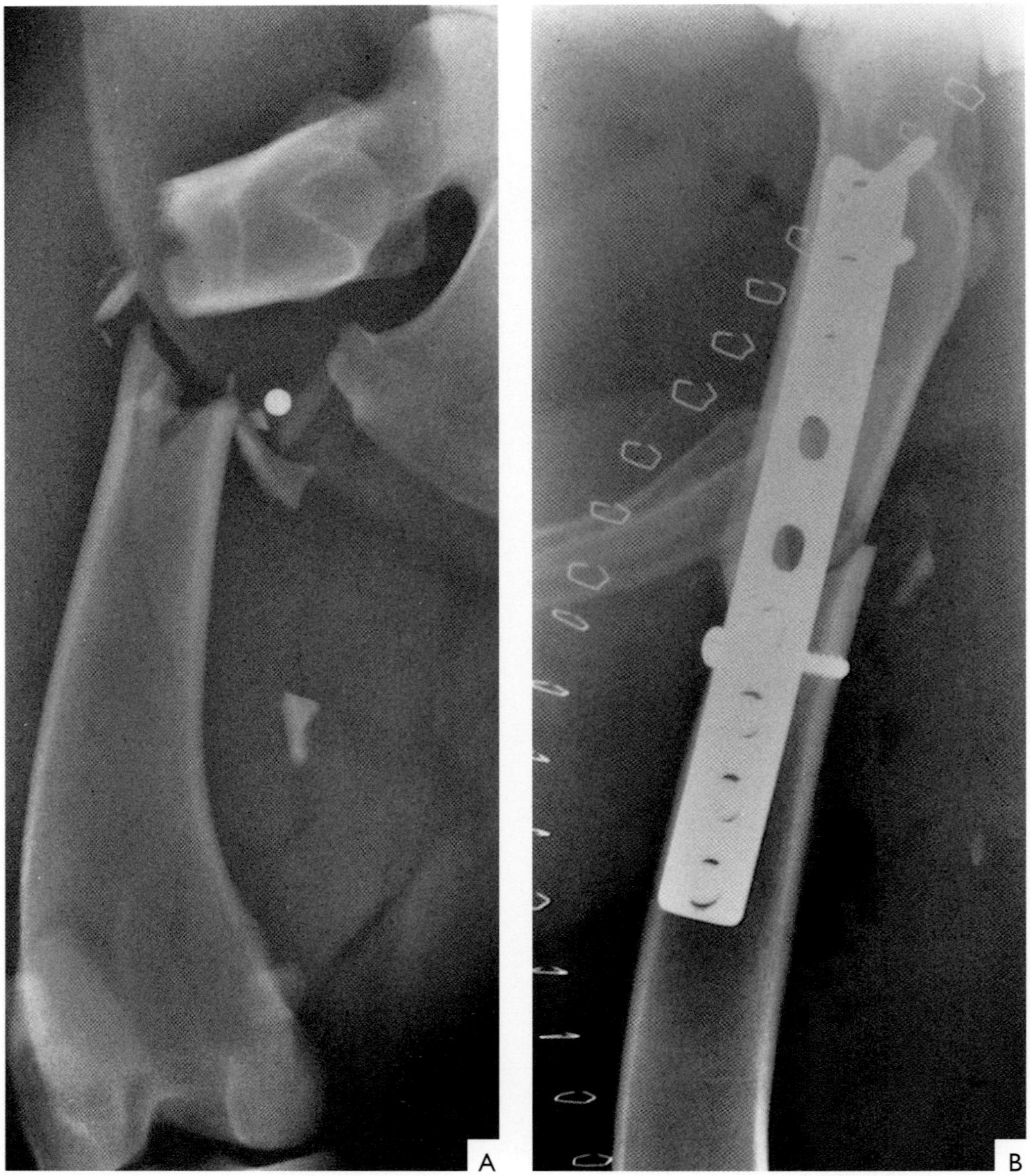

FIG. 3.55 (A) Short oblique proximal femoral fracture with small comminuted fragments. (B) Short oblique proximal femoral fracture, plated. A lag screw and a long screw into the femoral neck ensure interfragmentary compression and good proximal stability.

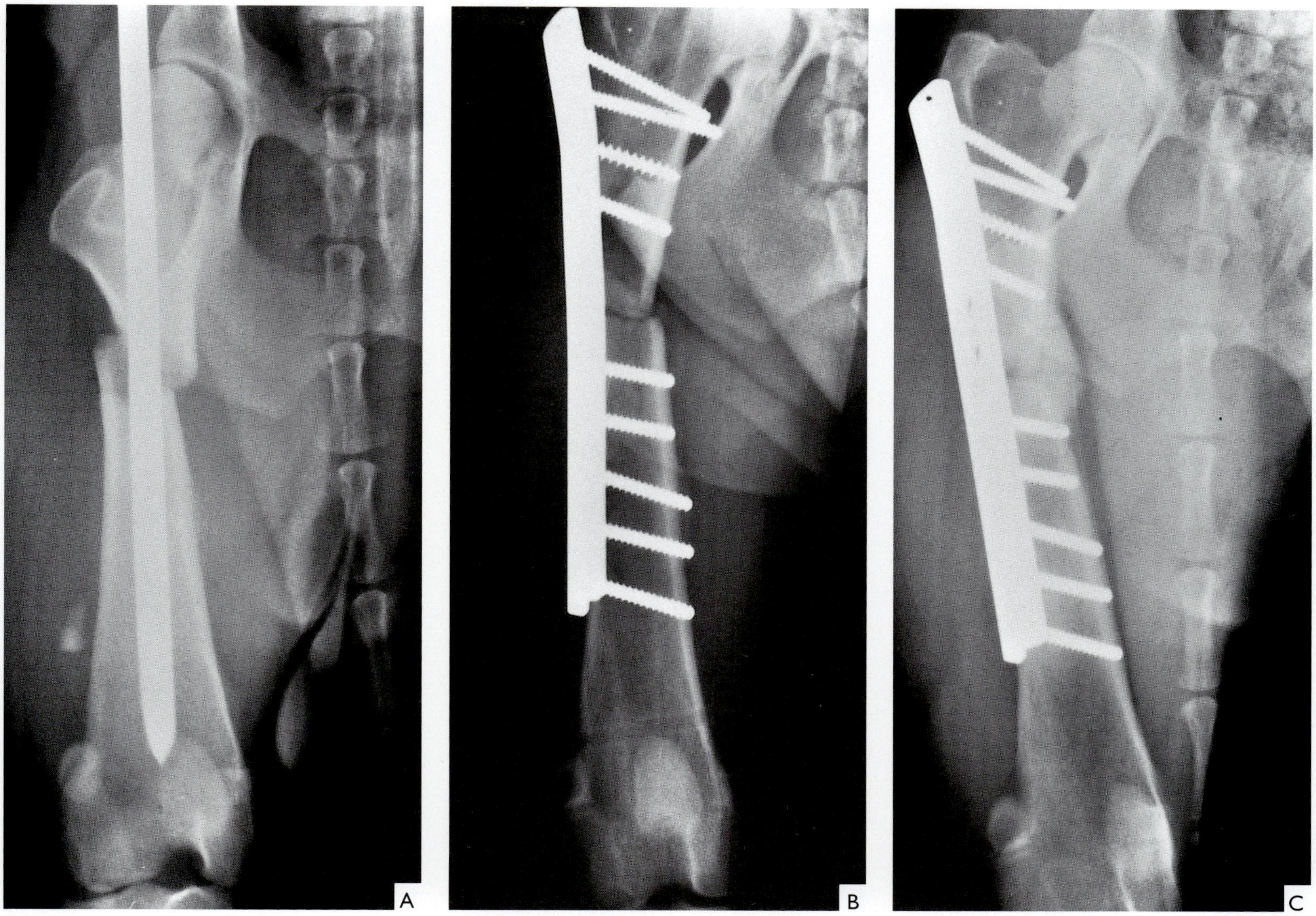

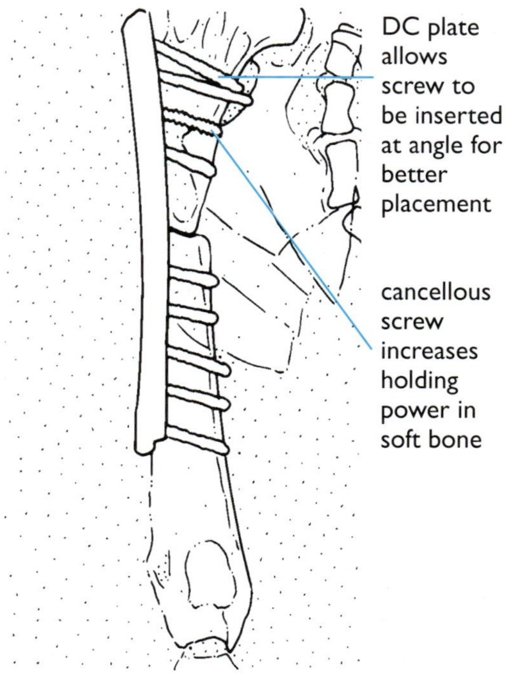

FIG. 3.56 (A) AP radiograph of a proximal femoral fracture treated with an IM pin. The pin has penetrated the knee joint and the fracture site is unstable. (B) In the same case, the pin has been removed and the plate applied. The long proximal screws were directed into the shaft because of weakening of the femoral neck from the previous pinning. The cancellous screw has increased holding power in the weakened bone. (C) AP radiograph shows good healing three months postoperatively.

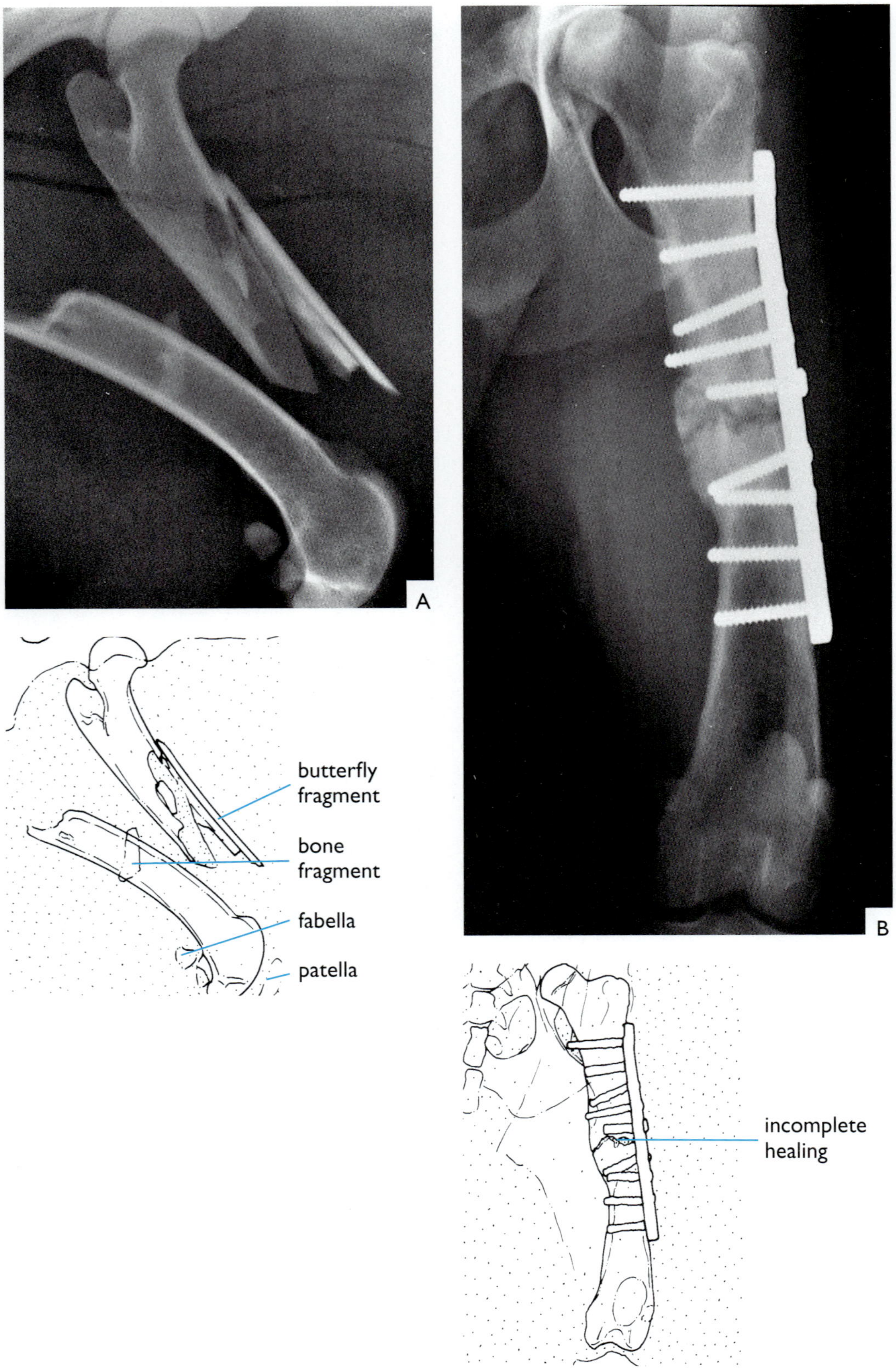

FIG. 3.57 (A) Comminuted midshaft femoral fracture with butterfly fragment. (B) Comminuted midshaft femoral fracture with butterfly fragment treated with a bone plate. Healing is progressing.

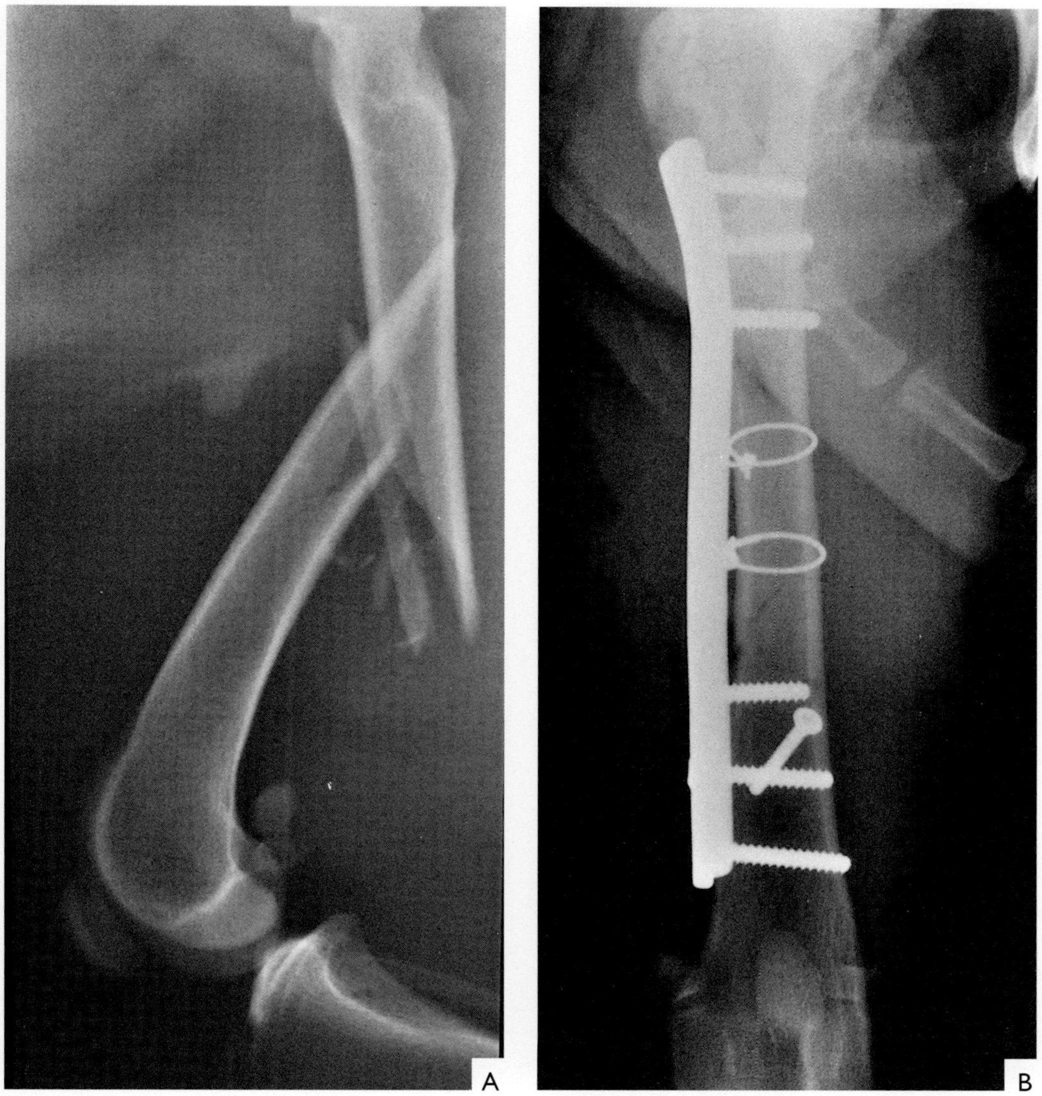

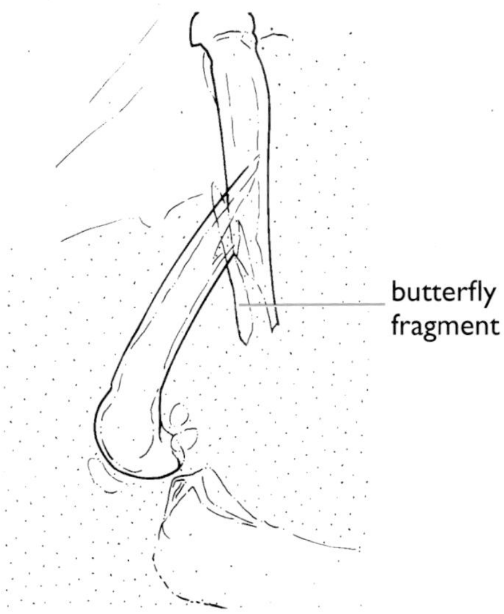

FIG. 3.58 (A) Midshaft femoral fracture with butterfly fragment. (B) Radiograph of a midshaft femoral fracture with a butterfly fragment treated with a bone plate. Cerclage wires were used to stabilize the large fragment. A lag screw controlled a fissure found at surgery.

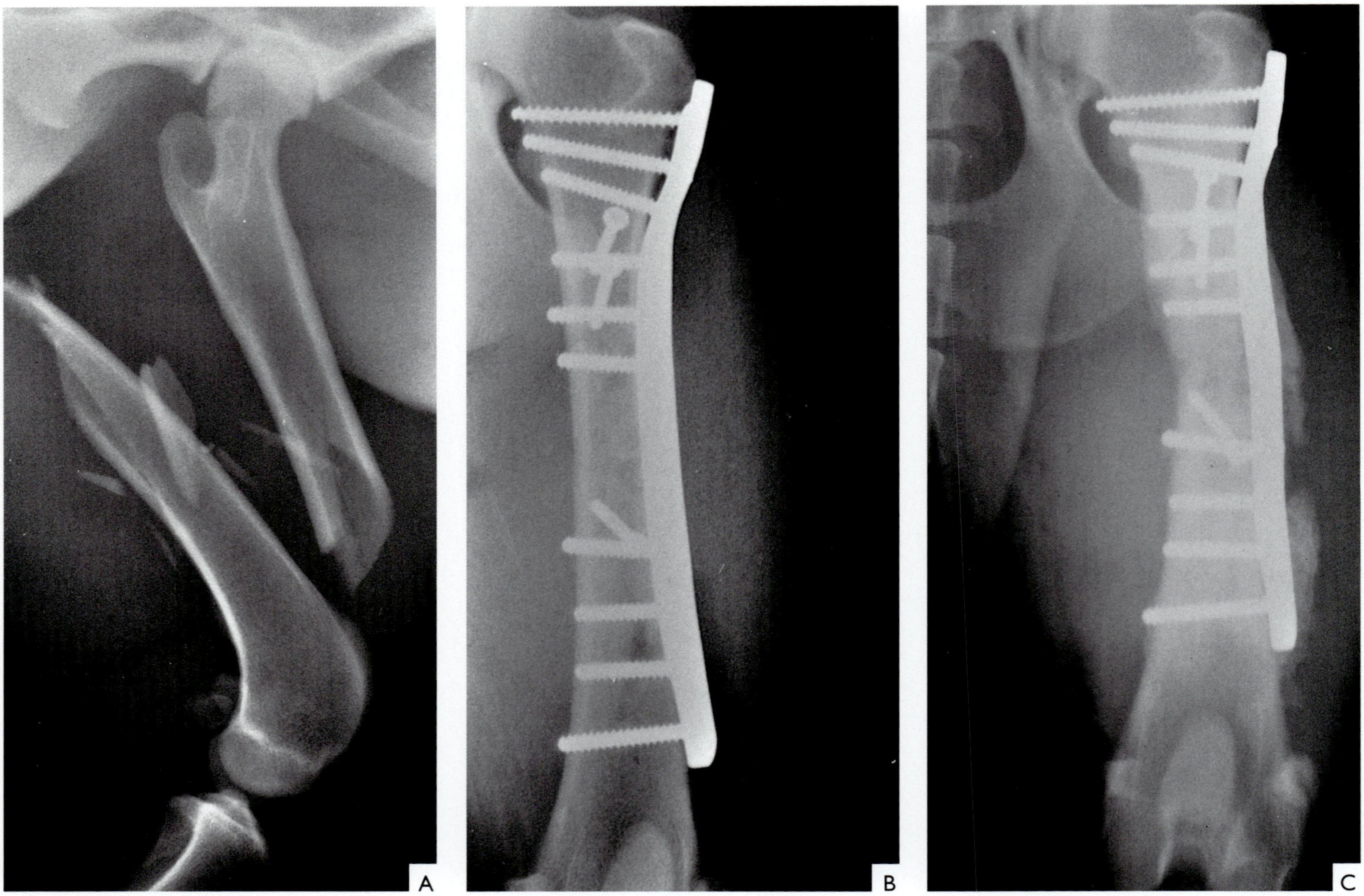

FIG. 3.59 (A) Midshaft femoral fracture. (B) Severe midshaft femoral fracture, plated. Lag screws were used for interfragmentary compression to form a stable fracture. A neutralization plate was applied. (C) Radiograph of (B) showing healing and bony overgrowth over the plate.

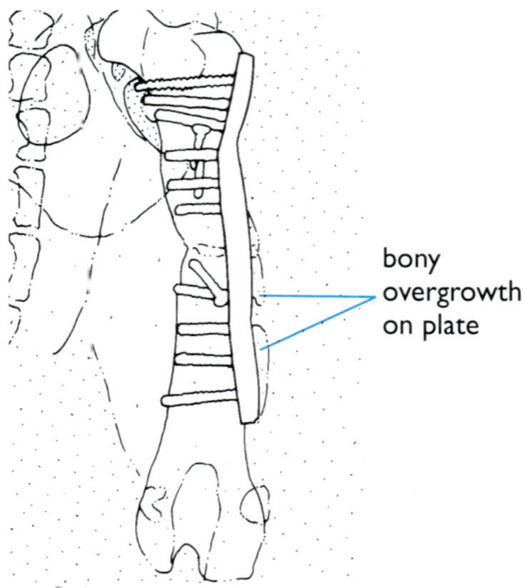

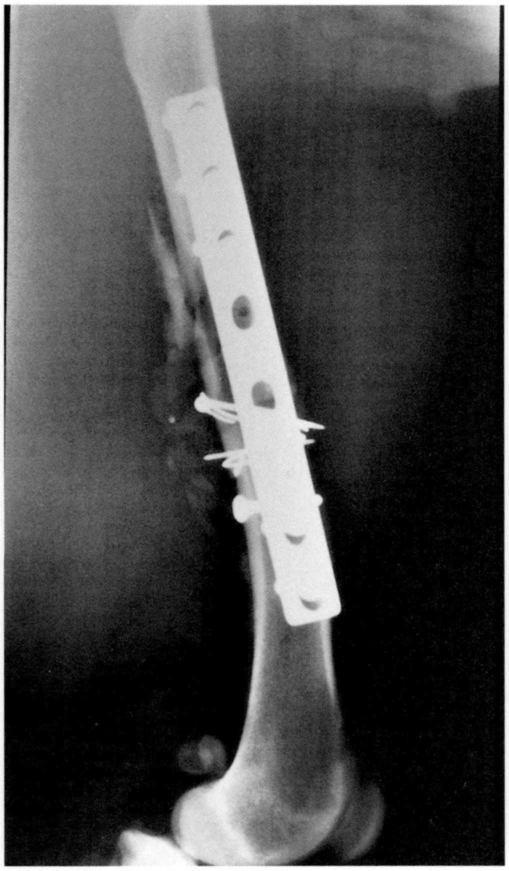

FIG. 3.60 Midshaft femoral fracture with lag screw and K-wires with cerclage wires. A bone plate has been applied.

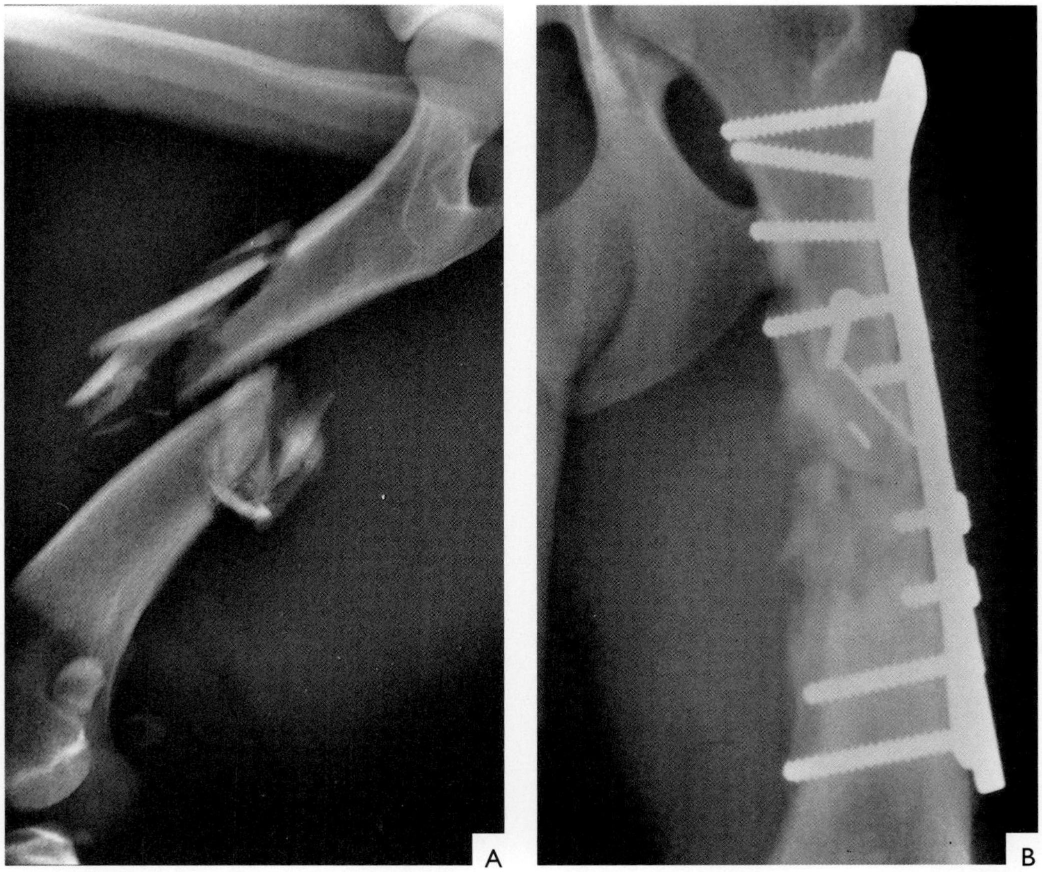

FIG. 3.61 (A) Comminuted midshaft femoral fracture. (B) Comminuted midshaft femoral fracture held in position by lag screw and K-wires. The plate acts as a buttress plate. Healing is progressing.

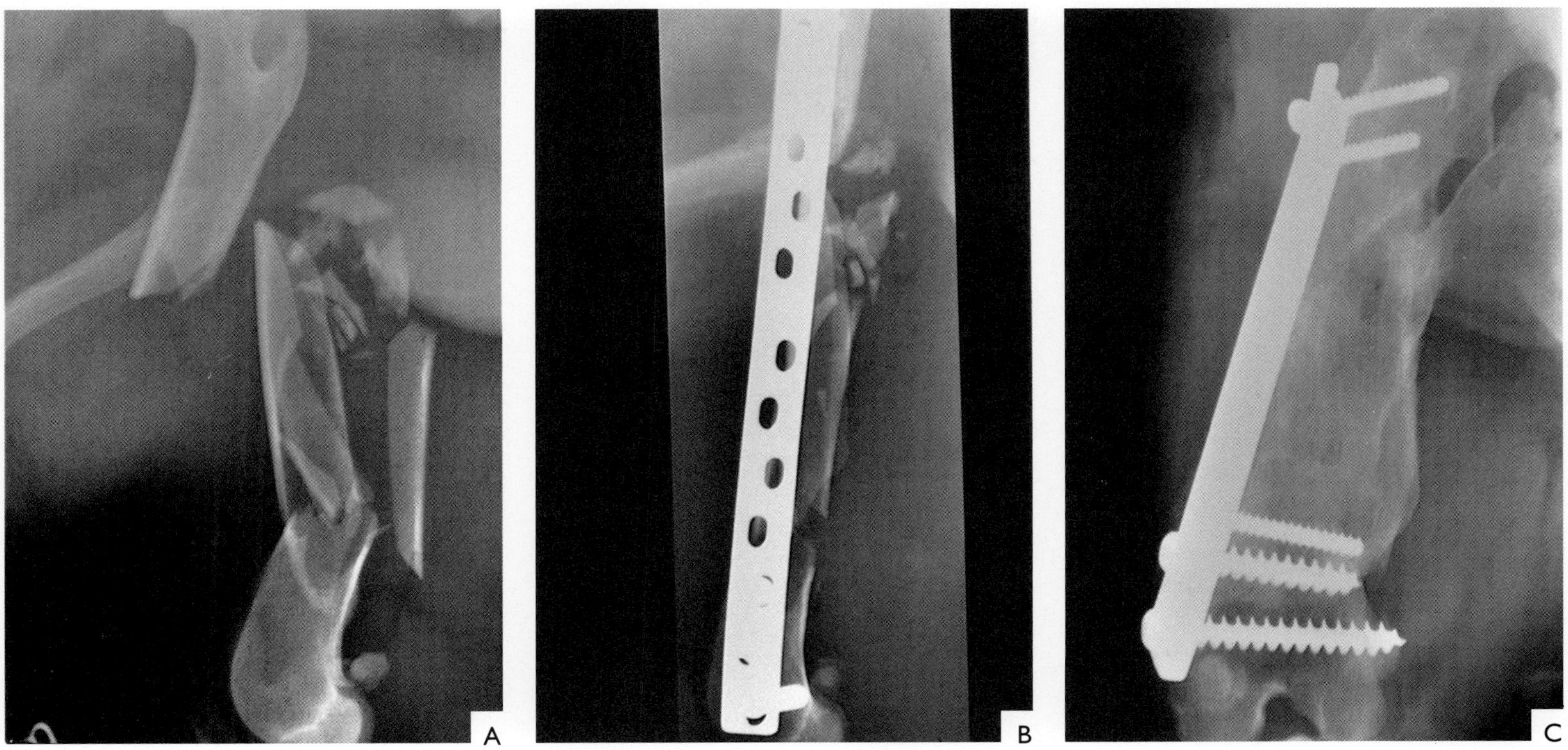

FIG. 3.62 (A) Radiograph of a severely comminuted midshaft femoral fracture. (B) Severely comminuted midshaft femoral fracture with the fragments packed in place. Some fragments are missing. A buttress plate has been applied. The screws could only be placed in the most proximal and distal fragments. (C) Very severely comminuted midshaft femoral fracture after the bone has healed. Cancellous screws were used to obtain a firm hold on the distal fragment. Note the large callus and bone mass as compared to where the fragments are repositioned with lag screws, cerclage wires, and K-wires.

The selection of the proper plate size is of concern, since one that is too heavy will remove all stress from the bone (stress protection), resulting in atrophy (osteoporosis). A plate that is too small will bend or break or the screws will pull out (Fig. 3.63).

After the plates are removed, some protection to the limb is provided for two weeks so that the bone can adapt to full stress and fully calcify.

As a last resort, a limb may be amputated.

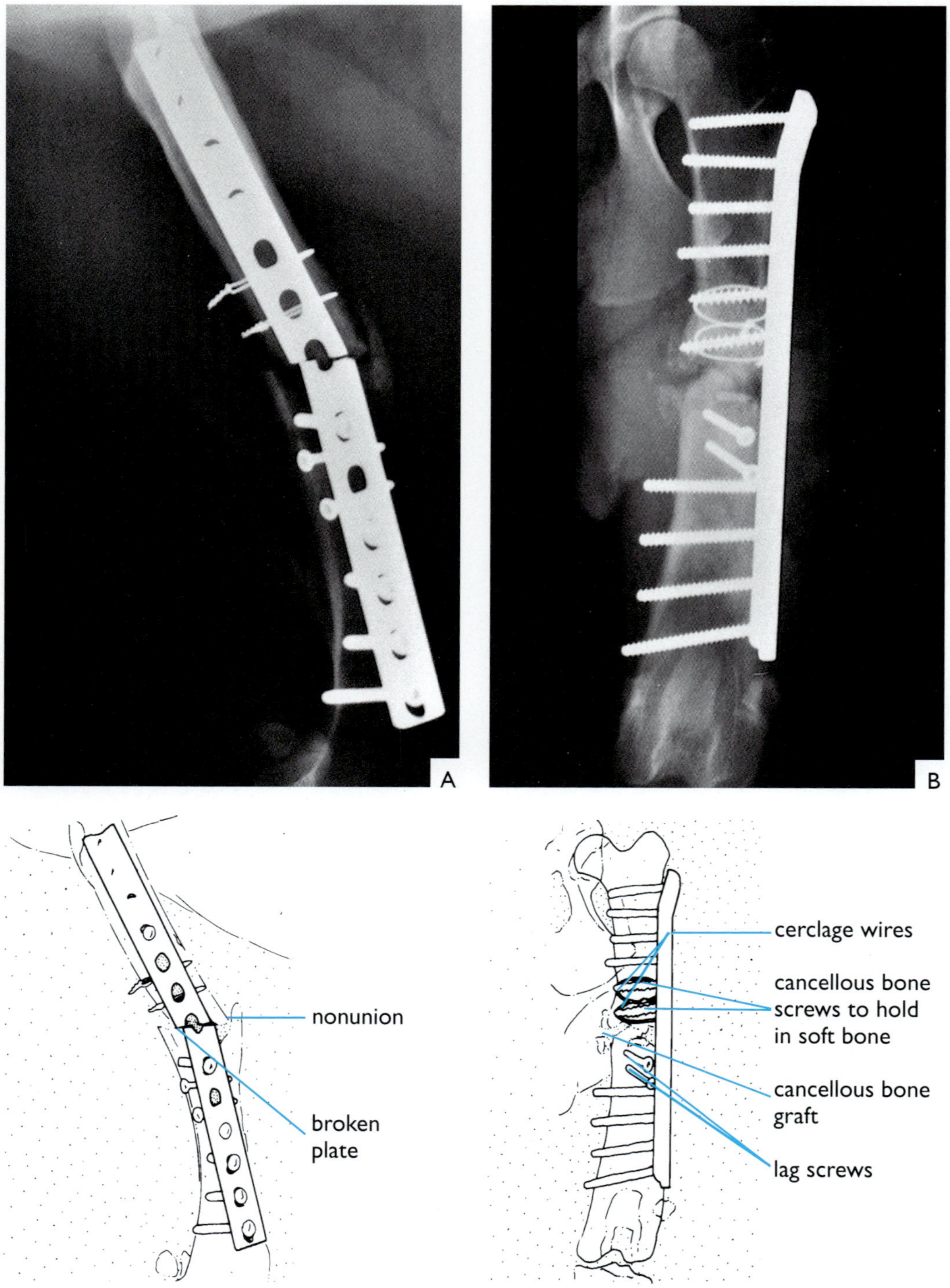

FIG. 3.63 (A) In this midshaft femoral fracture, the plate was too light for the dog's activity and it broke. (B) A broken plate was replaced with a heavier one in this midshaft femoral fracture. Centrally, cancellous bone screws were used for greater holding power in soft bone. The rest of the screws are finer, threaded cortical screws. Healing eventually resulted.

Midshaft Transverse or Short Oblique Femoral Fractures

Midshaft transverse or short oblique femoral fractures are most effectively treated with a dynamic compression plate. At least three screws should be located in each fragment. The holes in the plate are constructed so that an eccentrically-placed screw, when tightened, slides on an inclined plane between the neck of the screw and the plate to move the underlying fragment. These specially-designed holes also allow the screws to be placed at an angle rather than strictly perpendicular to the plate.

SURGICAL TECHNIQUE

The fracture is exposed through a cranio-lateral approach. The skin and subcutaneous tissues are incised parallel and cranial to the junction of the fascia lata and the biceps femoris. The fascia lata is incised along this same border, exposing the fracture. Blood clots and hematoma are cleared away. The proximal fragment rotates outwardly (Fig. 3.64). Reduction of the fracture is done by traction and angulation, and is maintained with a bone clamp. Two K-wires inserted across the fracture will help maintain the reduction temporarily. The plate should extend along the lateral surface of the femur. At least three or more screws should go into each fragment (Figs. 3.65, 3.66).

The plate is contoured to lie flat on the bone, with the area directly over the fracture line raised about 1 mm. The plate is applied to the femur. The hole nearest the fracture, but at least 1 cm away, is drilled, measured with a depth gauge, and tapped. The fragment with the greatest portion against the plate at the fracture line is drilled in the eccentric mode, using a special drill guide. The centrally located screw is inserted first. The off-center one is set in next. Clamps hold the plate proximally and distally. The K-wires are removed. The off-center screw is now tightened. As it slides into position, it moves the underlying bone fragment, compressing the fracture. The rest of the screws are inserted normally. The bone clamps are removed. All the screws are tightened. The screws must penetrate both cortices. The area is flushed with saline.

Closure is made by suturing the incision in the fascia lata, subcutaneous tissues, and skin in the usual manner.

Because of the rigid support, animals are eager to run and owners may permit uncontrolled activity too soon, causing the screws to be torn loose. Large breeds must be restrained.

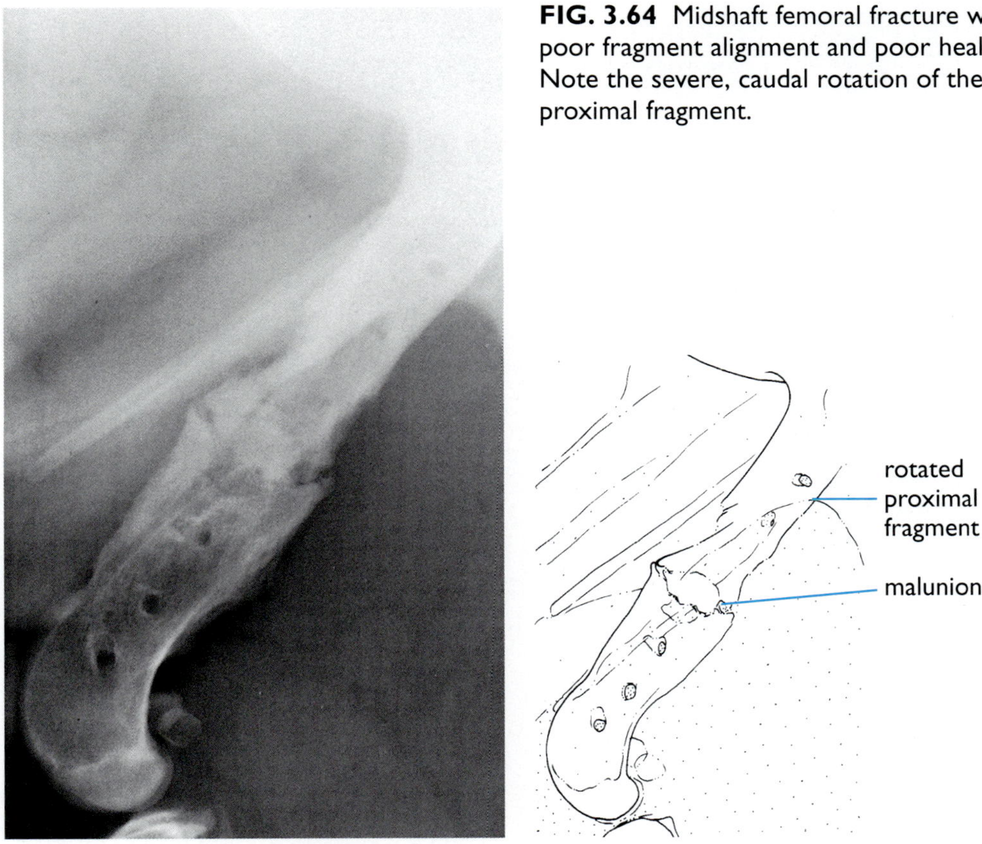

FIG. 3.64 Midshaft femoral fracture with poor fragment alignment and poor healing. Note the severe, caudal rotation of the proximal fragment.

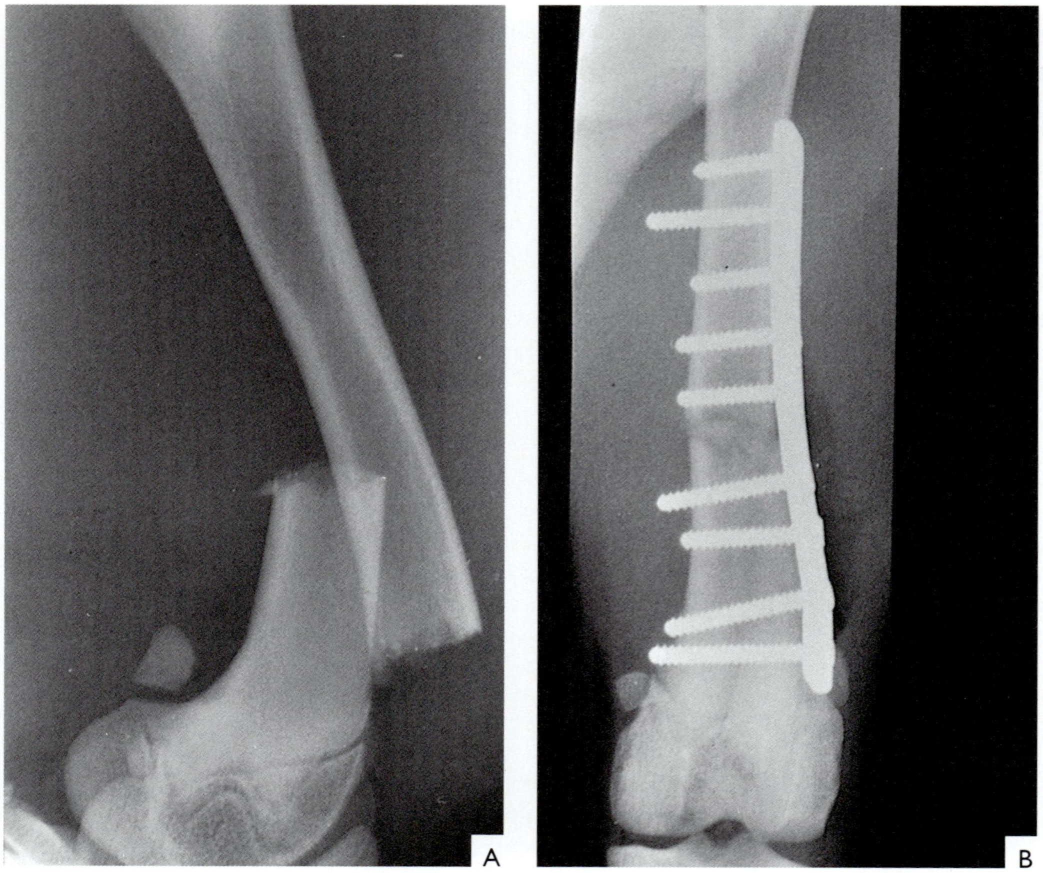

FIG. 3.65 (A) A fresh, fractured transverse distal femur. Note the outward rotation of the proximal fragment. (B) A transverse distal femoral fracture that was treated with a bone plate.

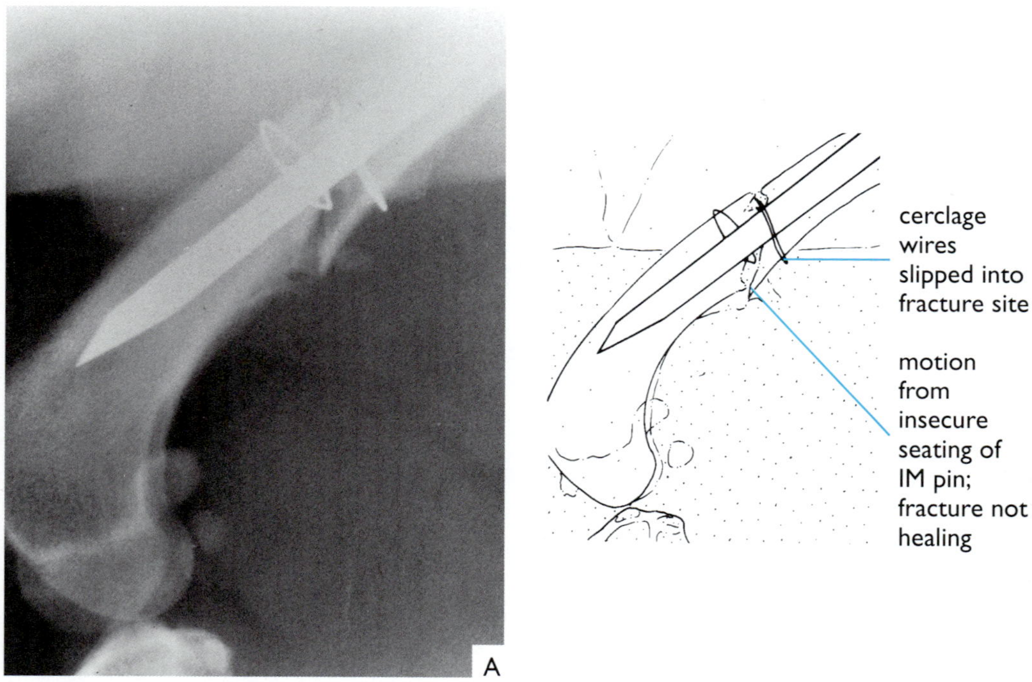

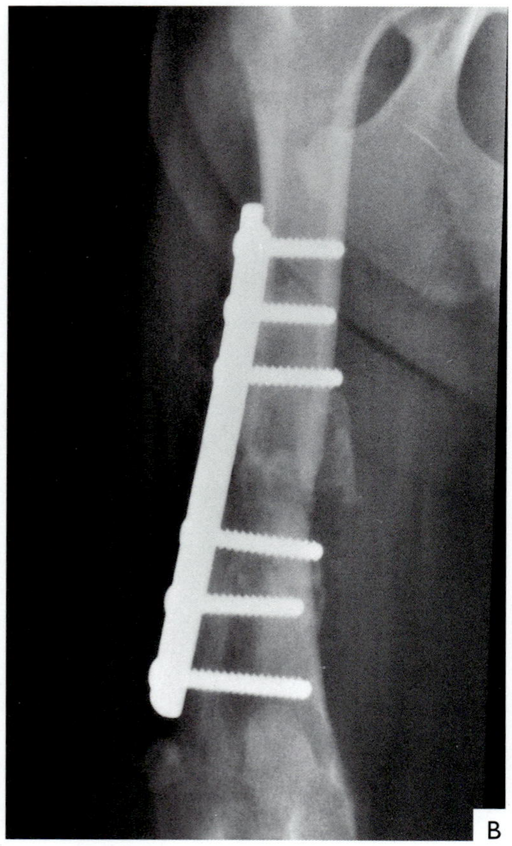

FIG. 3.66 (A) This distal transverse femoral fracture was treated with an IM pin and two cerclage wires. Incorrect pin placement and wiring resulted in nonunion. Some of the wires slipped into the fracture site. (B) In a similar case, the pin and wires were removed and the fracture was plated. A cancellous bone graft was applied. The fracture subsequently healed.

Midshaft Femoral Fractures with a Large Segmented Fragment

Midshaft femoral fractures frequently have a large caudal segment broken away from one or both fragments. Referred to as butterfly fragments, they are reattached to the segment from which they are mainly derived. Two K-wires are inserted to hold the fragment in position. A gliding hole is drilled in the near cortex of the butterfly fragment. The hole is countersunk to allow deeper seating of the screw head. A tubular guide is inserted and the opposite cortex of the segment from which it was detached is drilled for a threaded hole. The screw length is derived from the depth gauge. The far cortex hole is tapped. The guide is removed and the screw is seated, lagging the butterfly fragment in place. A long oblique split may require several screws for stability. The heads are seated in the countersunk holes. A lag screw inserted through a hole in the bone plate can be very effective.

The fracture now consists of two fragments that are reduced and held with two K-wires. An additional lag screw may be introduced or a pair of cerclage wires placed. The plate is a dynamic compression plate, but is used in the neutralization mode. It should extend over most of the femur's length. All the screws are seated in the centrally drilled holes. The most proximal and distal screws are inserted first. The rest are placed alternately. No screws are inserted where they might enter the fracture line. The fracture, which has been reduced and stabilized, is inherently stable. The plate protects it from undue stress.

Femoral shaft fractures with several fragments are reconstructed by means of K-wires, cerclage wires, and interfragmentary compression screws. The latter are preferable. Some fragments may be too small to be adequately replaced. Cancellous bone grafting material is situated around the fracture site and areas of missing bone. Cerclage wires must be tightly twisted and set into small grooves cut into the cortical bone, or secured over the slightly projecting ends of K-wires to prevent slippage and loosening. Doubled wire or wires with a prepared eye seem to hold the best. It is possible to apply a cerclage wire with a simple pair of pliers, depending on the surgeon's skill.

Distal Femur

Distal femoral epiphyseal fractures in immature dogs and cats are quite common. Supracondylar and condylar fractures are frequently seen in mature dogs and cats. Early intervention is needed before muscle spasm and fibrous proliferative tissues make reduction exceptionally difficult. Articular surfaces in condylar fractures must be congruent, especially in the patellar surface of the trochlear groove.

Epiphyseal fractures are fixed with a single pin. Screws, plates, or crossed pins can cause premature fusion and cessation of growth. Condylar fractures, whether single or bilateral, are treated with lag screws. Supracondylar fractures receive flexible intramedullary pins that are introduced retrograde or used in a Rush pin technique, or can be treated with crossed pins. Epiphyseal fractures usually need open reduction and a means of fixation. Closed reduction is often unsatisfactory.

Femoral Distal Epiphyseal Fracture

SURGICAL TECHNIQUE

The distal fragment is located caudally and proximally. A lateral approach through the stifle is taken. An incision is made parallel and slightly lateral to the patella and the straight patellar ligament, cutting through skin, subcutaneous tissues, retinaculum, and joint capsule. The incision is extended distally to the tibia and proximally into the fascia lata. The patella is luxated medially. It is often difficult to bring about reduction. The bones in young dogs and cats are soft and easily injured. Levers should be used cautiously; bone forceps can crush the condyles. Where reduction is very difficult, it is better to cut away a small portion of the distal end of the proximal fragment.

After reduction an intramedullary pin is introduced just beneath the trochlea's articular surface in the center of the condyle (Fig. 3.67). It is drilled through to exit in the center of the distal epiphysis. Further drilling places it into the proximal fragment until the point reaches the inner surface of the cortical bone cranially. The pin is withdrawn a short way and cut off. It is countersunk beneath the bone surface, which secures it in the cortical bone of the cranial portion of the proximal fragment. The particular shape of the physeal area prevents rotation. The pin prevents angulation and loss of reduction. It remains in place permanently, but can be removed if needed by cutting around the tip in the femoral shaft and withdrawing it.

The presence of a single round pin does not interfere with growth. Closure is done by replacing the patella and resuturing the retinaculum, joint capsule, subcutaneous tissues, and skin in the usual manner.

The leg is placed in a Robert Jones splint for a few days. The stifle is passively mobilized. Healing is usually rapid, with prompt return of function.

Supracondylar Fractures of the Femur

Supracondylar fractures of the femur are treated with crossed pins, modified Rush pins or two flexible intramedullary pins or, rarely, with a single intramedullary pin.

A lateral parapatellar incision is made and the patella is luxated medially. The fracture site is exposed and reduction is done by levering the fragments into position.

SURGICAL TECHNIQUE

CROSSED PINS An intramedullary pin is inserted through the skin and muscle tissue into the proximal fragment at an angle that passes through the fracture site and into the medial condyle. A pin cutter is introduced alongside the bone from the incision. The pin may be withdrawn a bit, cut off, and set into position with a pin setter. Using the same technique, another pin is inserted medially to lodge in the lateral condyle. These pins are permanent (Fig. 3.68).

FLEXIBLE INTRAMEDULLARY PINS A flexible intra-medullary pin is introduced retrograde up the proximal fragment to exit above the trochanteric fossa. A second pin is inserted in the same fashion. The pins are withdrawn until only the tips are present at the fracture site. The fracture is reduced. The pins are driven into the distal fragment, then cut off below the skin in the trochanteric area. They are removed after healing (Fig. 3.69).

MODIFIED RUSH PIN TECHNIQUE Flexible intramedullary pins are introduced into the medial and lateral surfaces of the condyles to be driven through the fracture site, up the medullary cavity of the proximal fragment. They do not penetrate the cortex. Their bending presses them against the medial surfaces of the cortical bone, lock-

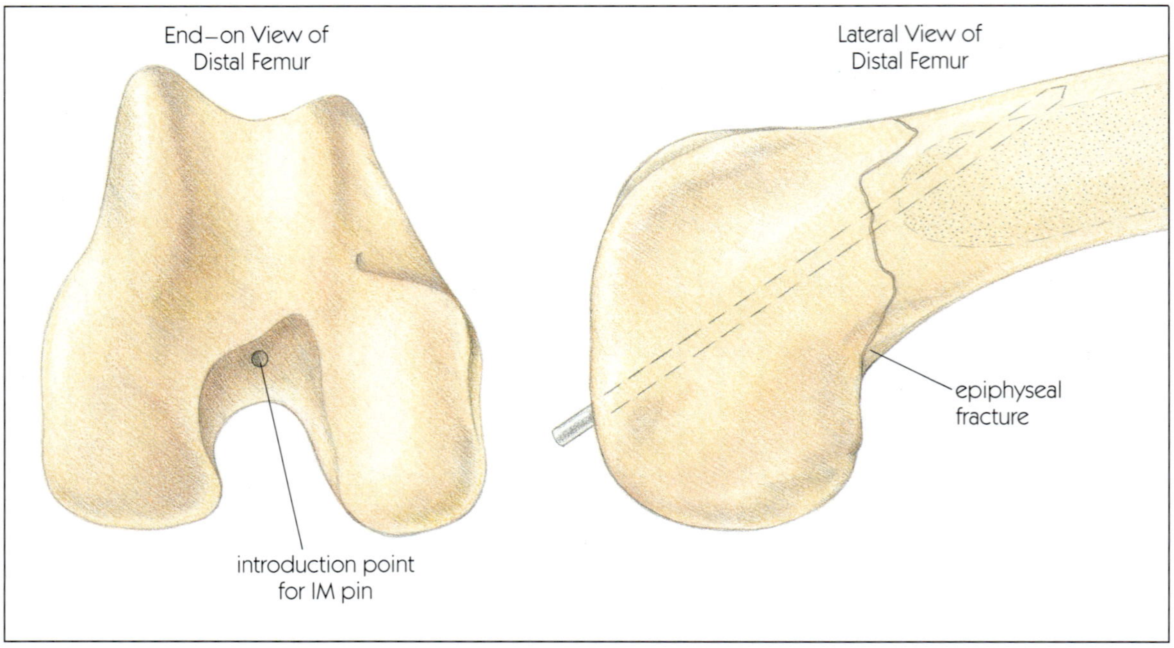

FIG. 3.67 Placement of a short IM pin for treatment of distal femoral epiphyseal fractures.

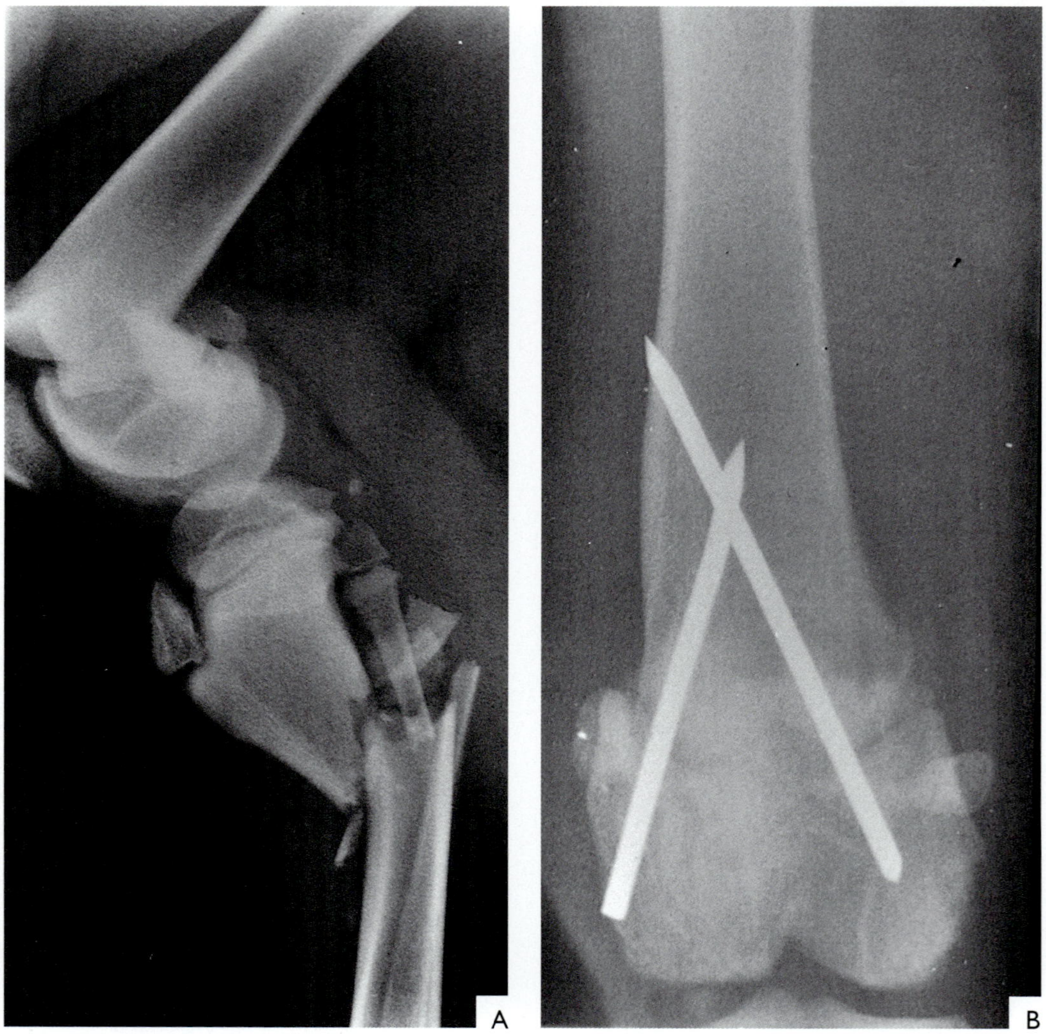

FIG. 3.68 (A) Radiograph of a distal femoral epiphyseal fracture. (B) A distal femoral epiphyseal fracture treated with crossed pins.

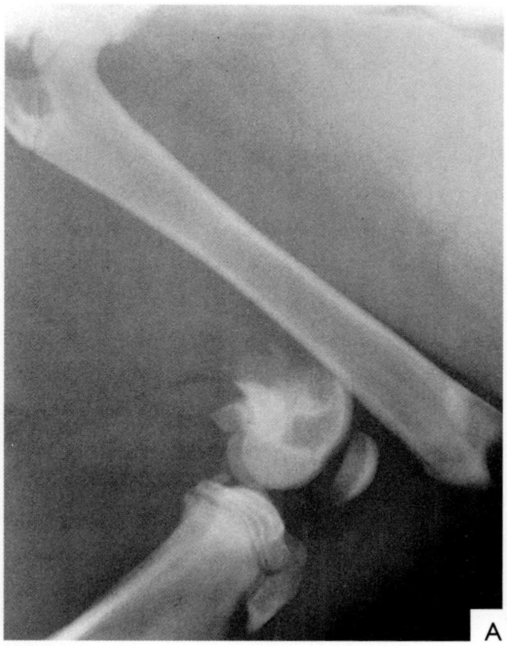

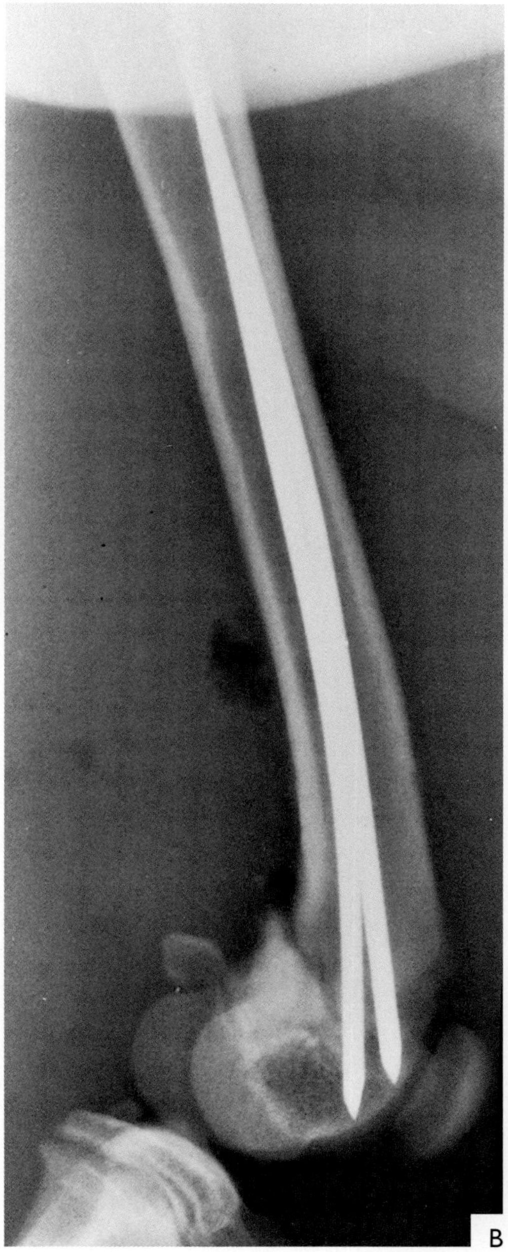

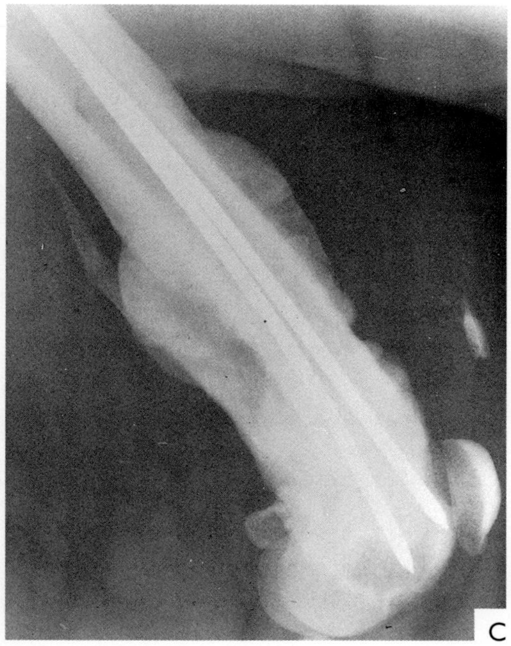

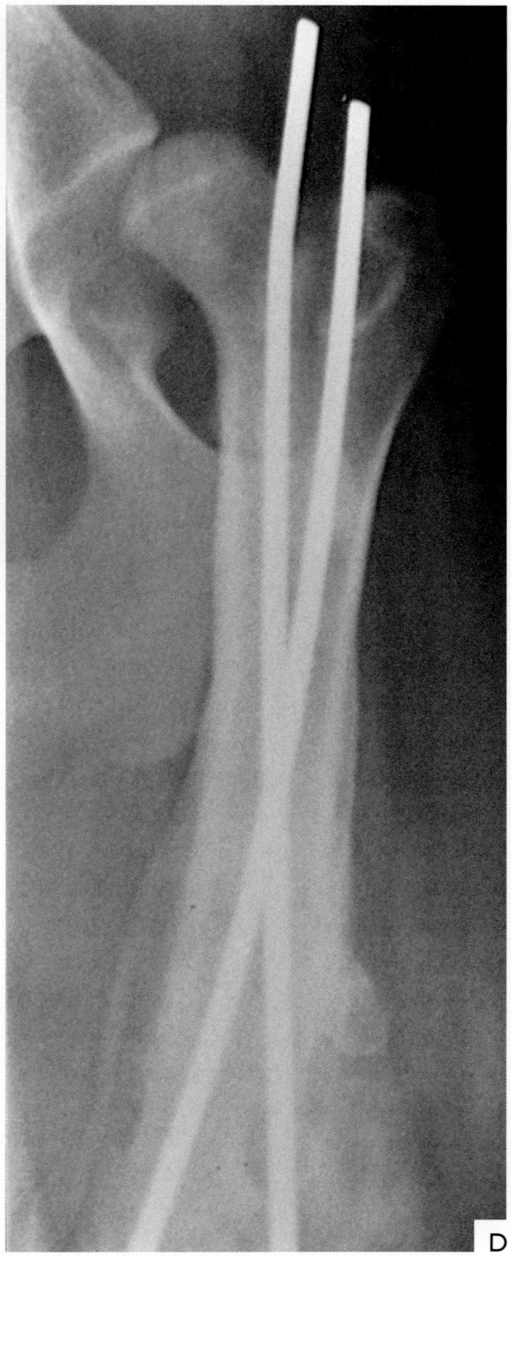

FIG. 3.69 (A) Distal femoral epiphyseal fracture, Salter II type. (B) This radiograph of a distal femoral epiphyseal fracture shows placement of double IM pins. (C) Lateral radiograph of a distal femoral epiphyseal fracture shows healing of the fracture and the heavy periosteal overgrowth common in immature patients. (D) AP radiograph of a distal femoral epiphyseal fracture shows healing. The pins will be withdrawn from the trochanteric fossa.

ing them in place. The ends at the condylar surfaces are bent at right angles and cut off. They are turned to lie against the bone (Fig. 3.70).

Closure is routine. The pins are removed after healing is definite, usually in about a month.

INTRAMEDULLARY PIN Due to the cranial bowing of the diaphysis, a single large intramedullary pin will ordinarily impinge on such a small portion of the condylar fracture surface that it will not be capable of good fixation. Depending upon the shape of the femur and size of the fragment, however, it is sometimes feasible (Fig. 3.71).

Fractures of the Femoral Condyles

Condylar fractures are relatively rare. Either condyle may be broken away, but it is usually the medial one. A supracondylar fracture combined with a central split is called a "T" fracture. There is always considerable soft-tissue damage. The stifle ligaments may be torn.

The articular surfaces must be congruent. Accurate reduction, compression and solid fixation is provided by lag screws. With T fractures, the condyles are fastened together with a transverse lag screw. The supracondylar fracture is then treated with cross pins or a modified Rush pinning technique (Fig. 3.72).

SURGICAL TECHNIQUE

For fractures of the medial condyle, a medial parapatellar incision is made. The incision is extended dorsally to permit luxation of the patella laterally. The fragment is replaced and secured temporarily with a K-wire or a bone forceps. A cancellous lag screw is applied in large dogs. A cortical screw is appropriate for small dogs. K-wires are used in smaller breeds.

The screw is inserted from the lateral surface of the proximal portion of the medial condyle into the center of the distal fragment. A portion of the insertion site is reamed to permit deep seating of the screw head (Fig. 3.73).

Fractures of the lateral condyle are approached by a lateral parapatellar incision and the fragment is secured with a lag screw.

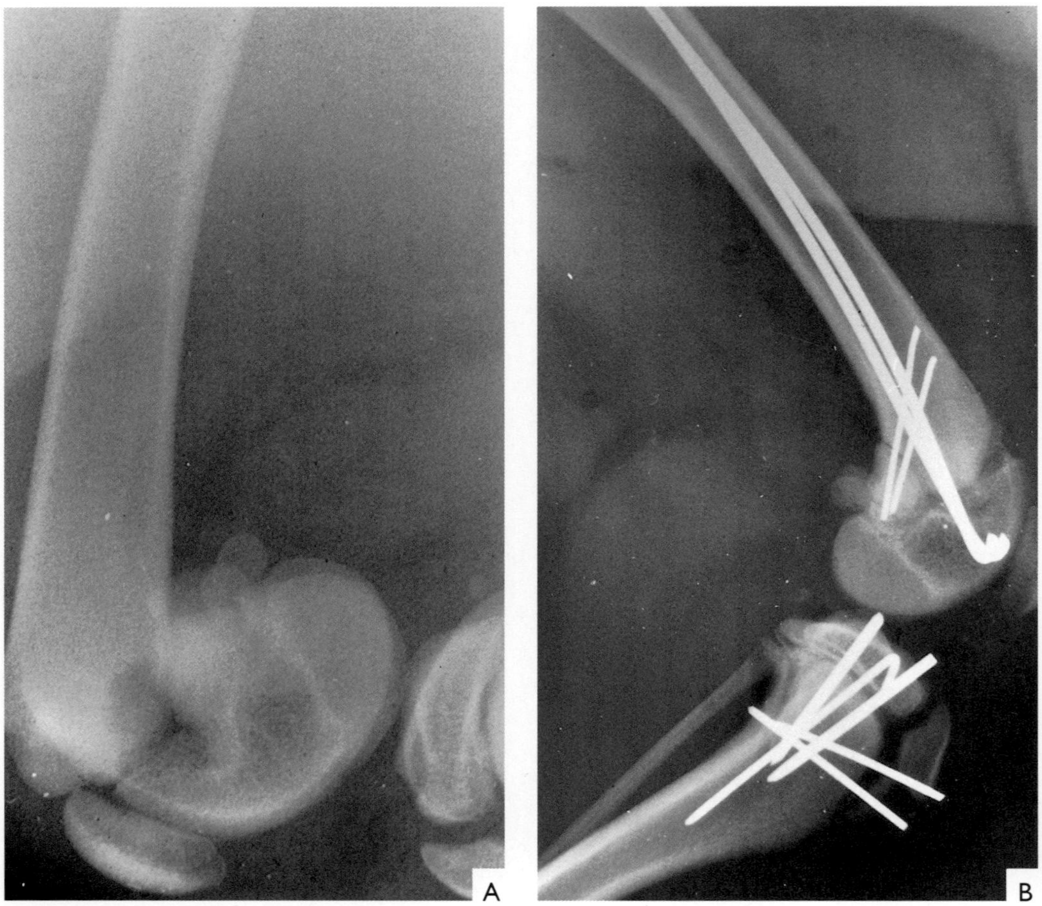

FIG. 3.70 (A) Distal femoral epiphyseal fracture. (B) Lateral view of a distal femoral epiphyseal fracture treated with modified Rush pin technique. Note the K-wires used to stabilize the distal fragment prior to insertion of the pins.

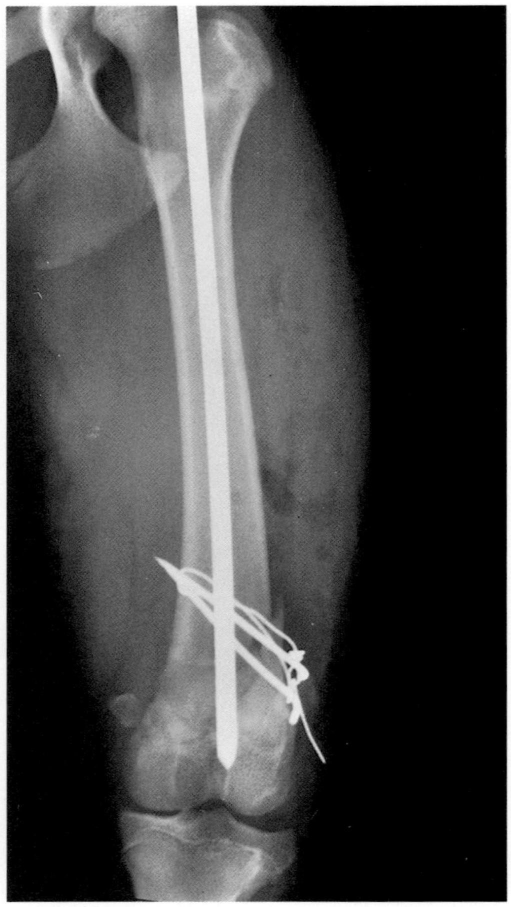

FIG. 3.71 A distal femoral epiphyseal fracture type Salter II, that was treated with an IM pin and K-wires, with a binding wire loop to stabilize the distal fragment.

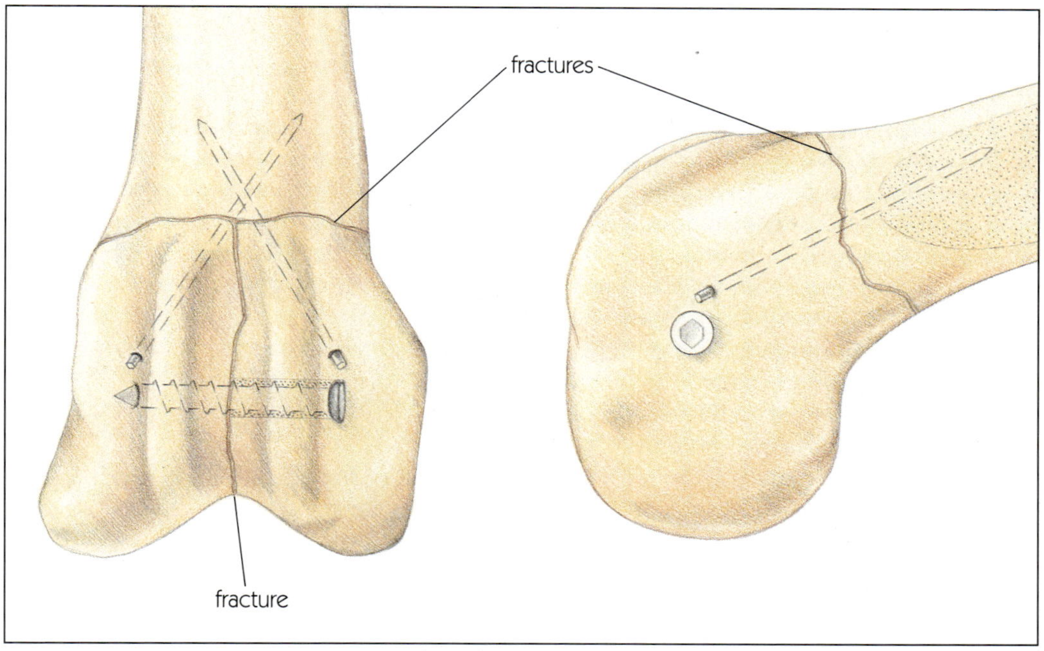

FIG. 3.72 T fracture of the distal femoral condyles treated with a lag screw and crossed pins. Location of insertions of lag screw and crossed pins.

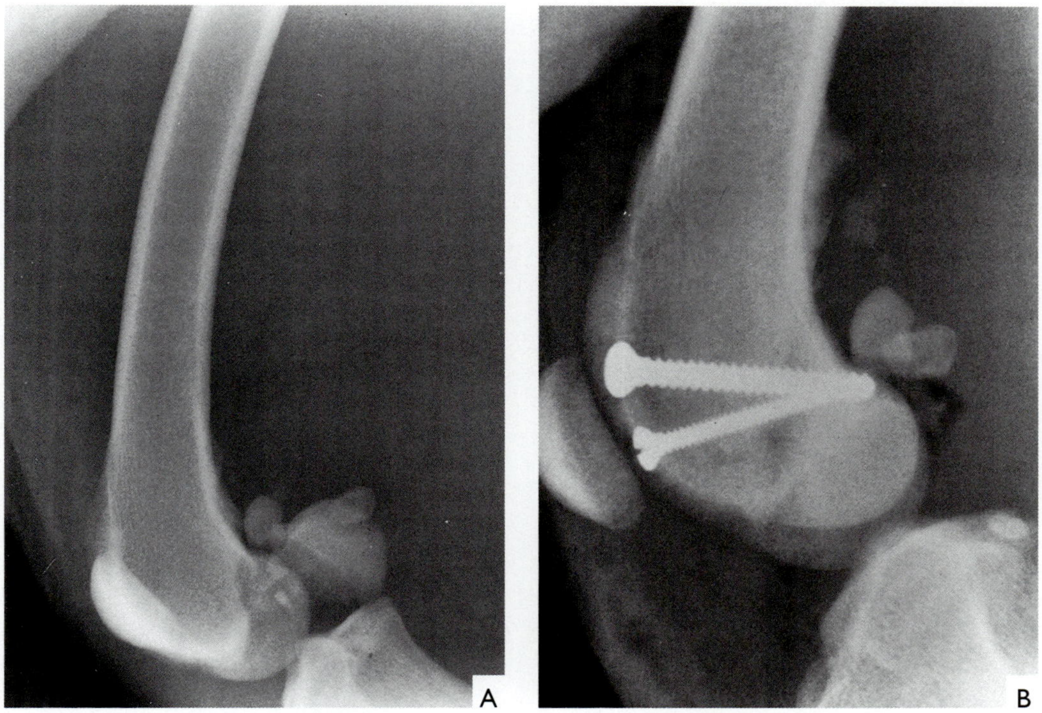

FIG. 3.73 (A) Medial femoral condylar fracture. (B) Medial femoral condylar fracture treated with bone screws.

T Fracture of the Distal Femur

T fractures of the distal femur are approached through a lateral parapatellar incision. This permits lagging the condylar halves together and treatment of the supracondylar fracture. The articular surface of the trochlear groove must be made congruent. A lag screw is applied to compress and control the condyles into one unit. The supracondylar fracture is then repaired.

Where the reduction is particularly difficult, an osteotomy of the tibial crest is performed (Fig. 3.74). Medial and lateral parapatellar incisions are made; the patella and patellar ligament are retracted dorsally, increasing access to the joint and the fractures. The tibial crest is replaced with two K-wires and a tension band figure-8 wire. The joint is inspected and flushed with saline.

Closure of the arthrotomy is done by suturing the retinacular structures, joint capsule fascias, subcutaneous tissues, and skin in the usual manner.

A modified Robert Jones splint is applied for a few days. Passive and active use of the joint is then begun. If Rush pins have been inserted, they are removed in about a month.

FRACTURES OF THE TIBIA AND FIBULA

Tibial fractures are very common. They vary from a simple greenstick, which can be adequately treated by a cast, to severely comminuted, contaminated, and infected fractures that require pins, external fixators, and bone plates. Proximally and distally, the joint surfaces must be preserved congruently to prevent degenerative joint disease.

In general, distal tibial fractures are more subject to stress and motion and seem to take longer to heal. Midshaft fractures are often severely damaged and, especially when mishandled, will take a long time to heal. There is no inherent problem with the bone itself.

The fibula rarely needs repair except at each end. The proximal portion is the site of insertion of the lateral collateral ligament of the stifle and the distal portion forms the lateral malleolus. Each is of great importance to its respective joint.

Avulsion of the Tibial Tubercle

Avulsion of the tibial tubercle is rarely seen in mature dogs and cats. In immature animals, the tubercle has a separate ossification center. Avulsion usually occurs as a physeal separation. The quadriceps muscles pull on the patella and the patellar ligament, which is attached to the tuberosity. Severe stress pulls the epiphysis away from its seat. Care must be taken not to damage the growth plate in younger patients, since premature fusion will result in a deformity (Fig. 3.75).

SURGICAL TECHNIQUE

There are several means of reattaching the avulsed fragment. In small dogs, two small wire sutures will suffice. Slightly larger dogs

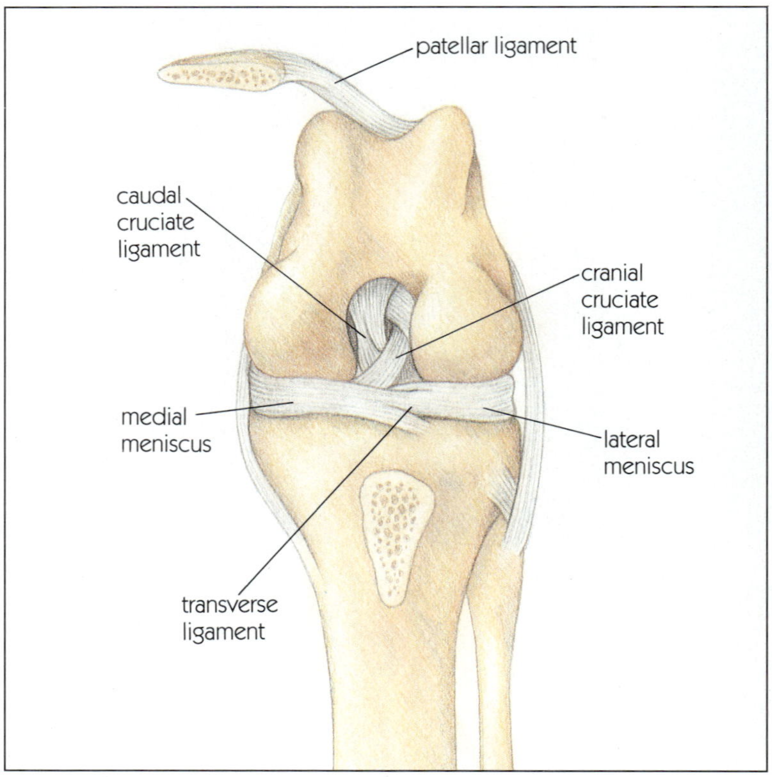

FIG. 3.74 Osteotomy of the tibial crest and reflection of the patellar ligament and the patella to provide extensive exposure of the stifle joint.

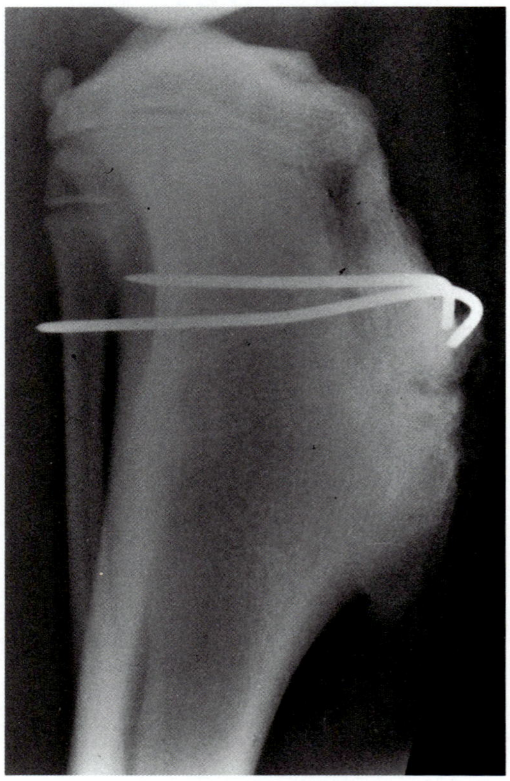

FIG. 3.75 Deformity due to premature fusion of the tibial tubercle physis after treatment for avulsion can be seen on the x-ray.

do well with two K-wires. Care must be taken not to split the fragment. Most dogs will do well with two K-wires and a tension band wire. A very large or older dog with a large piece torn away will do well with a K-wire and lag screw.

Spasms of the quadriceps muscle group frequently cause difficulties when reapproximating the fragment. Strong traction is applied to the patellar ligament—not to the bone fragment—while the leg is held in extension.

A lateral incision is made through the skin, subcutaneous tissues, and the fascia of the stifle. The incision travels close and parallel to the patellar ligament, down to the tibial crest area. The patella is found in a more proximal position. Sharp and blunt dissection is done. The fracture site is exposed and cleared of fibrous tissue and blood clots. The fragment and the attached patellar ligament are isolated. The bone fragment may split if traction is applied to it with forceps or if a pin is driven through it. Sustained traction is applied to the patellar ligament. The leg is held in extension. The fragment is secured in its proper position with a K-wire.

In toy breeds, two small holes are drilled through the fragment with a straight cutting-edge needle. Appositional holes are drilled in the fracture site so that when the fragment is properly positioned, wire sutures can be inserted in the medial and lateral pairs of holes and tightened to hold the fragment in place (Fig. 3.76).

In small dogs, two K-wires are inserted through the fragment and deep into the proximal tibial bone. The pin ends are bent at right angles and cut off. They are seated with a few taps of a bone mallet. It is important to bend the ends, since the straight pins can move distally, eventually penetrating the caudal aspect of the stifle (Fig. 3.77).

In most cases, K-wires are accompanied by a hole drilled transversely through the tibial crest about 1 or 2 cm below the fracture site. A figure-8 wire is inserted and placed over the ends of the K-wires, then twisted tightly, providing resistance to the pull of the quadriceps. In immature dogs, the device is removed as soon as healing begins so as not to injure the growth plate (Fig. 3.78).

With very large dogs, the fragment is secured with a K-wire. A lag screw is applied. This technique is usually used when a considerably large fragment is involved. Closure is routine. The leg is placed in a modified Robert Jones splint for ten days. Following this, the dog is allowed only restricted activity for three weeks (Fig. 3.79).

Proximal Epiphysis

While not common, fractures of the proximal epiphysis are disabling and require early repair. The proximal metaphysis is usually located craniomedially, with the epiphysis attached to the stifle joint. The tibial collateral (medial) ligament is often torn. Reduction is usually difficult, especially if there are blood clots or the surgery has been delayed. The proximal epiphysis also splits relatively easily, which limits the amount of force that can be applied in reducing the fracture. Once reduced, several methods of repair

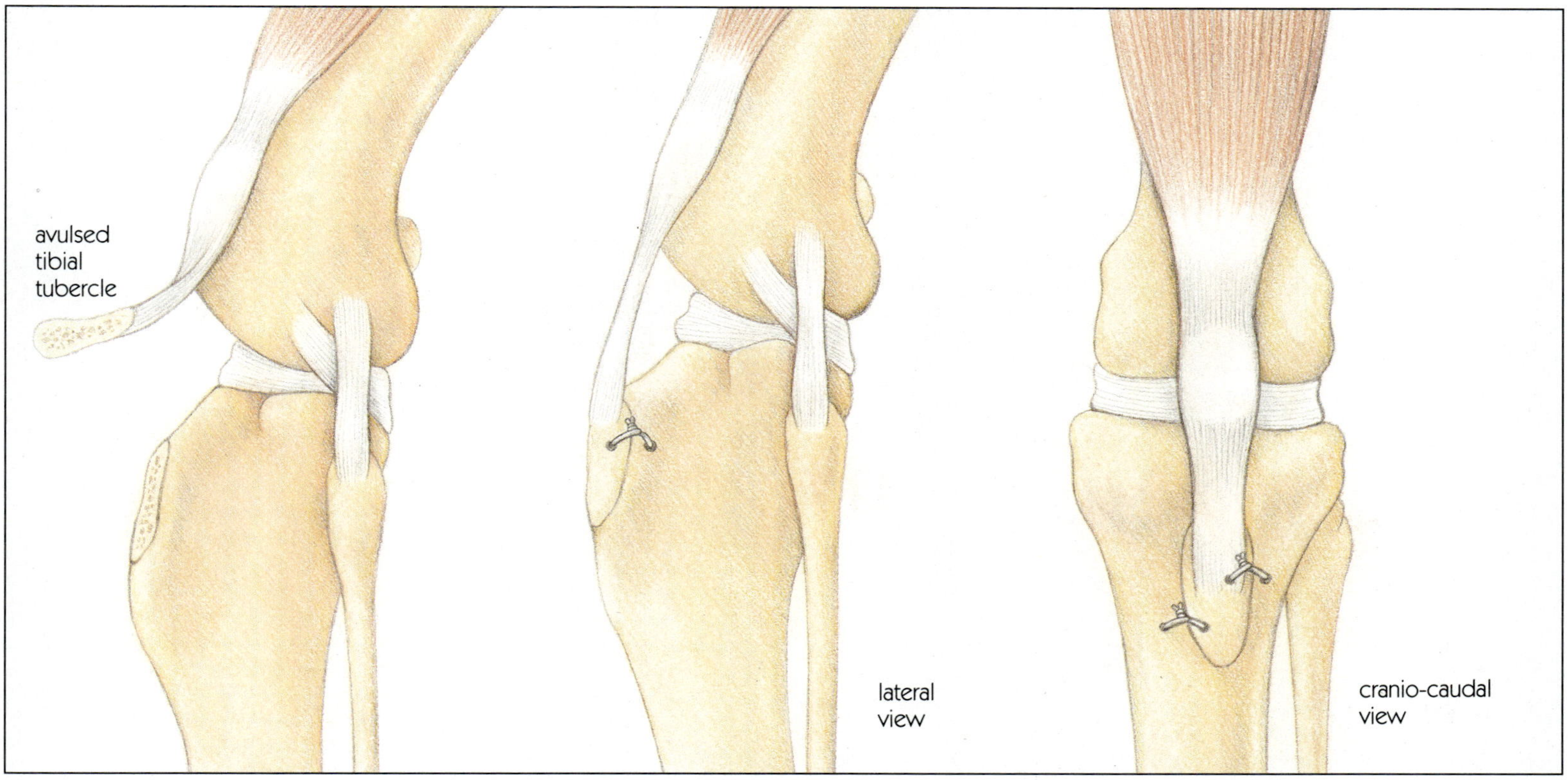

FIG. 3.76 An avulsed tibial tubercle is held in place with two orthopedic wire sutures.

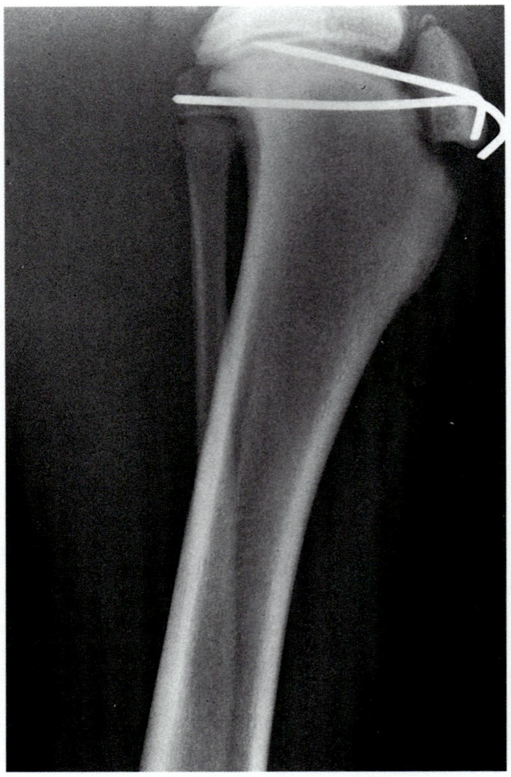

FIG. 3.77 An avulsed tibial tubercle held with two K-wires.

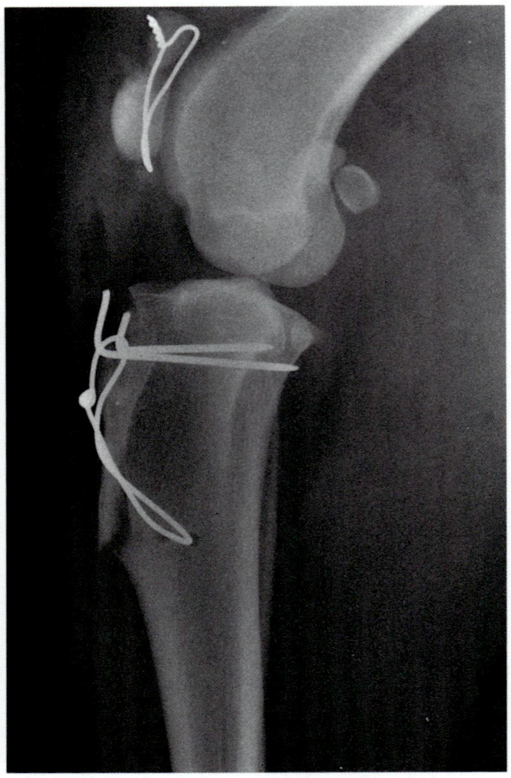

FIG. 3.78 An avulsed tibial tubercle held with K-wires and a figure-8 tension band wire.

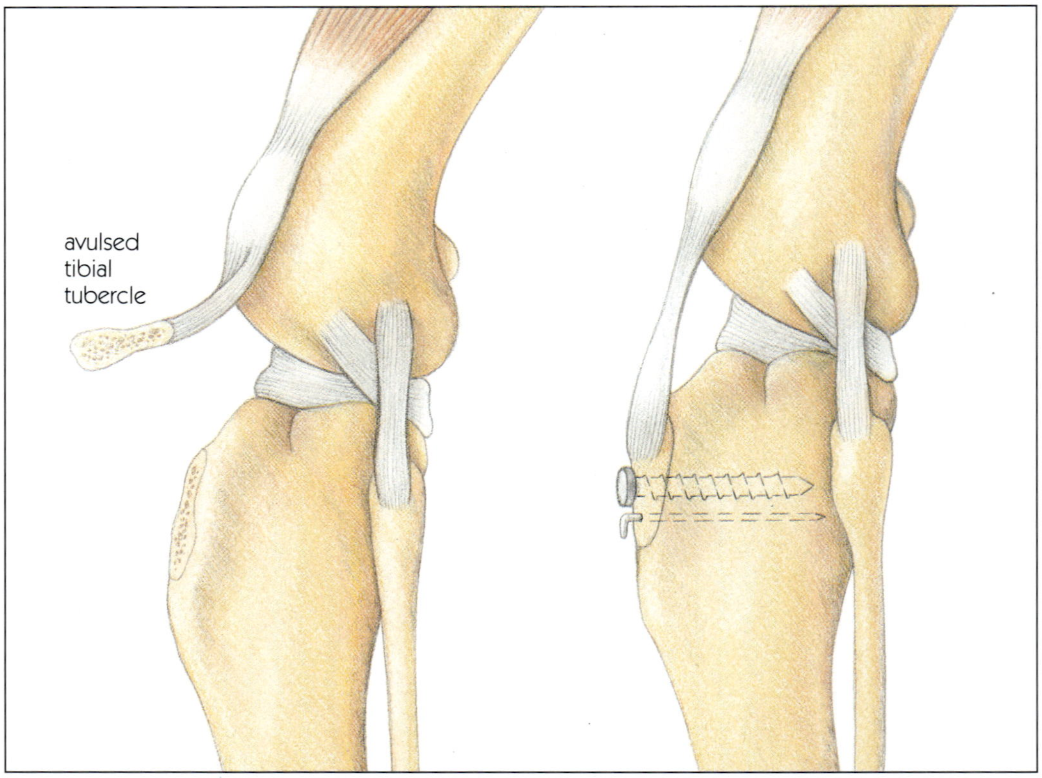

FIG. 3.79 The use of a K-wire and a bone screw in an avulsed tibial tubercle.

are available. Closed reduction is one possibility, but it may damage the epiphyseal fragment. Satisfactory control of the fracture by casts or splints is difficult.

In small dogs and cats, two K-wires are used. An intramedullary pin is used in larger immature dogs. The growth plate is not compromised with a single smooth pin. Where there is fragmentation and loss of supporting bone from the metaphyseal fragment, a small bone plate with a cancellous bone graft is used.

SURGICAL TECHNIQUE

A craniocaudal longitudinal incision is made in the medial or lateral surface of the proximal tibia. Medially, the bone and fracture site are found under the fascia. Laterally, the origin of the cranial tibial muscle is incised and the muscle is elevated from the underlying bone to expose the fracture.

The epiphysis is lifted carefully into position after the fracture site is cleared of blood clots and scar tissue. The reduction must be complete. In small breeds, a K-wire is inserted medially and laterally from the outer edges of the epiphysis through the fracture site, and seated into the diaphysis (Fig. 3.80). The ends are bent at right angles, cut off, and set to the bone surface. These pins remain permanently in place unless they become loose, in which case they should be removed. In larger breeds, an intramedullary pin is inserted from just medial to the patellar ligament through the epiphysis and deeply into the medullary canal of the distal fragment. The presence of a single smooth pin does not interfere with the epiphyseal

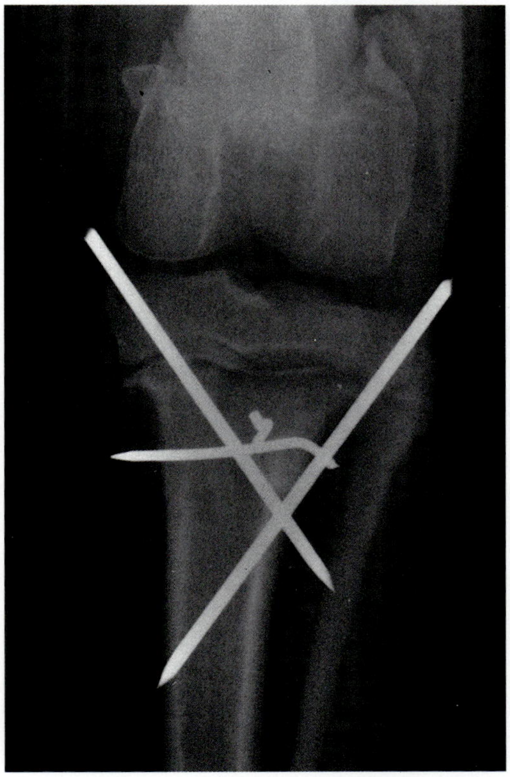

FIG. 3.80 This fractured proximal tibial epiphysis was treated with two crossed pins.

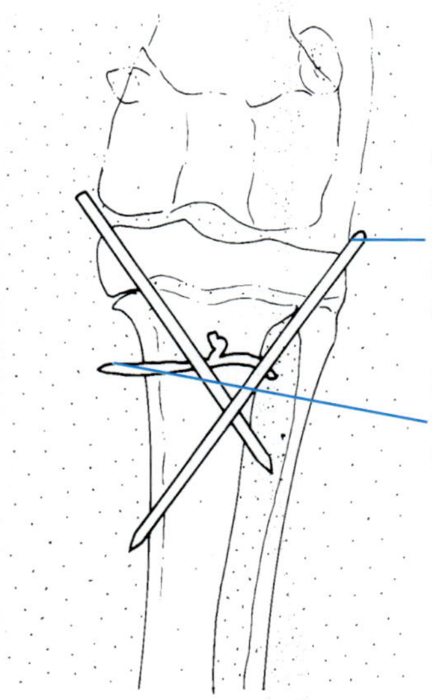

growth plate. The pin is withdrawn 1 cm, cut off, and seated with a pin setter (Fig. 3.81). The pin is removed after healing takes place.

A lag screw will compress the fracture site and is more liable to cause premature fusion and growth deformity, especially in the less mature animal.

When the proximal end of the metaphyseal fragment is comminuted, the epiphysis will lack support, usually on the lateral side. A T- or L-shaped small bone plate is applied, taking care not to injure the tendon of origin of the long digital extensor muscle. The comminuted area is packed with the fragments and a cancellous bone graft. The plate is used as a buttress to support the epiphysis until healing takes place (Fig. 3.82). It is usually left in place.

The leg is placed in a modified Robert Jones splint for about two weeks. Restricted activity is enforced for another two weeks.

Proximal Tibia

Fractures of the proximal tibia are frequent but not as common as those of the midshaft. They are often transverse or short oblique. A medial approach is taken. An intramedullary pin is often satisfac-

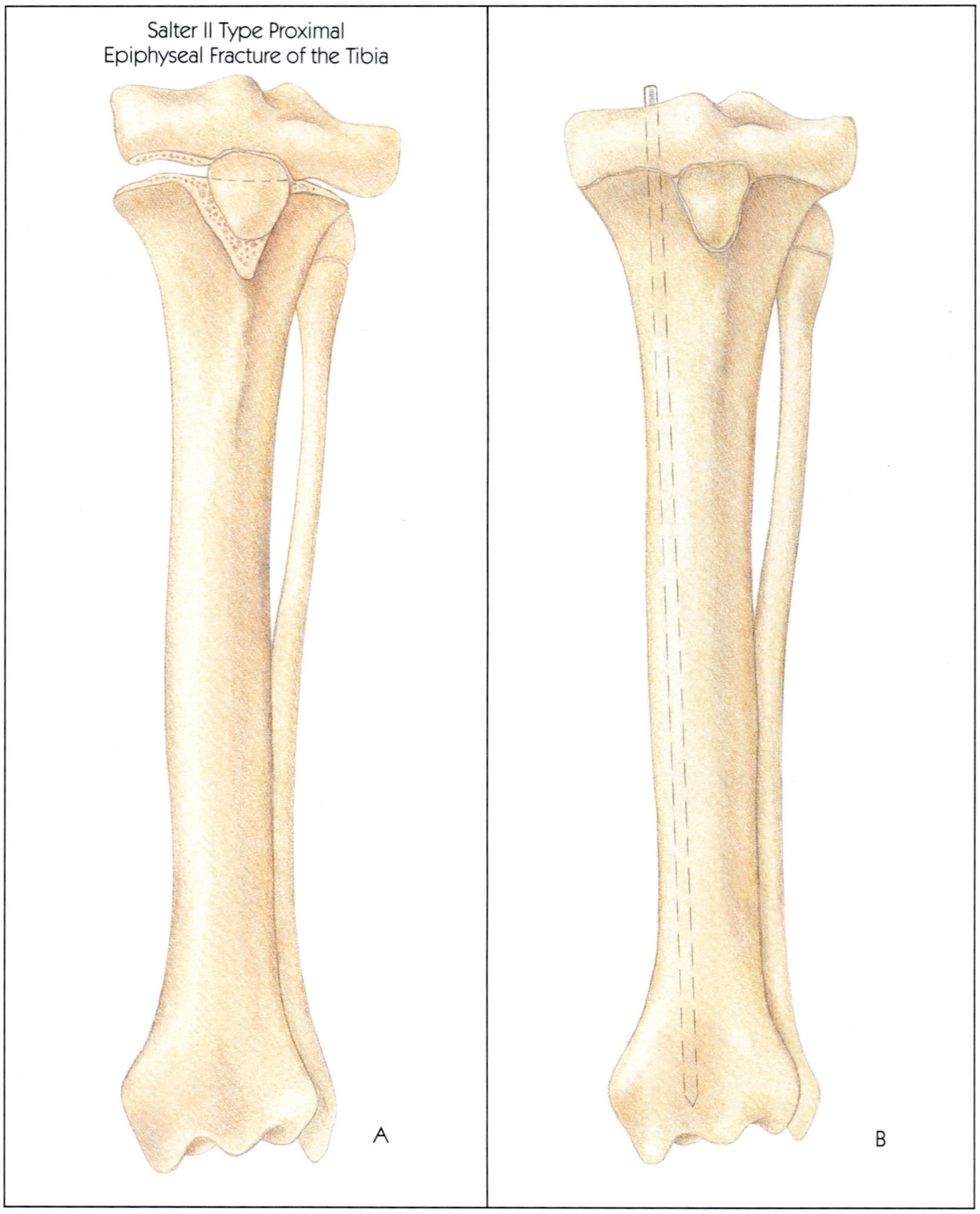

FIG. 3.81 (A) A Salter II type proximal epiphyseal fracture of the tibia. (B) Fixation of a proximal epiphyseal fracture of the tibia with an IM pin.

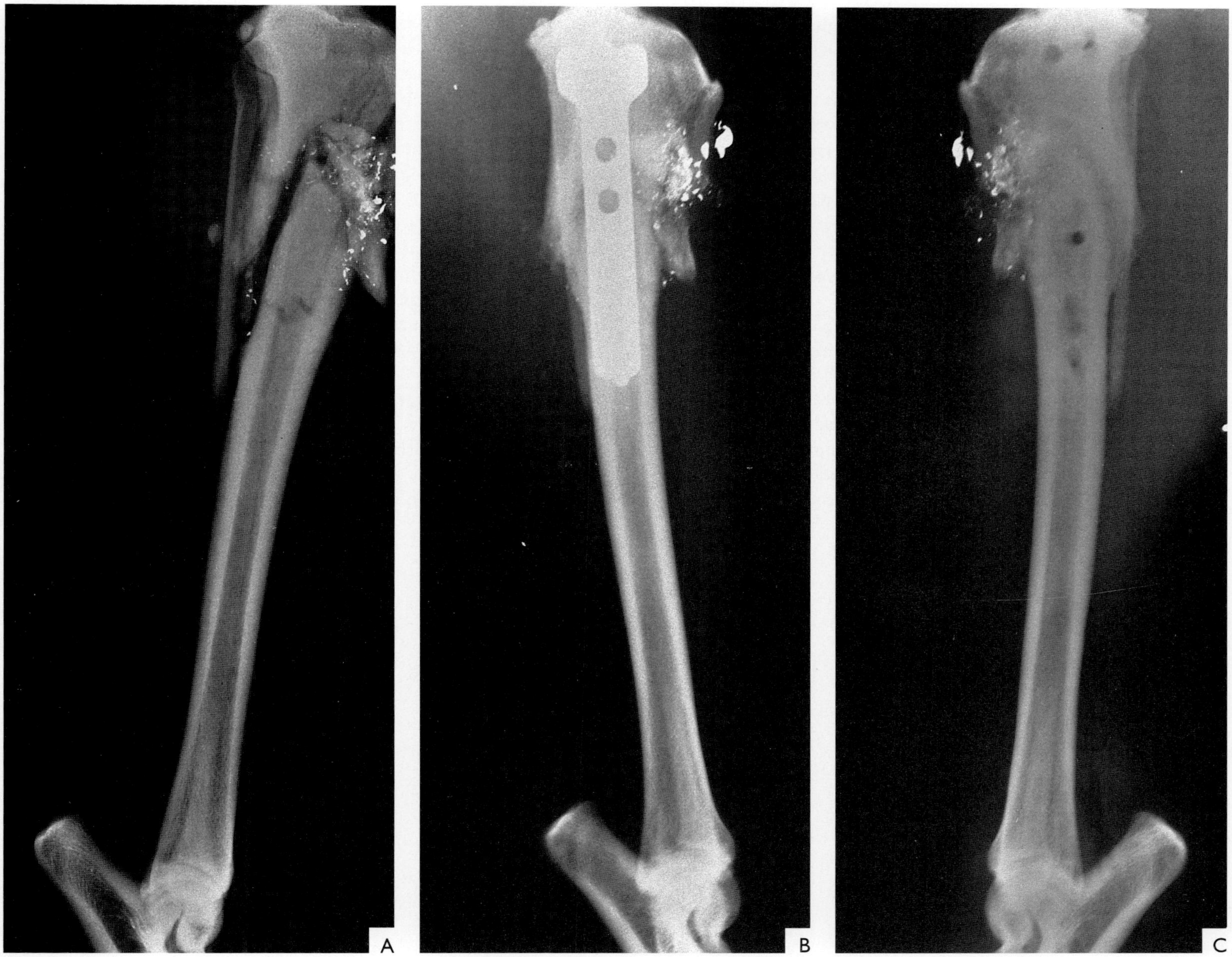

FIG. 3.82 (A) Gunshot fracture of the proximal tibia. (B) Radiograph of same patient, treated with a T-plate used as a buttress. (C) Healed fracture after plate removal.

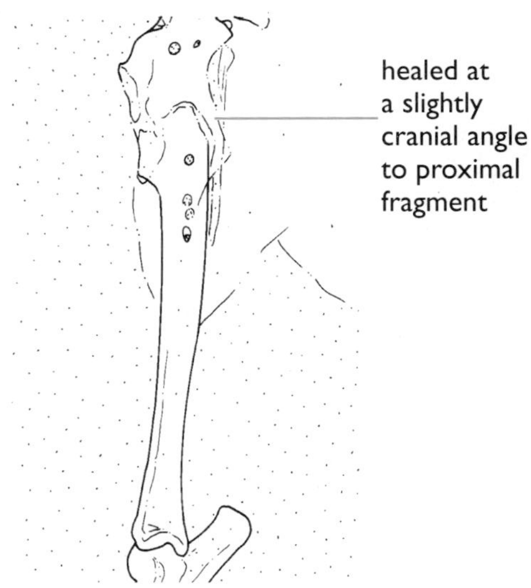

tory since the fractured ends tend to interdigitate and control rotation. External fixation is rarely needed. With a short oblique fracture, a lag screw is placed across the fracture but it cannot support the fracture by itself. A neutralization plate is applied. The fibula is usually also fractured. If only the shaft is involved, no treatment is required. However, if the fibular head is torn away, it must be replaced, since it is the location of the insertion of the fibular collateral (lateral) ligament of the stifle. A bone screw is used in larger dogs and a K-wire in small dogs. The end of the wire is bent at a right angle and cut off. The pin is seated with a few taps of a bone mallet, which will prevent the pin from moving.

SURGICAL TECHNIQUE

A longitudinal incision is made through the skin and subcutaneous tissues over the craniomedial aspect of the shaft of the tibia. Sharp and blunt dissection exposes the fracture site. Avoid incising damaged tissues. An intramedullary pin is selected that will fit into the medullary canal of the distal fragment. The pin is inserted from the proximal end of the tibia medial to the straight patellar ligament and about 1 cm caudal to the tibial crest. The stifle is held at a right angle. The pin is inserted until the tip is seen at the fracture site. A pin guide is often effective. The fracture is reduced. The pin is seated deeply into the distal fragment. It is then withdrawn about 1 cm, cut off and driven into place with a pin setter and mallet (Fig. 3.83). It should not be driven in so firmly that it distracts the fracture. Rotational movement is checked. A K-wire driven across the fracture site cranially helps control motion. The pin is removed after healing takes place. A plate may be used if there is room for two or more screws in the proximal fragment. The plate will require only a small amount of contouring. Dynamic compression is done if the fracture is not comminuted and is transverse or short oblique (Fig. 3.84). In longer oblique fractures, a lag screw across the fracture and a neutralization plate are applied. Closure is done by suturing fascia, subcutaneous tissue, and skin in the usual manner (Fig. 3.85).

Midshaft of the Tibia

Fractures of the midshaft of the tibia are very common. They vary from a greenstick to the most severely contaminated and infected fractures. The injury has often been made worse by the activity of

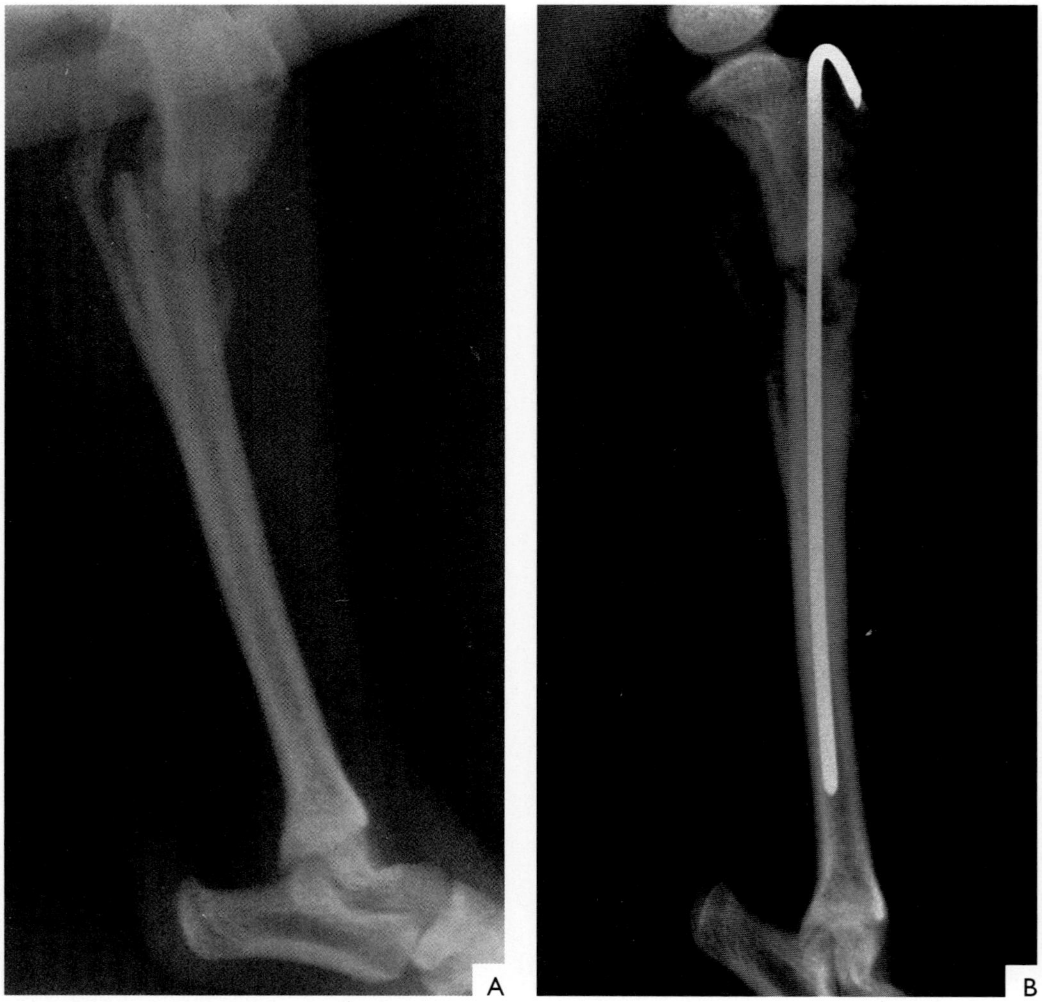

FIG. 3.83 (A) Proximal tibial fracture. (B) The same fracture, treated with an IM pin.

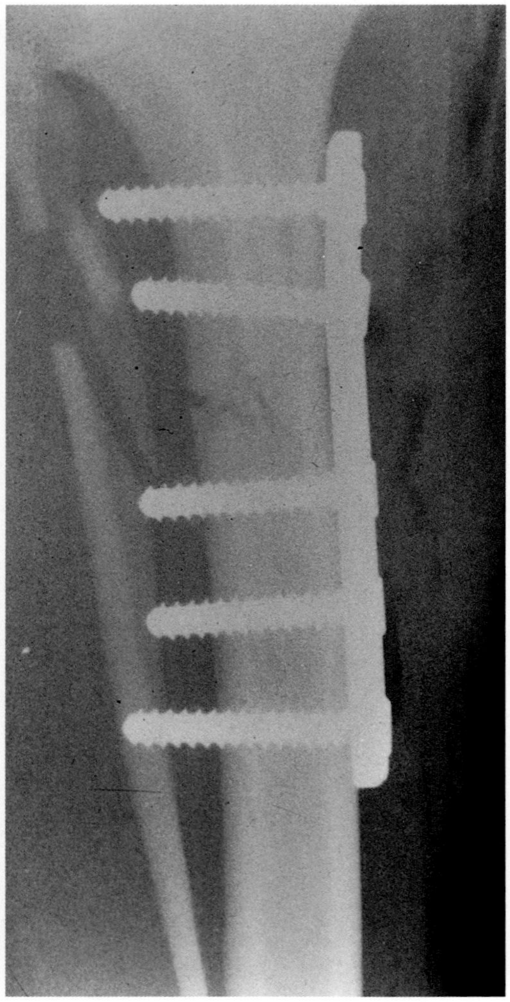

FIG. 3.84 A proximal tibial fracture treated with a compression bone plate.

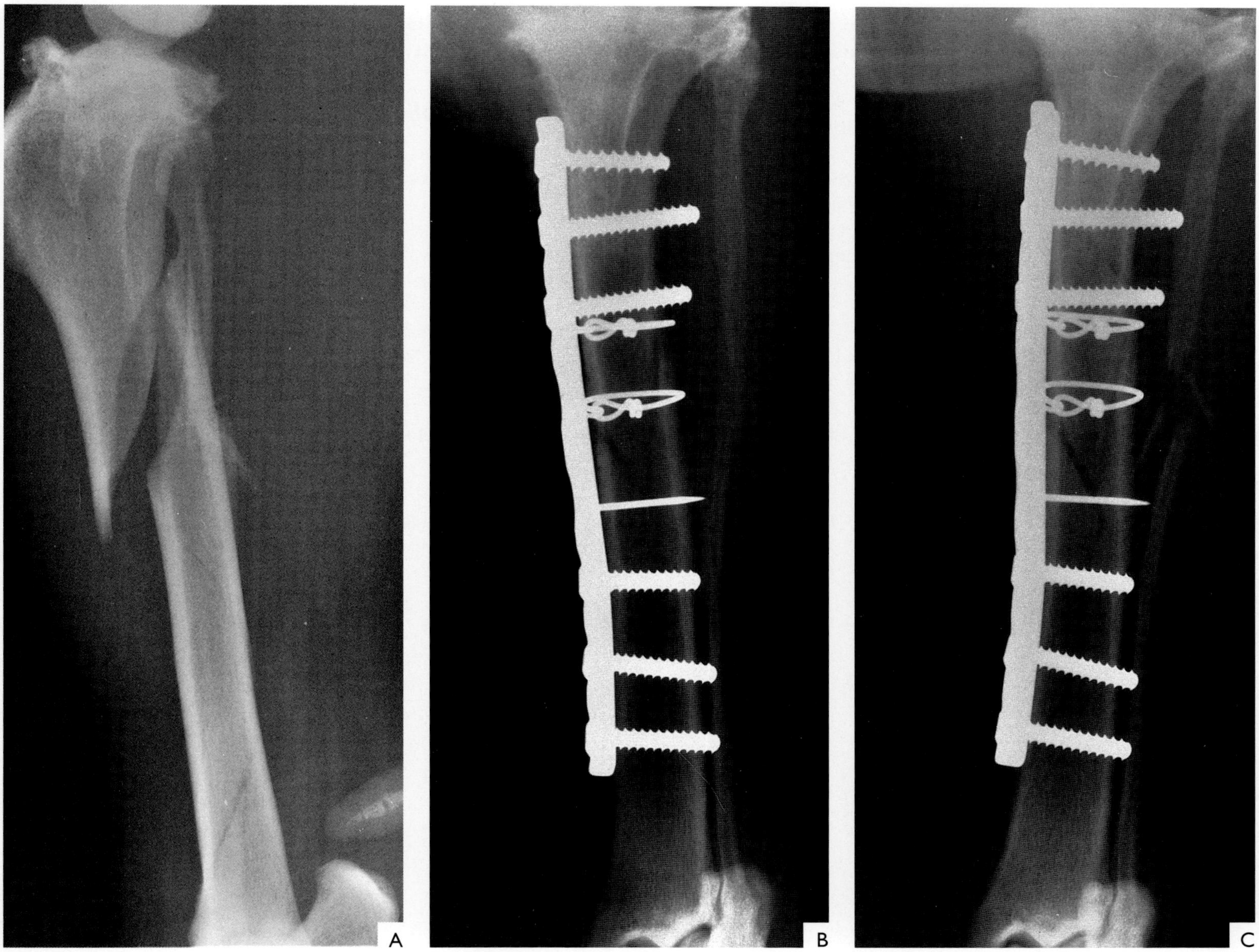

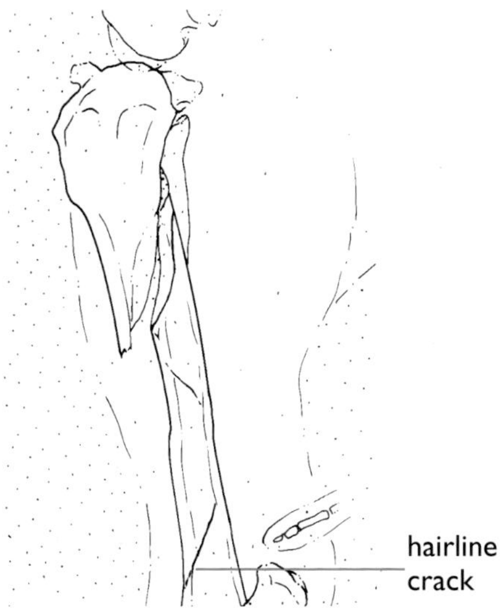

FIG. 3.85 (A) Proximal oblique fracture of a tibia. Note the hairline crack in the distal portion. (B) Same patient, treated with a bone plate. It does not protect the crack in the distal tibia. (C) The completely healed fracture. Note use of cerclage wires and K-wire.

the animal as the lower fragment dangles and exacerbates the soft-tissue injuries. Fragment ends may penetrate the skin and be exposed to every form of contamination. Thorough emergency debridement is essential. The surrounding tissues may be badly damaged. Immobilization is essential for bringing the infection under control and allowing healing to ensue.

Several modes of fixation are available: the intramedullary pin alone or with the use of external fixation, the modified Rush pin technique, external fixation in several configurations, and bone plating. The latter is especially useful in comminuted fractures in conjunction with interfragmentary compression.

SURGICAL TECHNIQUE

The tibial shaft is approached from the medial aspect. A longitudinal craniomedial incision sufficient to expose the fracture is made parallel to the tibial crest, from proximal to distal. Plates require extensive exposure. The cranial branches of the medial saphenous artery and vein and the superficial peroneal nerve cross the middle of the tibial shaft. They are preserved as much as possible.

Short Oblique or Transverse Fracture

With a short oblique or transverse fracture with minimum soft-tissue damage, an intramedullary pin is often satisfactory.

SURGICAL TECHNIQUE

A pin is selected that will just fit into the medullary canal of the distal fragment. The pin is introduced from the proximal end of the tibia, medial to the straight patellar ligament, about 1 cm from the tibial crest. The pin is driven in until the tip emerges from the distal end of the proximal fragment. The stifle is held at a right angle. The fracture is reduced by angulation and the pin is driven into the distal fragment. It is withdrawn 1 cm, cut off, and again impacted with a pin setter and mallet. Due to the bowing of the tibia, seating

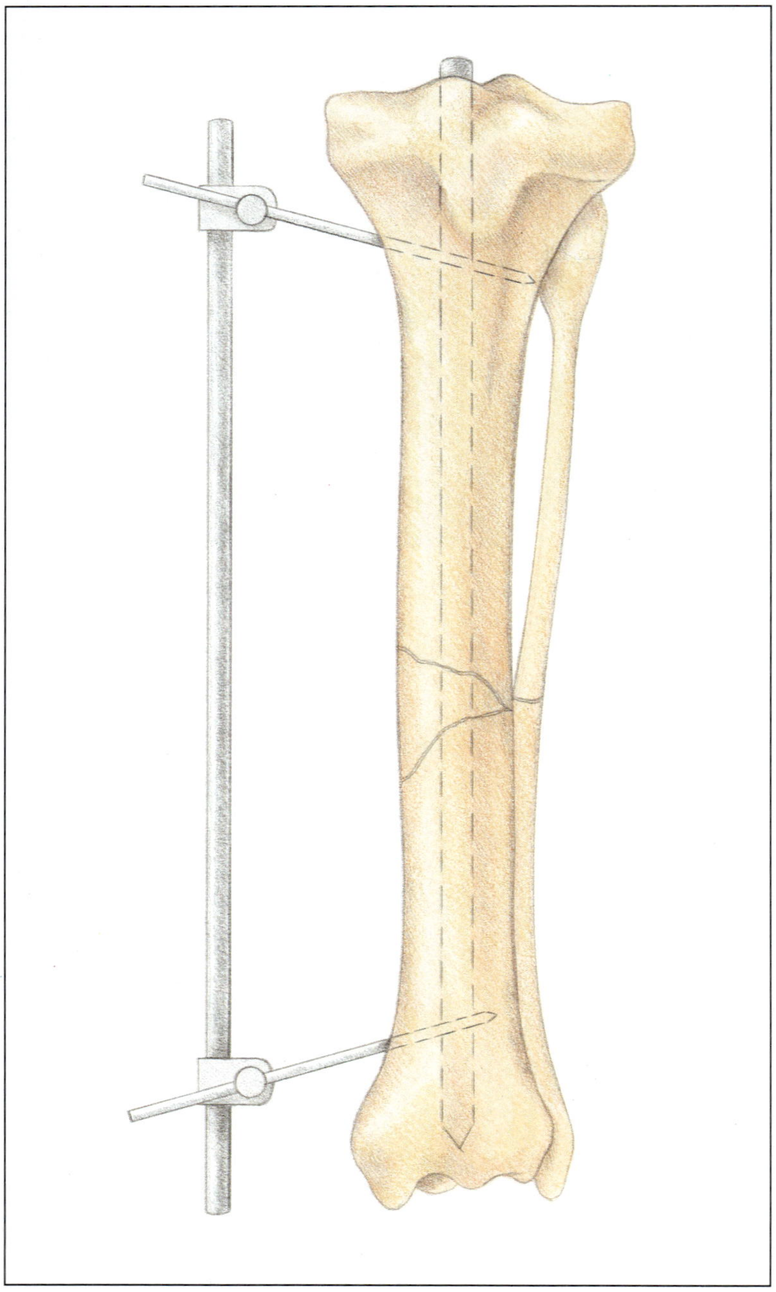

FIG. 3.86 Intramedullary pin in tibia, with additional support from an external fixator.

the pin in the distal fragment will align the fragments with a slight appositional gap, but this will not interfere with healing. Closure is done by suturing the fascia, subcutaneous tissues, and skin in the usual manner. A Robert Jones splint is applied and kept on for two weeks. Restricted activity is enforced for two more weeks. The pin is removed when healing is apparent. The very short distorted tibias in the chondrodystrophoid breeds are not easily pinned. An external fixator is used.

Intramedullary Pin and External Fixator If the tibial fracture is transverse or long oblique and would be unstable with an intramedullary pin as the sole means of fixation, an external fixator is applied to provide additional support. A single connecting bar is used with a pin in the most proximal and distal ends of the bone. It is applied on the medial side of the bone (Fig. 3.86). Extra support for larger dogs is provided by a single connecting bar with two pins in each fragment. An additional supporting connecting bar is applied above the first.

Modified Rush Pin Technique The fracture is exposed, reduced, and held with bone forceps. The lateral and medial surfaces of the tibial crest area are exposed. A drill hole is made on each side, equidistant from the proximal surface of the tibia. Flexible pins are introduced and driven down the medullary canal to seat distally. The bowing spring action of the pins pressing against the inner walls of the bone holds them firmly. The ends are bent at a right angle, cut off, and pressed against the bone surface. The pins are removed after the fracture heals. The bent ends offer a grip for the extraction with a vise grip. There is some danger in splitting the bone when applying these pins (Fig. 3.87).

External Fixation Midshaft tibial fractures, especially those that require dressings and treatment for tissue loss and infection, are particularly suited to external fixation. Pins and plates are not well tolerated in the presence of infection. The device is applied to the medial side of the limb. Several configurations may be used depending upon the severity of the fracture as well as the size and activity of the patient.

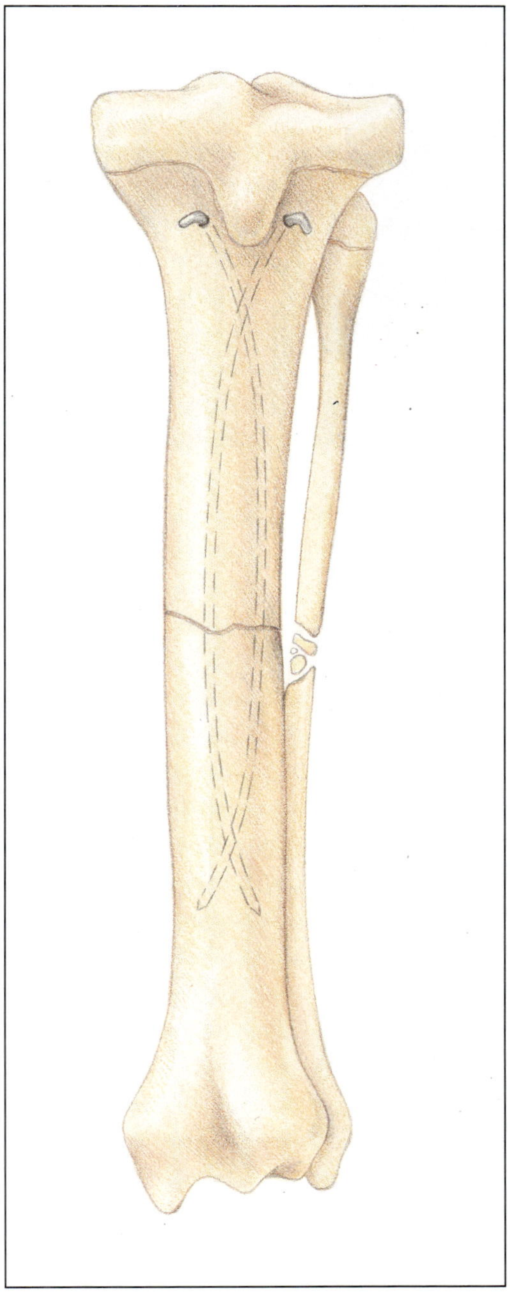

FIG. 3.87 Midshaft tibial fracture treated with a modified Rush pin technique.

A single connecting bar with two pins in the upper fragment and two in the lower is applied. These pins are inserted to penetrate both cortices but not to transfix the leg. They are inserted at an angle, with the points of each pair of pins angled towards each other. Three or even four pins may be used in each fragment or to stabilize a loose fragment. Where there is no contamination, interfragmentary compression can be done with lag screws or K-wires and cerclage wires, followed by an application of the external fixation splint. These devices are less expensive than bone plates. Where infection and tissue damage are present, the pins are inserted away from the affected area and reduction is obtained as much as possible without entering the contaminated area. Another connecting bar is applied above the first for extra strength.

Transfixing pins are used with medial and lateral connecting bars, plus additional pins either transfixing the limb or inserted into both cortices of the bone only (Fig. 3.88, 3.89).

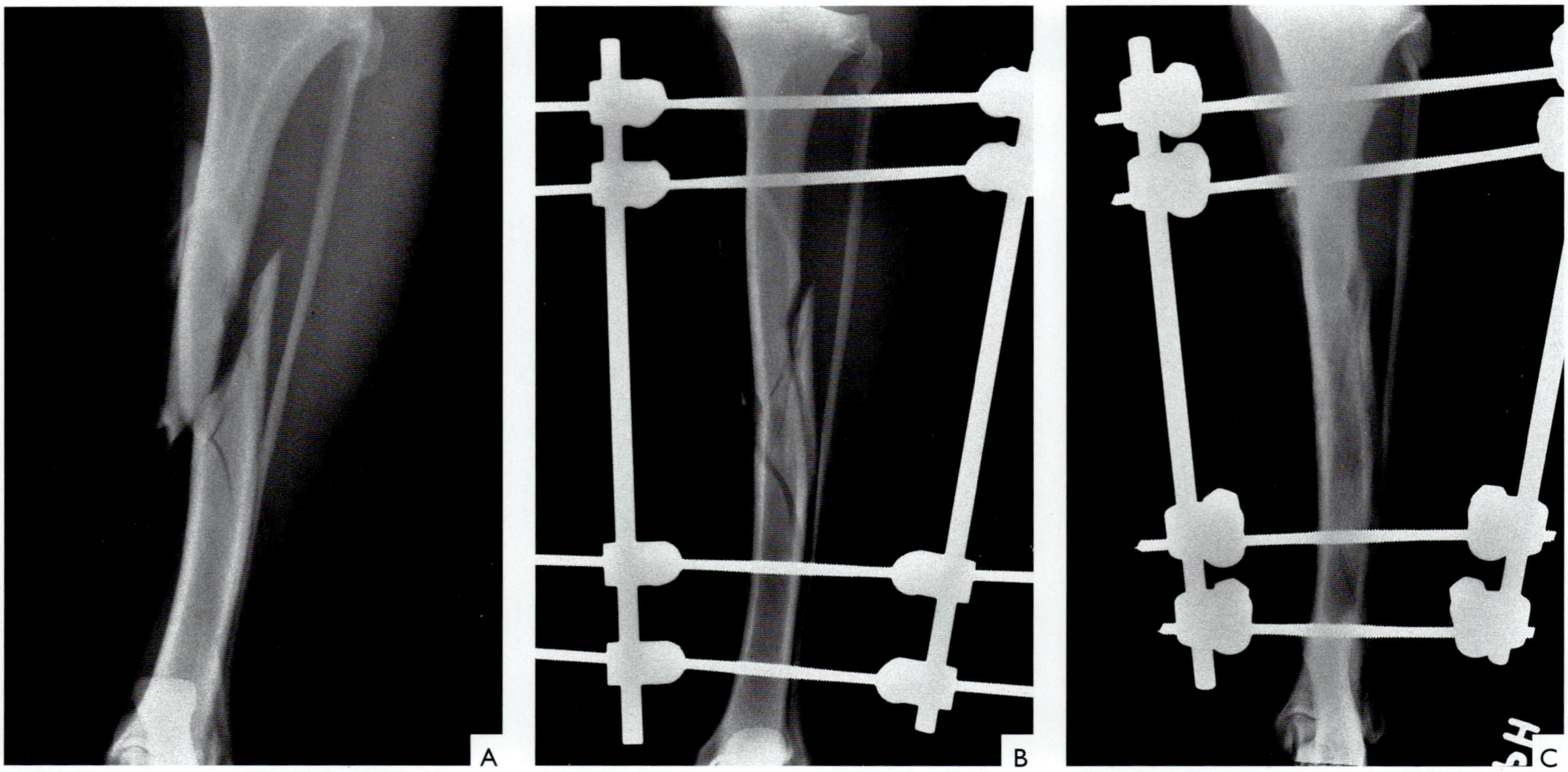

FIG. 3.88 (A) Radiograph of a midshaft tibial fracture. The slender fibula has remained intact. (B) Treatment consisted of a full K/E external fixator with two pins in the proximal and two pins in the distal fragments. The pins pass completely through the leg. (C) The fracture healed nicely in 2½ months. Note the periosteal stimulation around the top pins on the medial side.

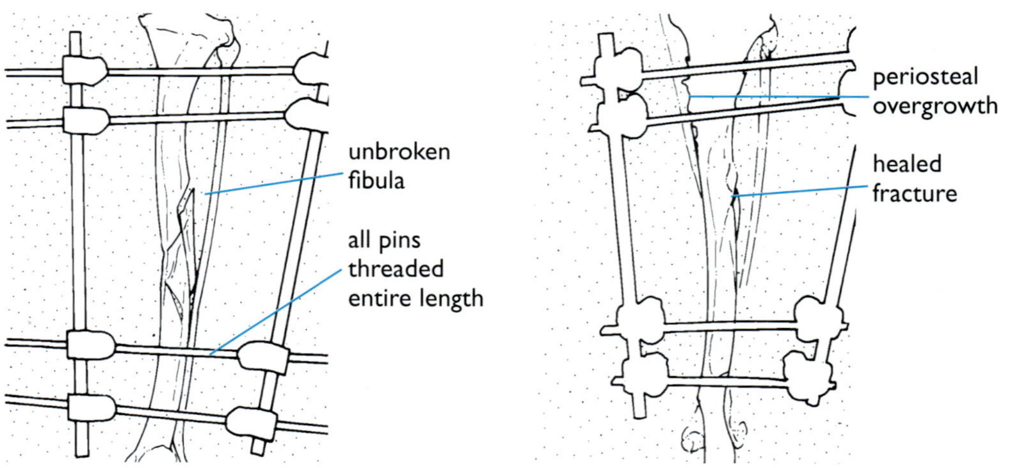

When the midshaft fracture is comminuted and unstable, pins are inserted completely through the limb proximally and distally. Connecting bars are attached medially and laterally. Additional pins may transfix or extend only through the bone. These latter are inserted at an angle, usually to control fragments. Transfixing pins are placed at right angles to the bone. Compression of the fracture site can be obtained by forcing the proximal and distal bars towards each other and securing the clamps while they are under tension.

Additional strength is obtained by adding another connecting bar, which extends longitudinally and is cranial to the limb. Short connecting bars are attached to the other connecting bars and pins are inserted from it into the bone to control the fragments. Modifications are made according to the needs of the fracture and the ingenuity of the surgeon (Fig. 3.90).

An improvement on the pins commonly used in transfixing the bone is to have them threaded entirely (Fig. 3.91) or in a portion of the center (center-face pins) (Fig. 3.92). The insertion holes are drilled. There are self-tapping threads on the central portion. The pins are threaded into the bone so that both cortices are involved. This prevents the bone from the sliding that can occur

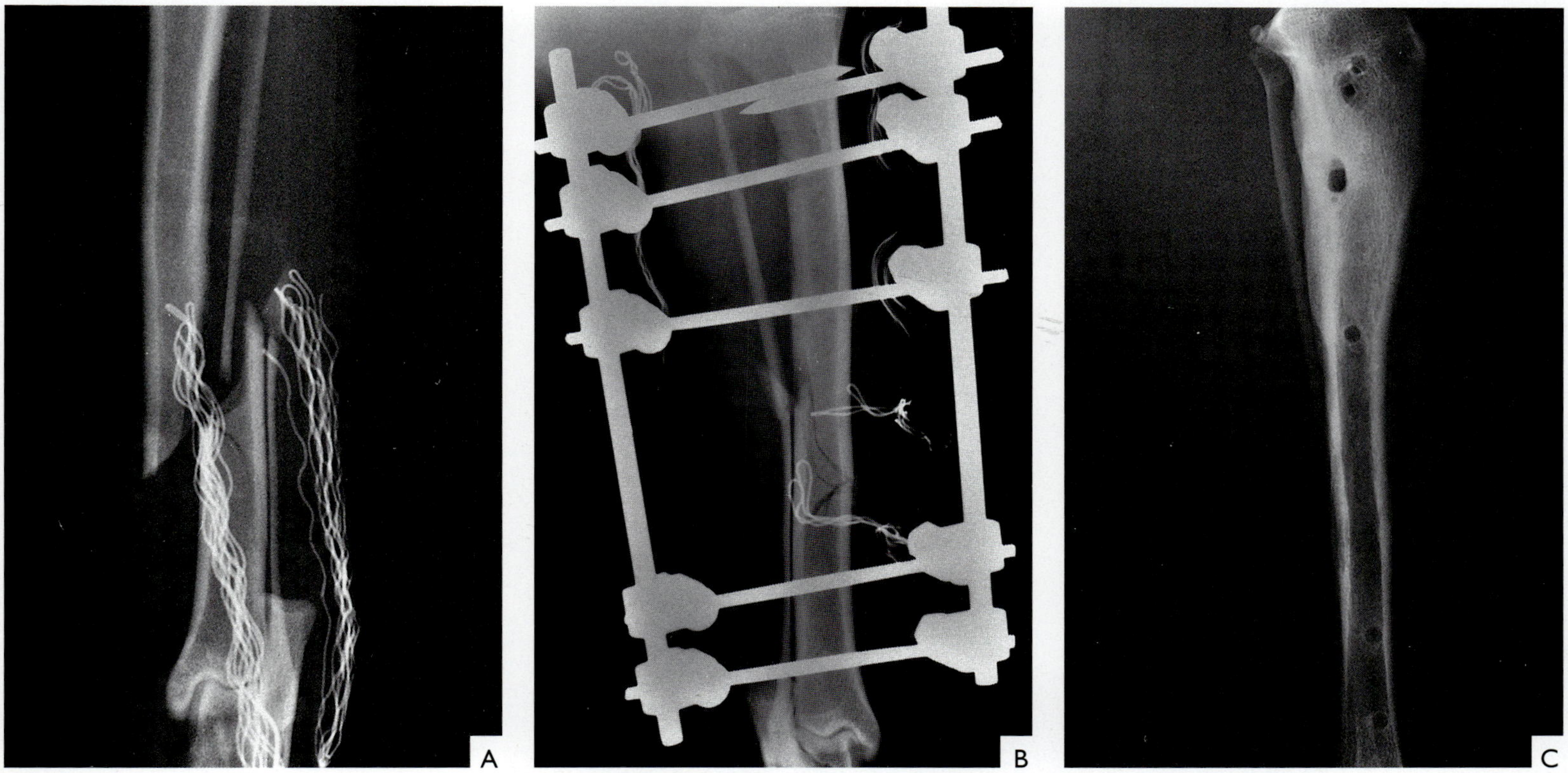

FIG. 3.89 (A) Short oblique midshaft tibial fracture. Radiopaque threads are from a sterile sponge. (B) Above treated with a full K/E external fixator. The two proximal pins do not penetrate the leg completely. (C) Completely healed fracture. The dark holes are where the pins were seated. Some bone erosion around the pins is seen.

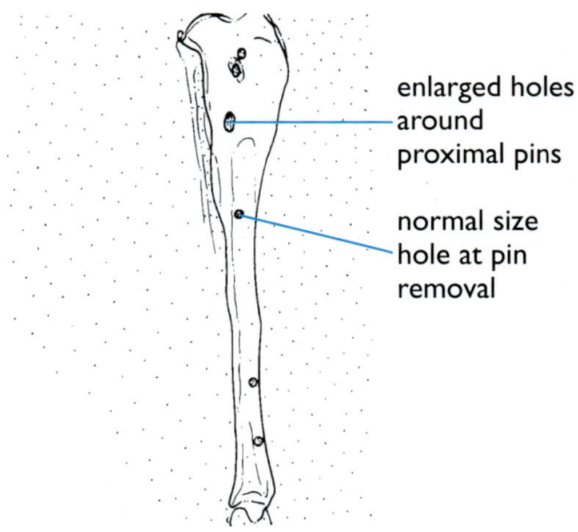

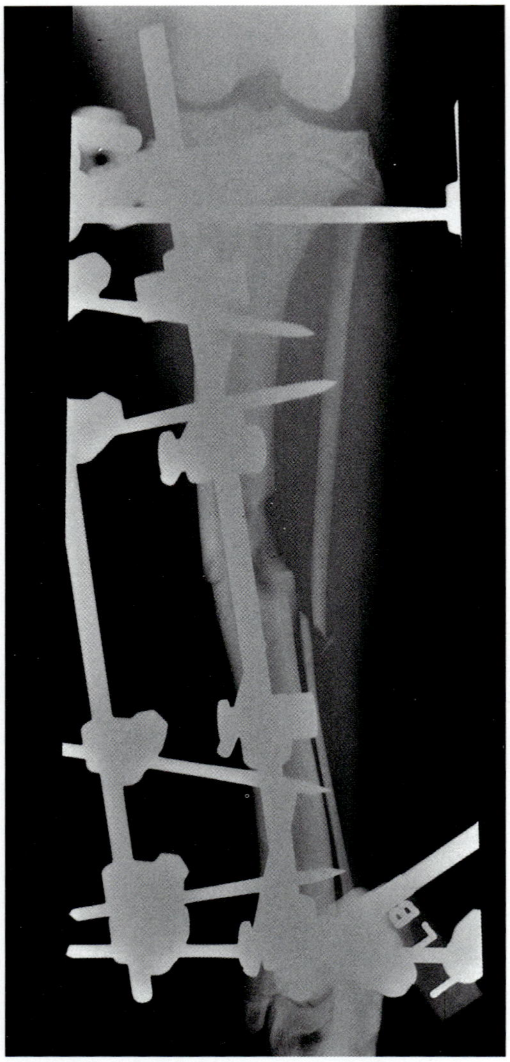

FIG. 3.90 A tibial fracture treated with a full K/E fixator, plus a cranial bar for additional rigidity. This configuration is called a tent.

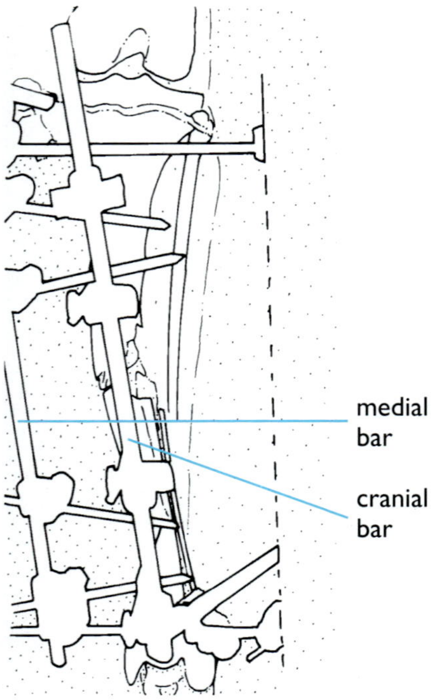

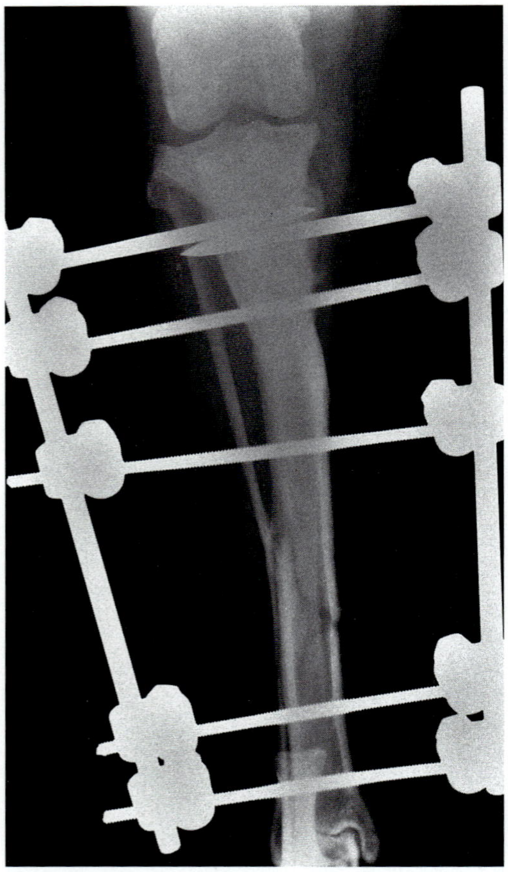

FIG. 3.91 A midshaft tibial fracture that was treated with a full K/E fixator and additional proximal pins. The full transfixion pins are fully threaded, improving their holding power by preventing slipping.

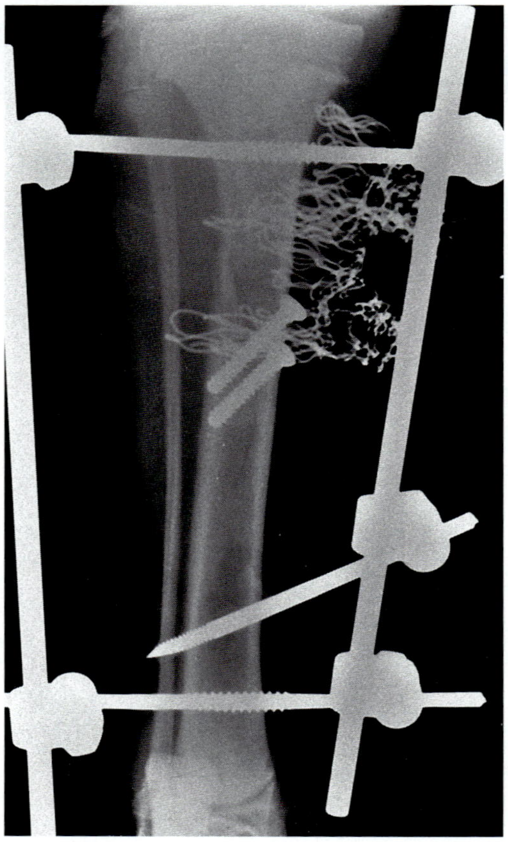

FIG. 3.92 A tibial fracture treated with a full K/E fixator, using pins with central threading (centerface pins). The radiopaque threads from a sterile sponge are visible.

with a smooth pin. The use of methylmethacrylate as a rigid substitute for the connecting bars establishes excellent rigidity at lower cost. The APEF system provides a kit containing all of the necessary equipment to apply external fixation. A temporary alignment frame is used to reduce and maintain the fracture. The incision is closed. Special plastic acrylic column tubes are filled with methylmethacrylate. Once the cement has hardened, the pins are cut off close to the outer faces of the columns. The alignment frame components are saved for the next application.

All of the pins transfix the limb. The flexibility of the plastic acrylic columns allows leeway in the direction of the pins.

The device is extremely strong and rigid. Removal is accomplished by cutting the pins, disposing of the bars, and withdrawing them. The cut pin ends are surgically prepared before they are withdrawn through the bone. A modified Robert Jones splint is applied for a week.

Bone Plates Bone plates offer an excellent means of treating midshaft tibial fractures. There must be sufficient tissue to cover the plate completely. They are especially useful in medium to large dogs with comminuted fractures. They permit improved healing and quick return of function.

The tibia is approached by an incision on the medial side extending longitudinally from medial to the tibial crest, curving cranially along the tibial crest, then curving caudally and distally toward the medial malleolus. Centrally, the cranial branch of the medial saphenous artery and vein in addition to the superficial peroneal nerve are exposed and preserved. The curved incision keeps the closure from being directly over the bone plate.

When the length of the fracture is less than twice the diameter of the bone, a dynamic compression plate is used. It should be long enough to allow several screws to be placed proximal and distal to the fracture. The fracture is reduced by angulation and held in reduction by bone forceps.

The plate is contoured to fit the bone surface. The plate is bent slightly, approximately one 1 mm, where it is to be located over the fracture (overbending). The plate is slipped under the nerve artery and vein and clamped to the bone. The first screw is inserted neutrally in the static fragment, in the screw hole nearest the fracture and about 1 cm from it. The second screw is inserted eccentrically in the movable fragment with the greater surface, next to the plate. As the second screw is tightened, it slides down the inclined plane in the dynamic plate's special screw holes. This draws the bone tightly against the plate and the opposing portion of the fracture. The plate is adjusted to seat in the best position and alternating screws are neutrally placed. The end screws extend only through the near cortex to allow a bit of bone flexibility, lessening the chance of bone fracture at the end of the rigid plate. All of the screws are tightened. The area is flushed with saline and suctioned dry. Alternatively, the second screw is placed in the eccentric mode in the second hole from the fracture site, and is tightened to compress the fracture. Additional compression is gained by drilling a hole in the first hole from the fracture site that transects the fracture. The near cortex is overdrilled for a gliding hole. The far cortex is drilled and tapped. A screw is placed that lags the two fragments together (Figs. 3.93–3.95).

Closure is by resuturing any fascial attachments of muscles that might have been incised to obtain better exposure. Closure of the subcutaneous tissues and the skin is routine. A modified Robert Jones splint protects the limb from stress for a week. Restricted activity is required for three weeks.

Long Oblique Midshaft Tibial Fractures

Long oblique fractures of the tibia are reduced, held with K-wires, and secured with cerclage wires or more securely with interfragmentary lag screws. These are inserted at various locations, central to the fragments they will be drawing together. They should not be in line.

The near cortex is drilled through a drill guide with a hole larger than the thread size of the screw. A guide is inserted in this hole to direct the drill for a hole that is to be tapped to receive the seated screw. The depth gauge determines the length of the screw prior to tapping. The near cortex hole is countersunk to allow the head of the screw to seat more deeply into the bone. The screw is inserted and tightened finger tight. The other lag screws are similarly inserted. When all are in place, the screws are tightened. A stable reduction is produced. In some cases, this may be all that is required.

Usually, it is wise to apply a bone plate as a neutralization plate (Figs. 3.96, 3.97). A plate long enough to provide at least three screw holes beyond the fracture site is selected and contoured to the bone. While the plate is held onto the bone with clamps, the screws are placed using a neutral drill guide. Screws are inserted at each end, alternating until all the screws are installed. None should enter the fracture.

A routine closure of the incision is done. The leg is placed in a Robert Jones splint for a week and restricted movement is enforced for three weeks.

Comminuted Fractures

Comminuted fractures are common. They are best treated, if possible, with interfragmentary compression and a bone plate. The fracture is reconstituted by securing one fragment to another with K-wires, cerclage wires or, preferably, with lag screws. A power drill is helpful when inserting K-wires into fragments because it is quite often difficult to do by hand. Once the fracture has been secured by K-wires, it is much easier to drill the holes and place the lag screws.

The near cortex of the fragment is drilled through a drill guide with a guide hole that is the diameter of the screw threads. The far cortex is drilled through an inserted drill guide with a hole the diameter of a screw shaft. The near cortex hole is countersunk. The hole is measured with a depth gauge.

The near cortex hole is countersunk to permit deeper seating of the screw head. A cortical screw 2 mm longer than the measured depth is selected. The far hole is tapped through the inserted drill guide. The screw is inserted and tightened. The holding K-wires are cut off close to the bone surface. They will remain permanently.

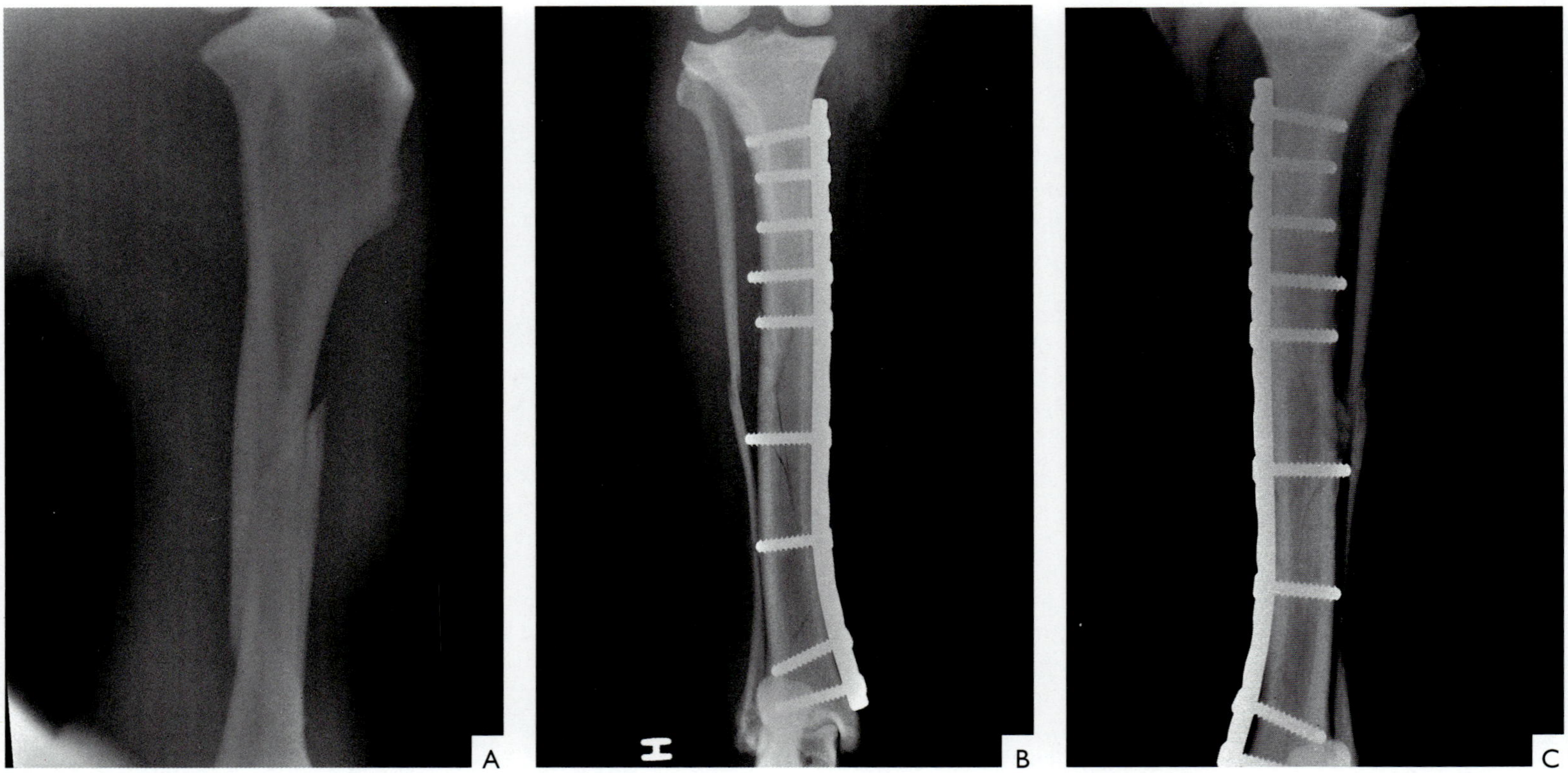

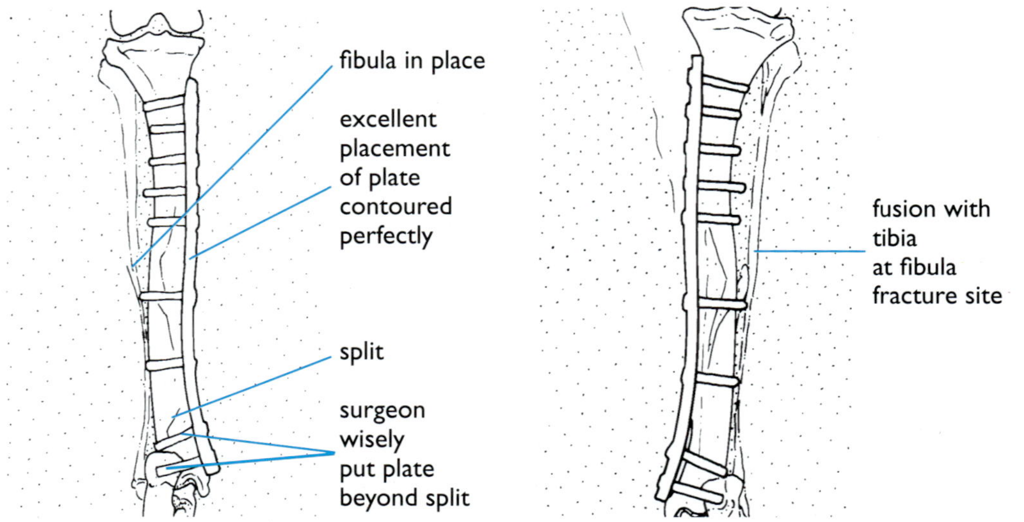

FIG. 3.93 (A) Short oblique midshaft tibial fracture. (B) After treatment with a neutralization plate. Note the excellent reduction. The plate extends properly beyond the distal hairline crack. (C) Completely healed fracture. The fusion of the fibula to the tibia is not unusual and is of no consequence.

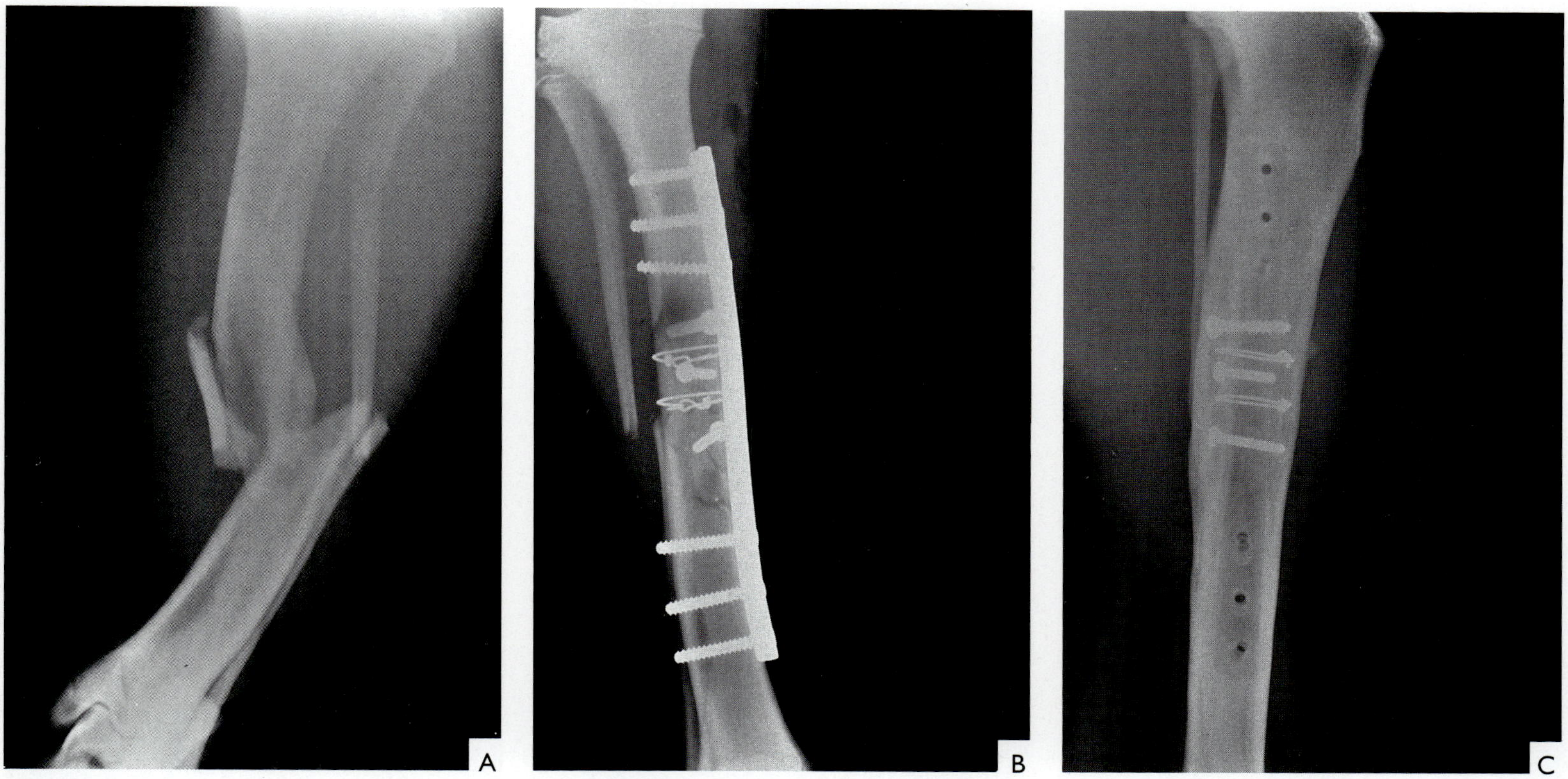

FIG. 3.94 (A) Comminuted short oblique tibial fracture. (B) Above treated with a neutralization plate. Note excellent use of interfragmentary screws and cerclage wires. (C) After plate removal, healing is complete with minimal callus. The bed in the bone where the plate was seated is visible on this radiograph.

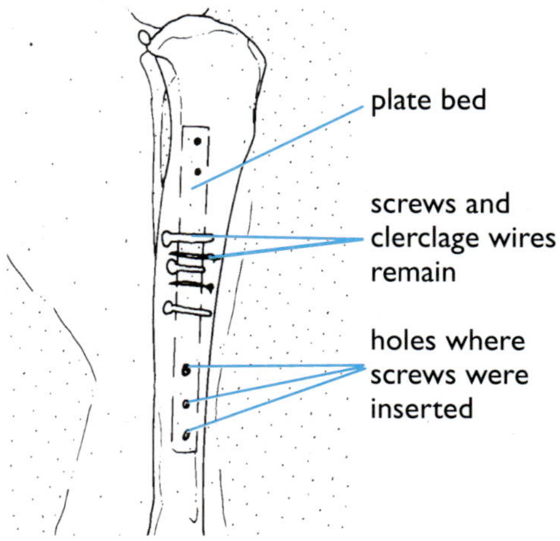

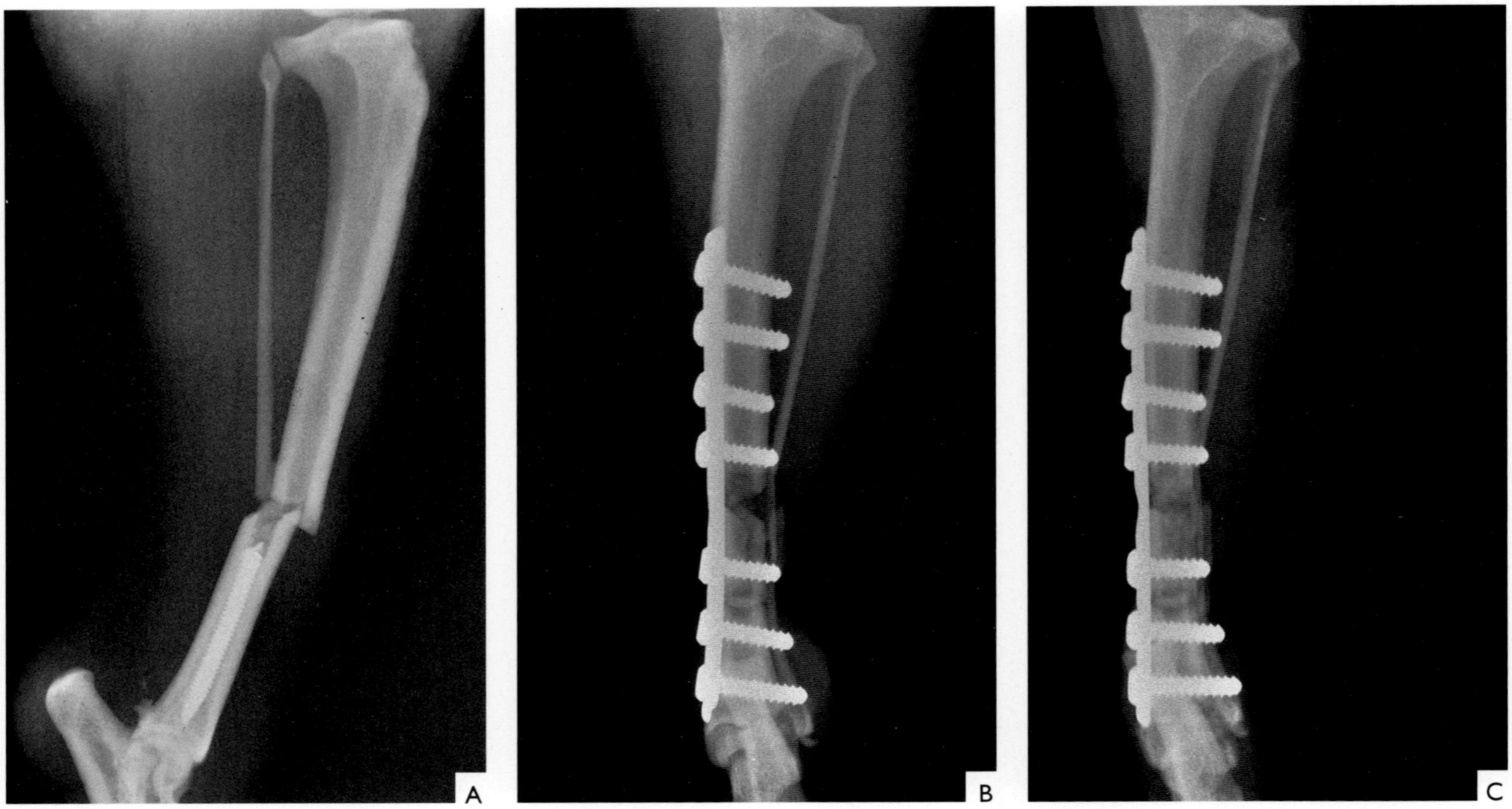

FIG 3.95 (A) A midshaft transverse fracture that was treated with an IM pin. The pin broke at the threaded portion, a common occurrence. (B) The pin fragment was removed and the fracture was plated. Healing has begun. (C) The fracture healed with a lateral tilt to the distal fragment.

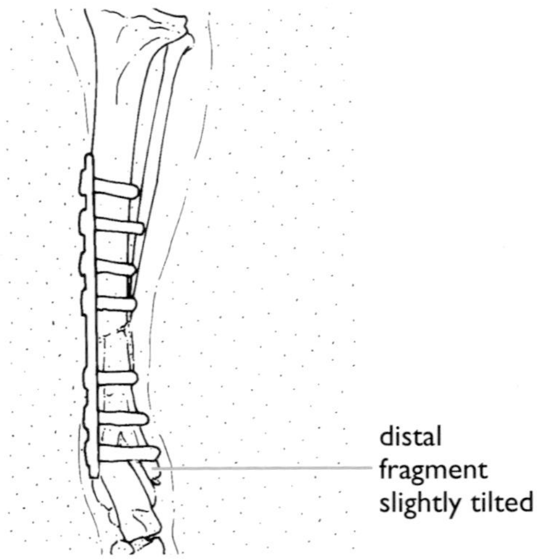

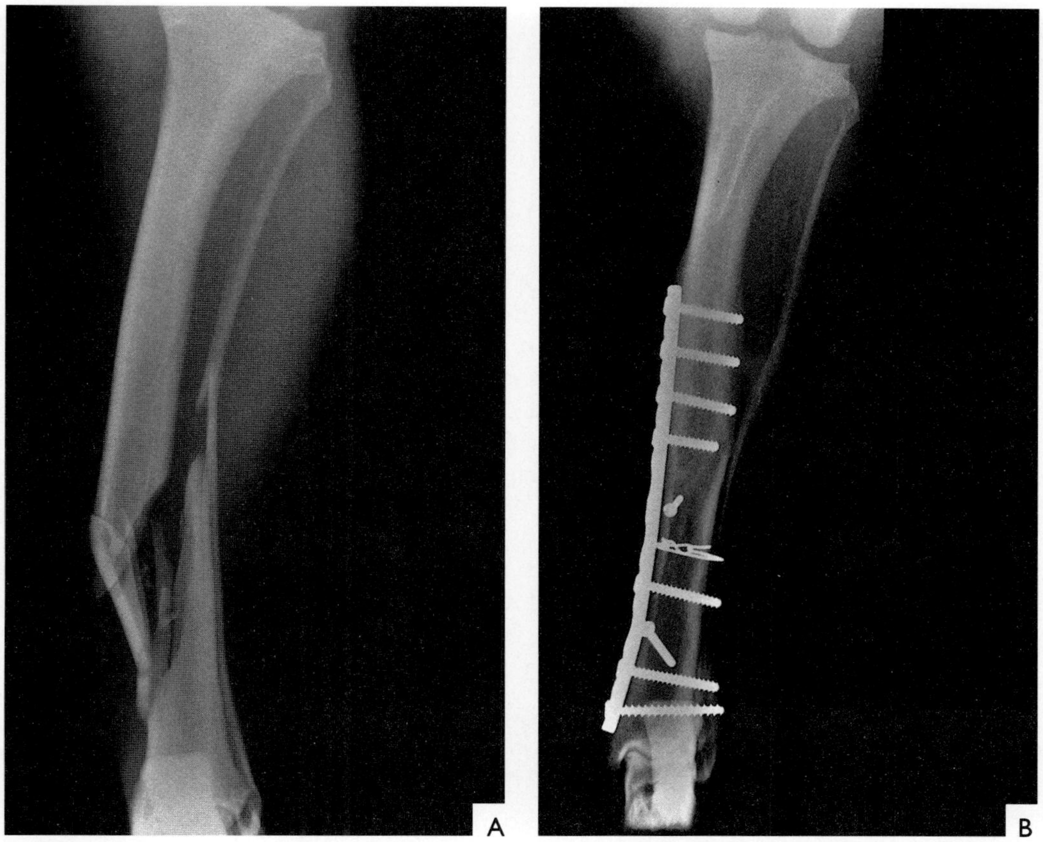

FIG. 3.96 (A) Oblique comminuted tibial fracture. (B) Healed fracture after treatment with a bone plate. Fusion of the fibula to tibia is common at fracture site.

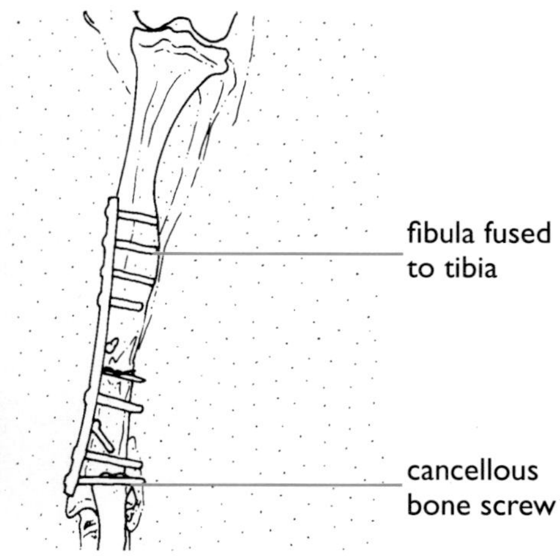

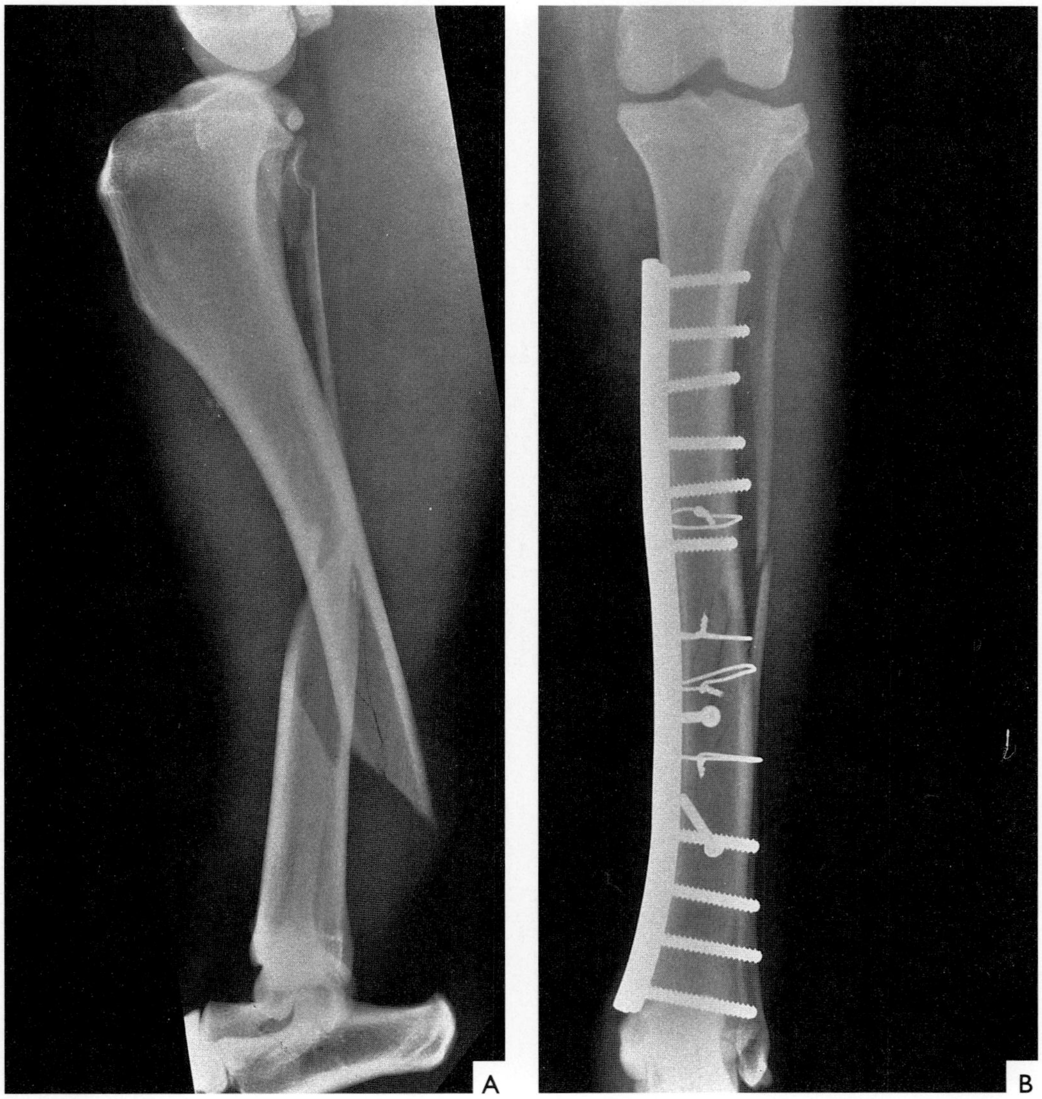

FIG. 3.97 (A) Long oblique midshaft tibial fracture. (B) Treatment with a bone plate.

Smaller fragments are held in place with inserted K-wires and a cerclage wire. Another cerclage wire is tightened around the bone using the slightly projecting K-wire ends to prevent slippage. Many cerclage wires may be used.

On occasion, a small fragment that would be displaced by the lag screw technique is held in place by threading both the near and far holes in the cortices. The fragment is held by the threads in the near hole and is positioned by the threads in the far hole.

When the shaft has been reconstituted, a neutralization plate is applied. The plate should be longer than the fracture by three holes. It is contoured to the bone surface and is placed over the cerclage wires. No screws should penetrate the fracture site. In some cases, a short screw into the near cortex is inserted where a long one would penetrate the fracture site in the far cortex. Screws can be angled to achieve placement away from the fracture line or to act as lag screws (Figs. 3.98, 3.99).

When a solid repositioning of the fragments is impossible, the plate is applied as a buttress plate. The area of missing or finely comminuted fragments is packed with a cancellous bone graft.

Closure is routine. Protection is provided by a modified Robert Jones splint for two weeks followed by restricted activity for one month.

Distal Tibia

Fractures of the distal tibia are often epiphyseal separations in immature animals. In adults, they are most often associated with injuries involving the hock. Open reduction is usually necessary to obtain the required apposition. Immobilization is provided by crossed pins or an intramedullary pin introduced proximally, either to be seated in the fragment or to penetrate it and the hock joint. Additional support is provided by a cast. The distal fibula, while still adherent to the tibia, becomes thicker and is involved in these fractures. Reducing the tibial fracture usually brings the fibula into place.

SURGICAL TECHNIQUE

The fracture is approached by a longitudinal incision on the medial surface of the distal tibia. The proximal transverse ligament may be

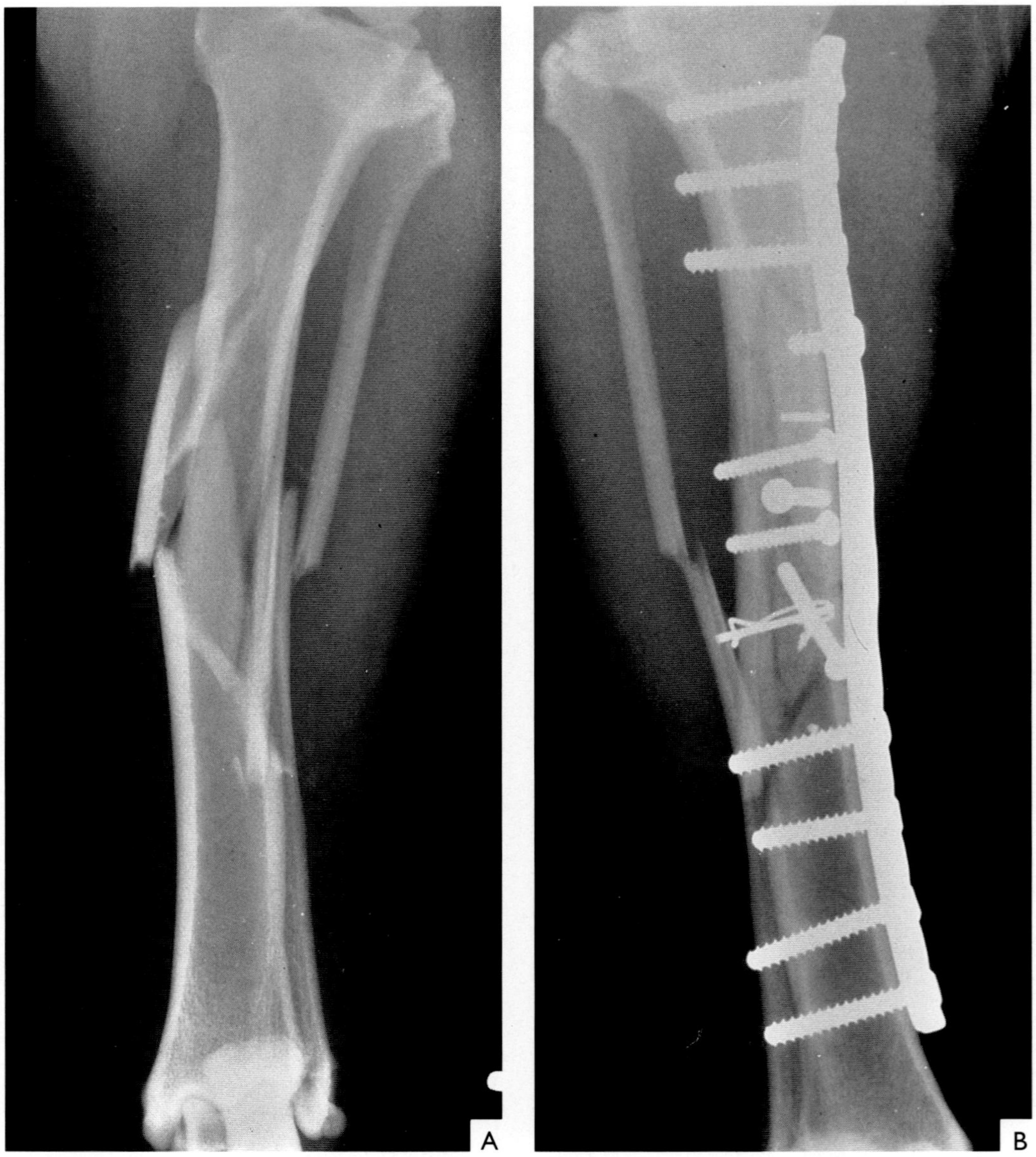

FIG. 3.98 (A) Comminuted shaft fracture of the tibia. (B) Treatment with a bone plate.

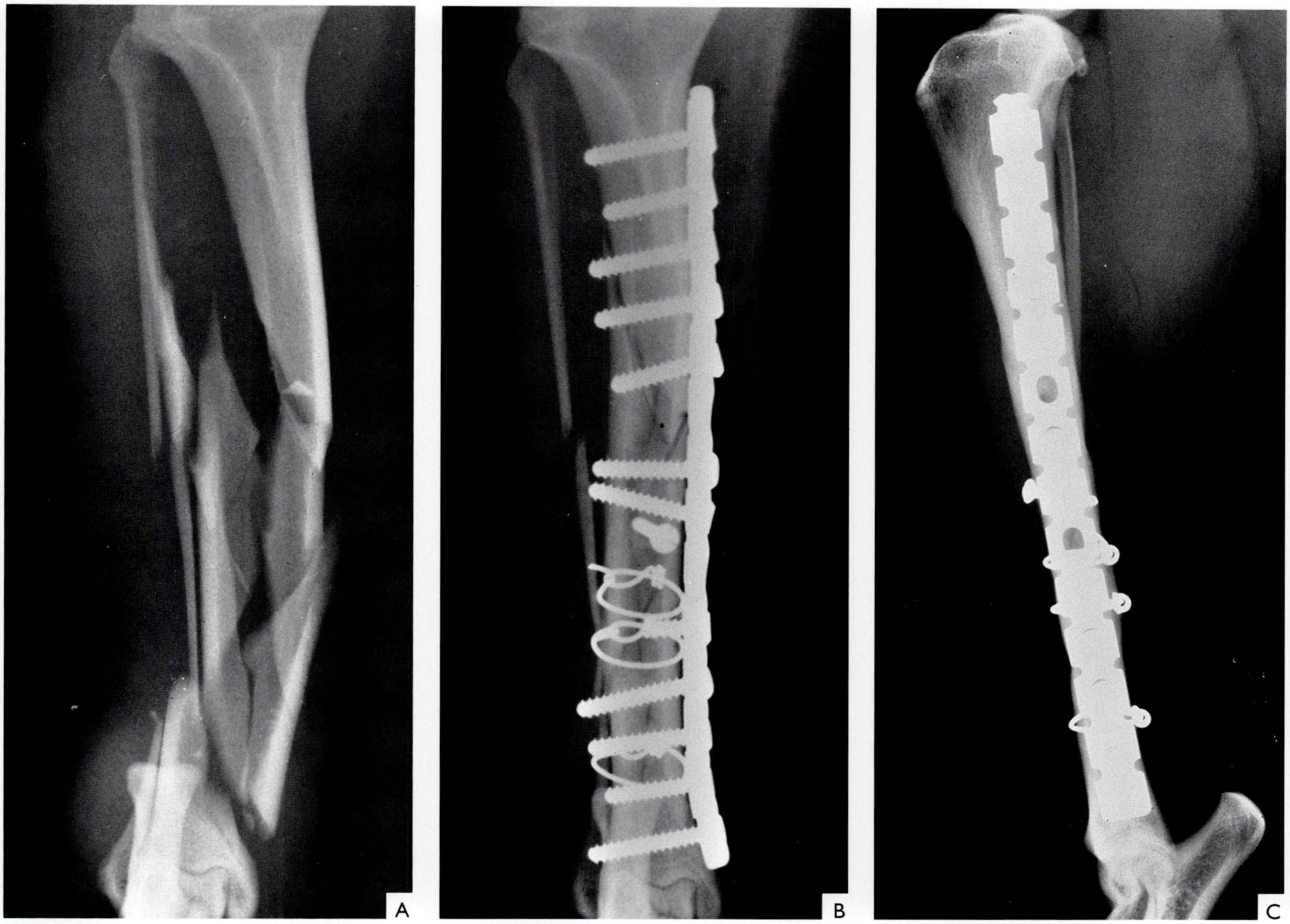

FIG. 3.99 (A) Radiograph of a severely comminuted tibial fracture. (B) Same injury treated with a reconstruction plate, interfragmentary screws, and cerclage wires. (C) After healing.

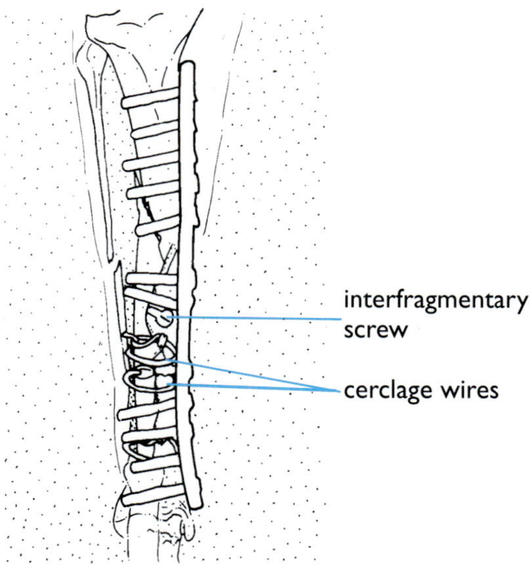

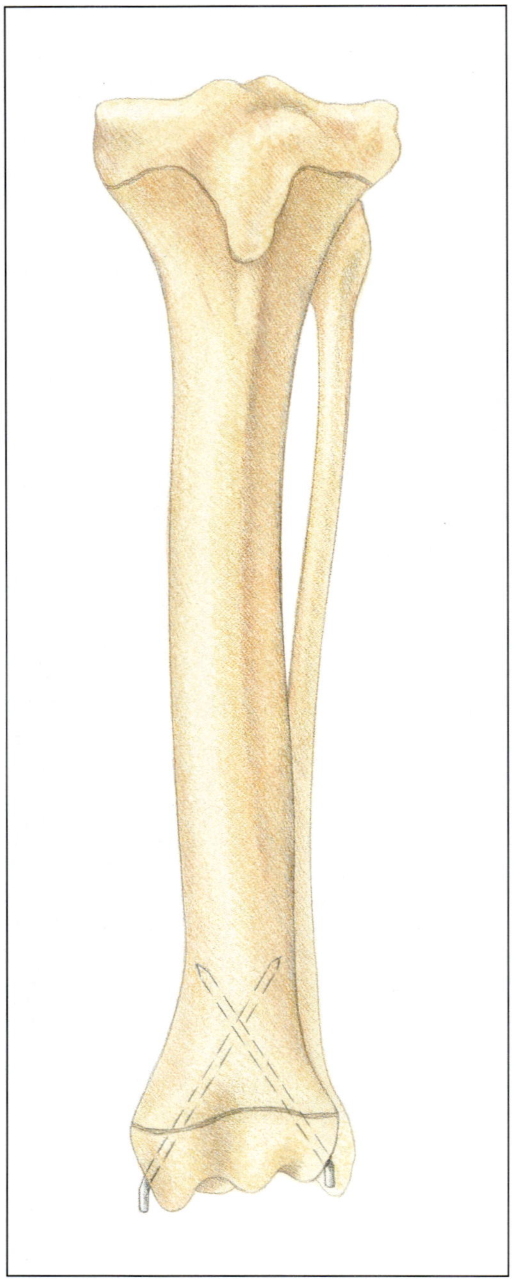

FIG. 3.100 Crossed pins in the treatment of a distal epiphyseal tibial fracture.

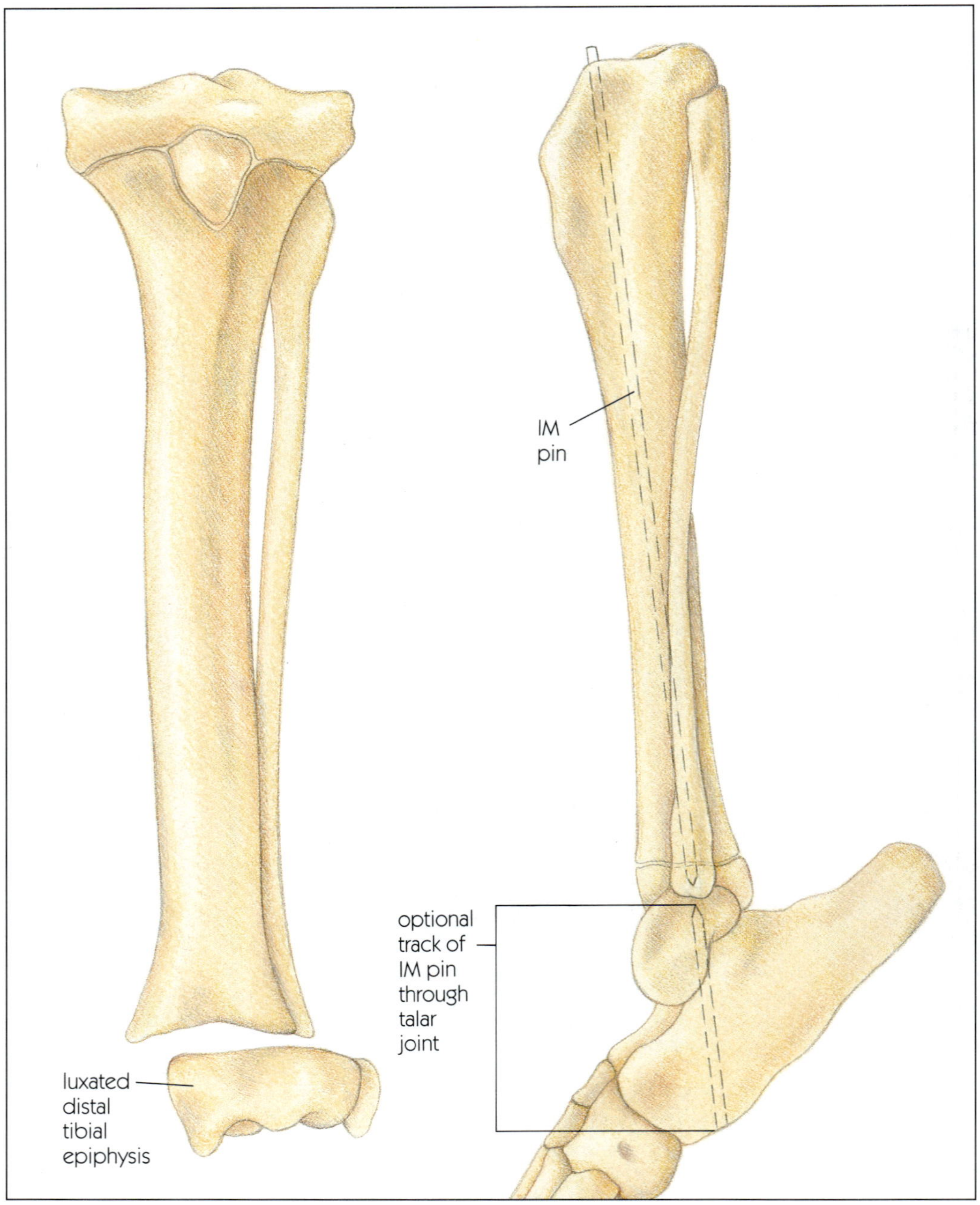

FIG. 3.101 An IM pin used for treatment of a distal epiphyseal fracture. The pin is inserted into the epiphysis. Alternatively, the pin may be inserted through the tarsus and the talar joint to be seated in the medullary cavity of the tibia.

torn. The fracture is reduced by angulation. Fixation can be obtained by introducing short pins from the medial and lateral malleolar area to cross the line of fracture and be seated firmly in the cortex of the distal tibia (Figs. 3.100, 3.101).

In physeal separations, a single intramedullary pin is introduced from the proximal tibia to insert into the distal fragment. The growth plate will tolerate a single smooth pin. Usually, the pin needs only to penetrate the fragment enough to prevent it from moving. The shape of the physeal plate will prevent rotation. If needed, the pin may be inserted from the tarsus through the hock joint, into the medullary cavity of the tibia. The joint is held in the standing position (Fig. 3.102).

It would appear that the joint surfaces would be severely damaged, but good recovery is the rule. In general, however, penetrating the joint should be avoided. A cast of light plastic extending to the stifle is applied (Scotch Cast Plus, St. Paul, MN). The cast must be closely monitored; if initial swelling goes down, the cast must be reapplied. Pressure sores, injuries to the toes and insufficient protection to the fracture can result from loose, inadequate casts. Chewing the cast is a sign of something wrong with it, not a behavioral problem of the patient. The cast is removed in three weeks. Intramedullary pins are removed after healing takes place, usually in four weeks.

Malleolar Fractures

Fractures of the medial, lateral, or both malleoli result in an unstable or luxated joint. In some instances, the disruption is so complete and the damage apparently so severe that it seems unlikely that anything can be done to restore function. The mortise and tenon-type joint needs to be exactly repositioned. With the fractured bone replaced, the joint is restored and results are usually better than expected (Fig. 3.103).

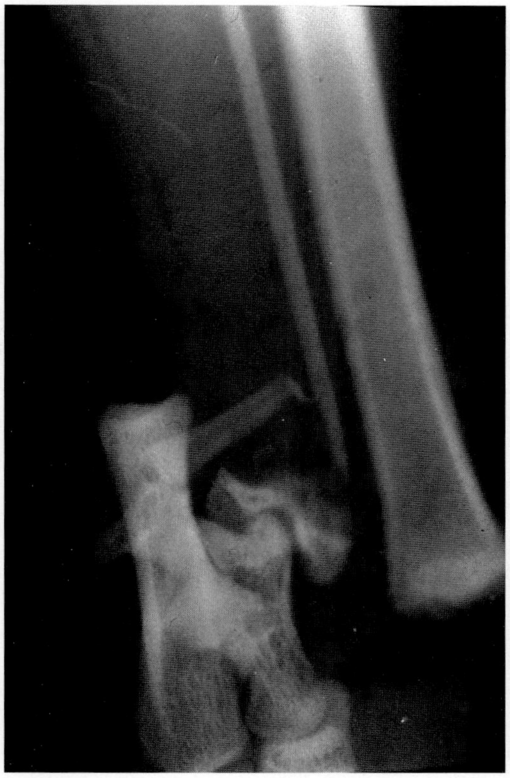

FIG. 3.102 Radiograph of a very severely injured distal tibia.

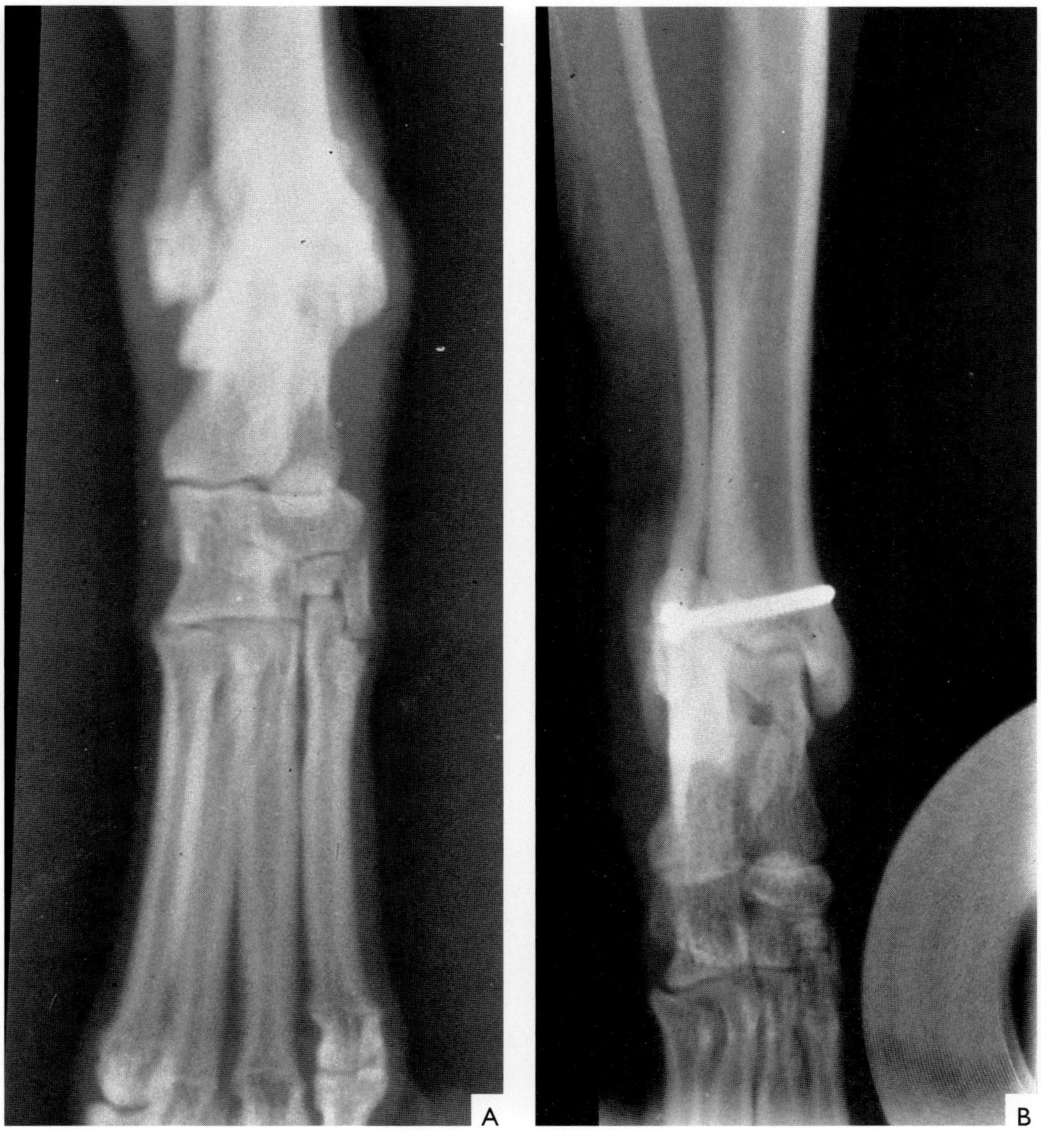

FIG. 3.103 (A) Fractured lateral malleolus. (B) Treatment with a bone screw.

SURGICAL TECHNIQUE

The lateral malleolus is approached by an incision through the skin and subcutaneous tissues over the lateral surface of the joint, starting below the lateral saphenous vein. The heavy fascia is exposed. The proximal transverse ligament is identified and carefully transected so as not to injure the tendon of the peroneus longus muscle, which lies under it. The caudal portion of the ligament and the surrounding fascia are elevated subperiosteally, exposing the lateral malleolus. In medium to large size dogs, the malleolar fragment is replaced and a bone screw is inserted to secure it. The screw should be long enough to engage the medial cortex (Fig. 3.104).

In most cases, the fragment is secured with a K-wire (Fig. 3.105) or threaded-tipped small intramedullary pin. The exposed end is bent at a right angle and cut off. A hole is drilled through a lateral portion of the tibial shaft, 1 cm or so above the line of fracture. A figure-8 tension band of orthopedic wire is inserted through

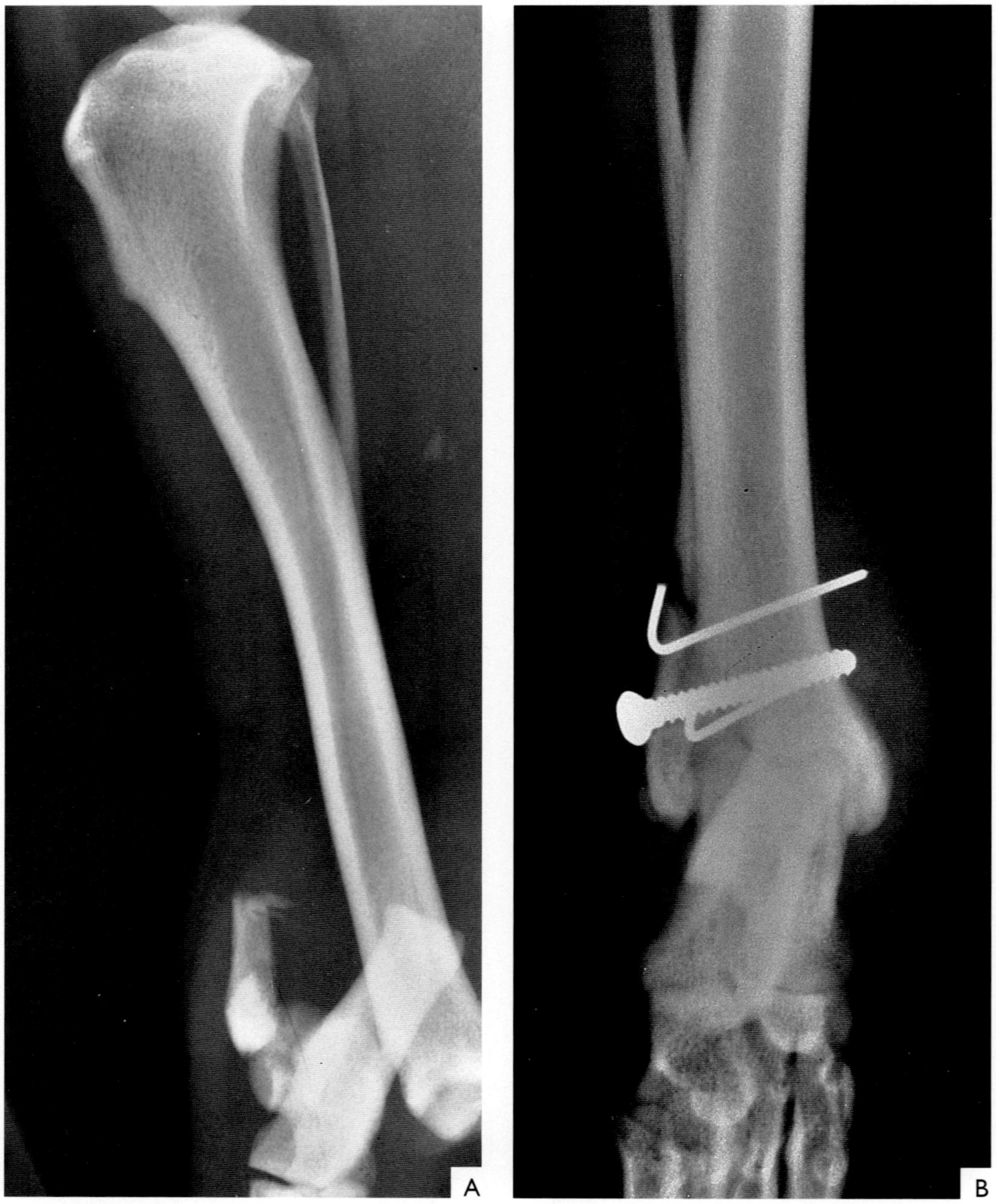

FIG. 3.104 (A,B) This lateral malleolar fracture was treated with a K-wire and a bone

the hole, under the K-wire or pin, and twisted tightly. The pin or wire is tapped firmly against the bone with a bone mallet (Fig. 3.106).

Closure is done by resuturing the proximal transverse ligament and fascia. Closure of the subcutaneous tissue and skin is routine.

The medial malleolus is approached by an incision through the skin and subcutaneous tissues directly over the fracture site. An incision is made through the deep fascia to the bone just cranial to the medial malleolus. It is necessary to elevate this fascia to expose the malleolus. The fragment is replaced and secured with a screw, threaded pin, or K-wire, as well as a figure-8 tension band.

Closure is made by resuturing the heavy fascia, subcutaneous tissues, and skin. A padded splint is put on for a week. Both malleoli can be fractured, each requiring repair. Even with obvious severe injuries, if the malleoli are accurately replaced, what appeared to be an incurable disaster will most often result in a functional joint.

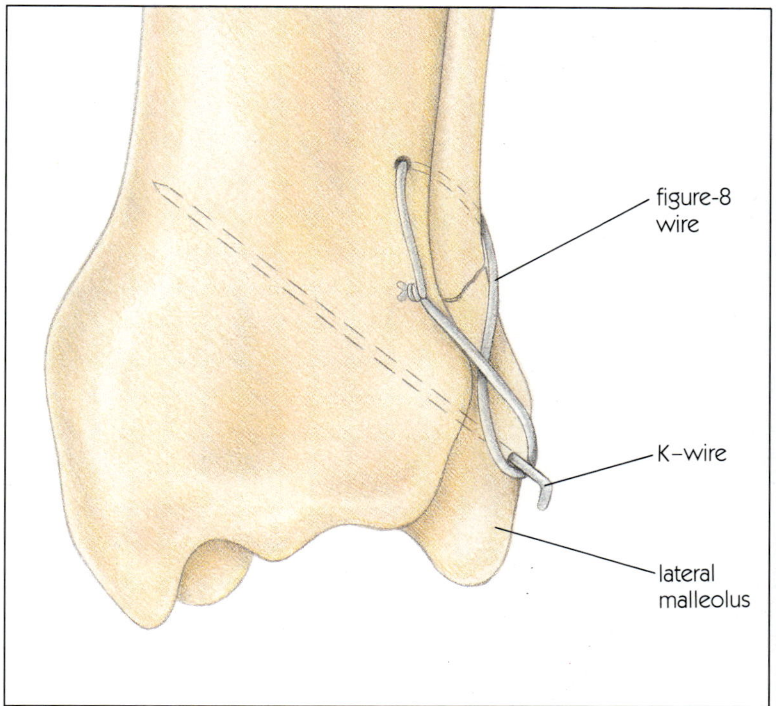

FIG. 3.105 A K-wire and figure-8 tension band in treatment of a fracture of the lateral malleolus.

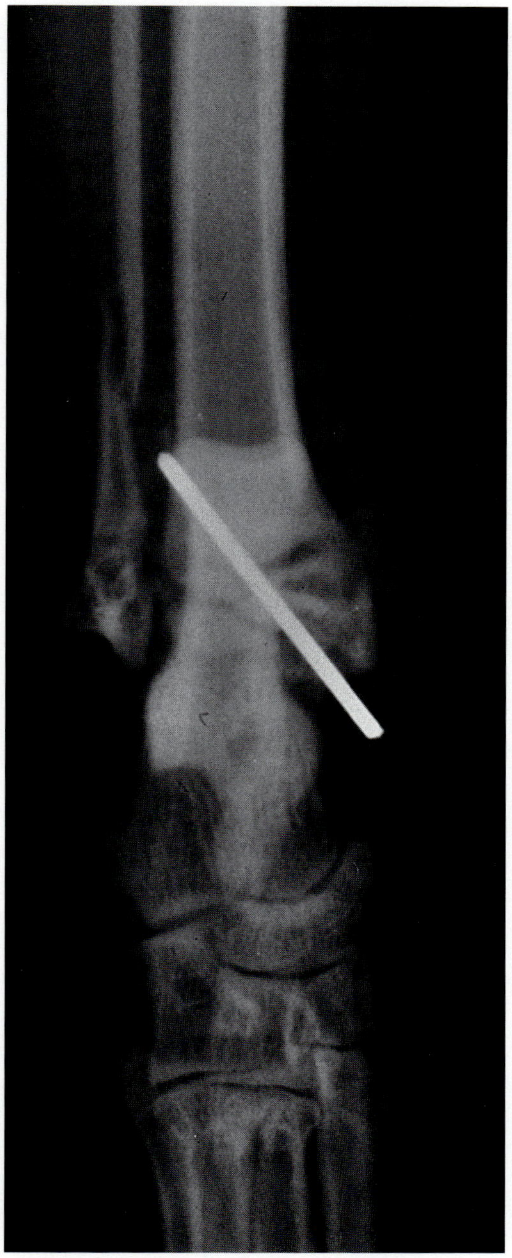

FIG. 3.106 A medial malleolar fracture treated with a K-wire.

CHAPTER 4

FOOT

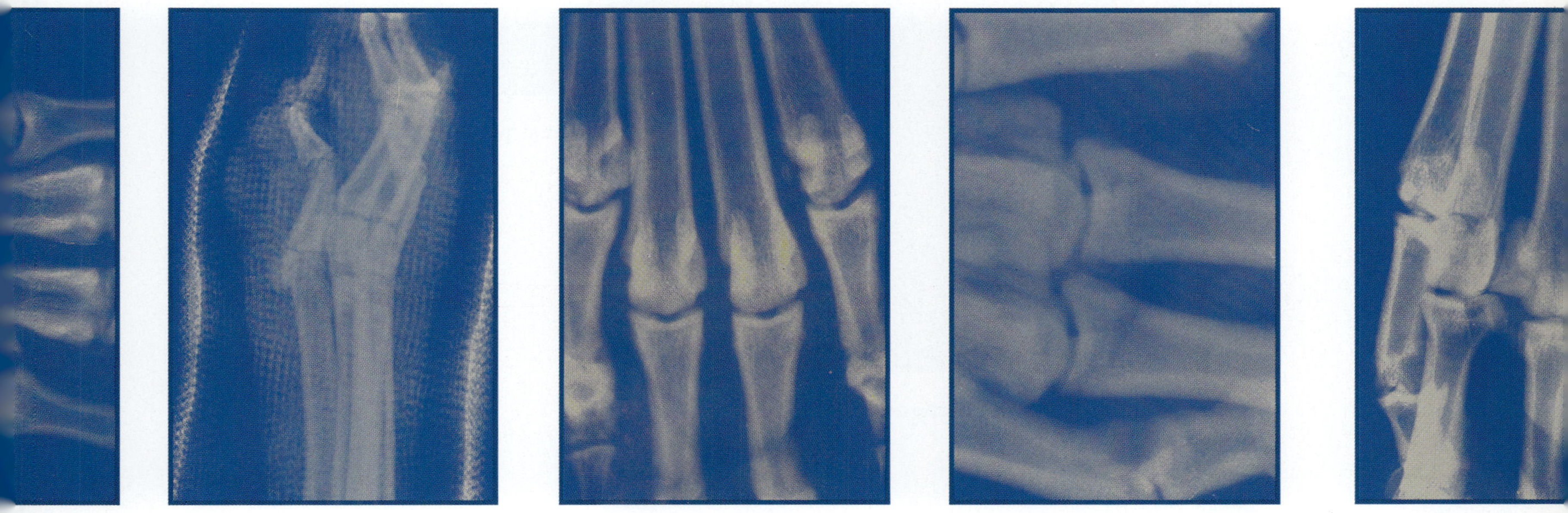

FRACTURES OF THE METACARPALS/METATARSALS

Surgical procedures for the metatarsals and metacarpals are essentially the same.

Fractures of the metacarpals are relatively common in the dog and cat. They may involve one (Fig. 4.1) or all four of the bones (Fig. 4.2), and vary in severity from greenstick to severely comminuted with contamination or infection. The second and fifth metacarpals (medial and lateral) are more commonly affected. There is usually considerable swelling and soft-tissue damage. The skin may be torn away, exposing the tendons and bones. Total degloving is sometimes seen, especially in cats.

Surgical approaches vary according to the number of bones involved and the location of the fractures. *Greenstick fractures* and those involving the medial or lateral bones with minor displacement

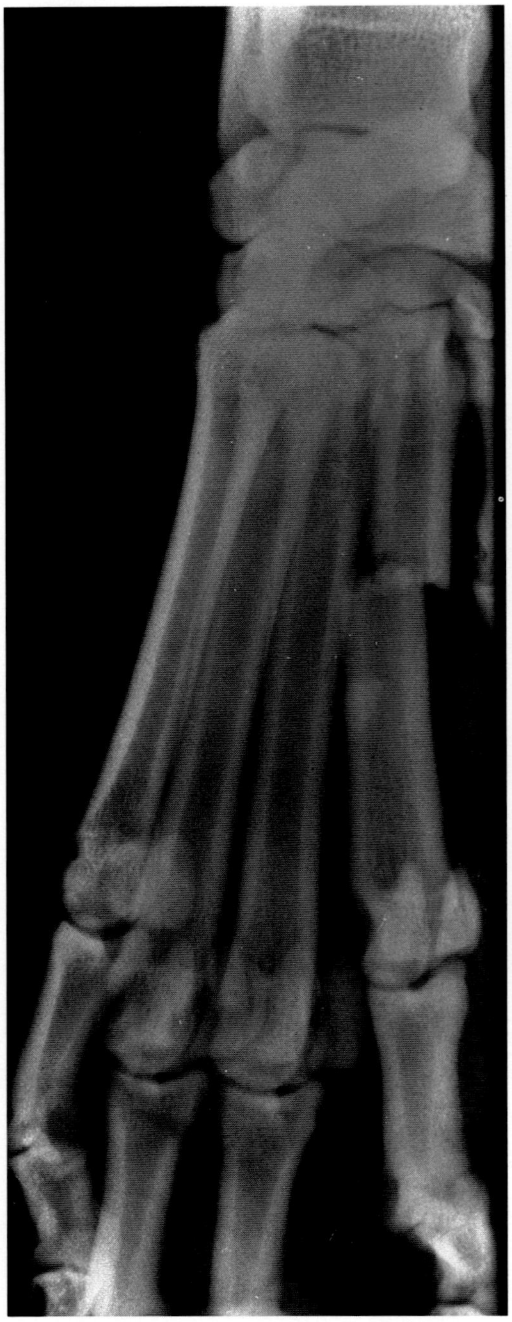

FIGURE 4.1 A single fracture of metacarpal II.

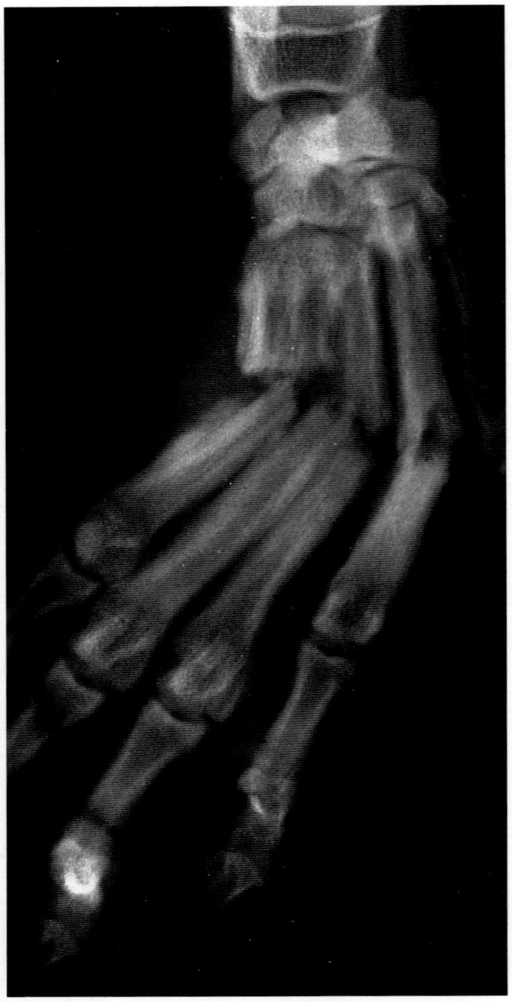

FIGURE 4.2 All four metacarpals are fractured.

are treated with a cast (Figs. 4.3, 4.4). The spoon splint does not appear to offer enough rigidity to control motion. *Very proximal fractures* involving the carpometacarpal joints require surgical intervention for joint congruency and stabilization. *Midshaft fractures,* especially those that involve most or all of the bones, do best with intramedullary fixation or small plates. Nonunions and malunions are treated with small plates.

Cerclage wires and interfragmentary compression with small lag screws are applied at all appropriate locations (Fig. 4.5). Because the foot is also placed in a cast, no other fixation may be needed. Cerclage wires are often used with intramedullary (IM) pins. Care must be taken to ensure that only bone is encompassed and that the wire is securely tightened. In large and very active dogs, pinning or plating is advisable even if only one bone is affected. If the fracture is slightly to moderately separated, the reduction is maintained by transfixing the fracture site with K-wires (Fig. 4.6).

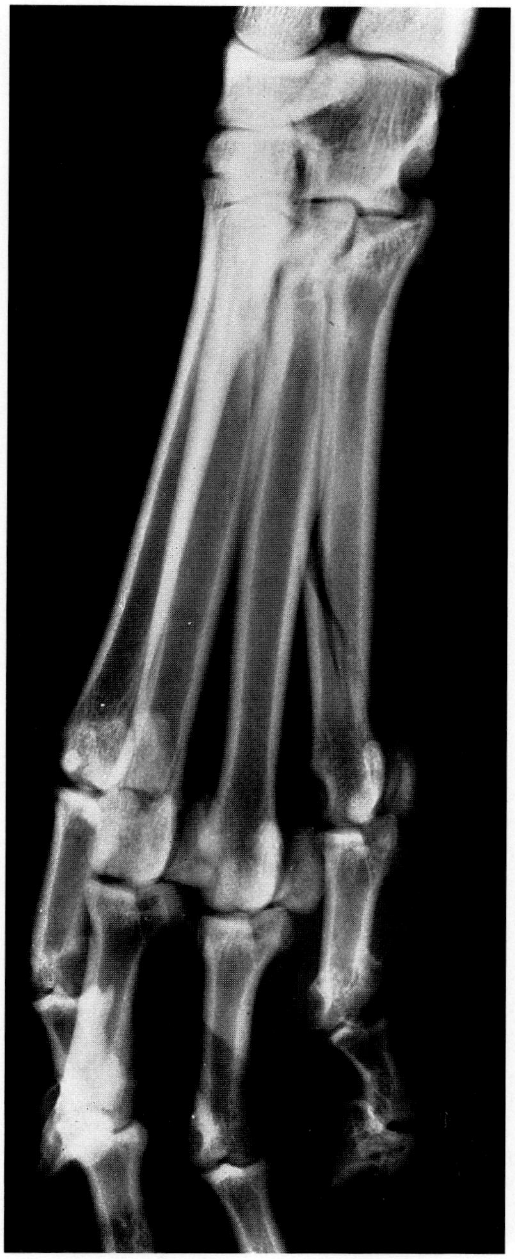

FIGURE 4.3 This metatarsal fracture shows minimal displacement.

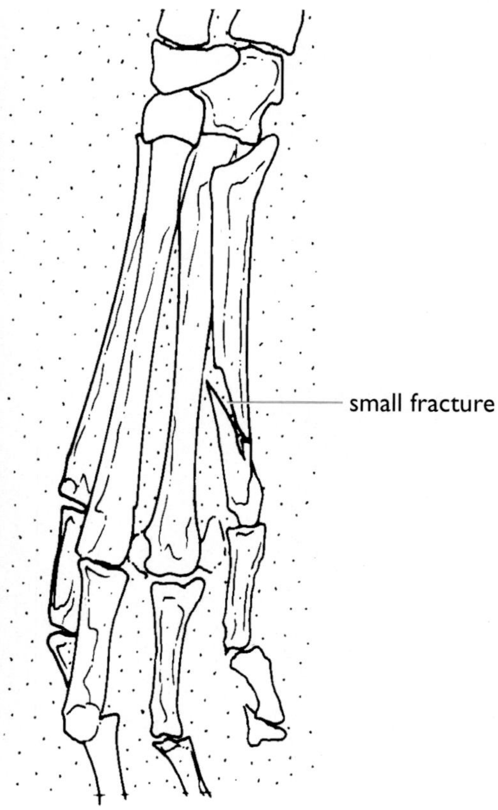

All fractures of the metacarpals/metatarsals or phalanges are supported in a cast, whether or not they have been treated by internal fixation. In the forelimb, the cast is applied with the carpus moderately flexed. Casts are kept on for 4 to 6 weeks. They require frequent inspection, repair, and replacement. A period of 2 to 4 weeks of restricted activity is advisable after cast removal.

Proximal and Distal Metacarpal/Metatarsal Fractures

Proximal and distal metacarpal fractures involving the carpometacarpal or metacarpal-proximal phalangeal joints are treated by open reduction and fixation.

A firm bandage is applied, starting at the toes, to compress the blood out of the limb. Because of the many small blood vessels encountered, a tourniquet on the leg is necessary. The bandage is then removed and the surgical field is prepared. The tourniquet limits the length of surgery to one hour.

SURGICAL TECHNIQUE

The surgical approach is made dorsally, directly over the bone at the fracture site. The skin is freed by sharp and blunt dissection, then retracted. The heavy fascia is incised. The tendons of the lateral and common digital extensors are isolated and retracted. The fracture site is exposed. The fragment is reduced and gripped with a small bone-holding forceps with sharp ends. A cerclage

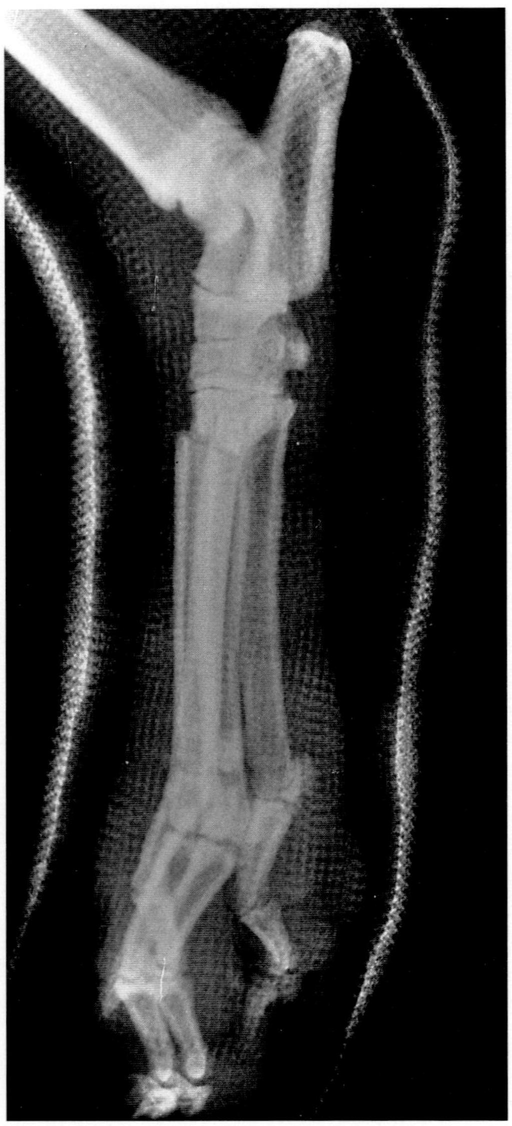

FIGURE 4.4 This proximal metatarsal fracture in a cast exhibits minimal displacement.

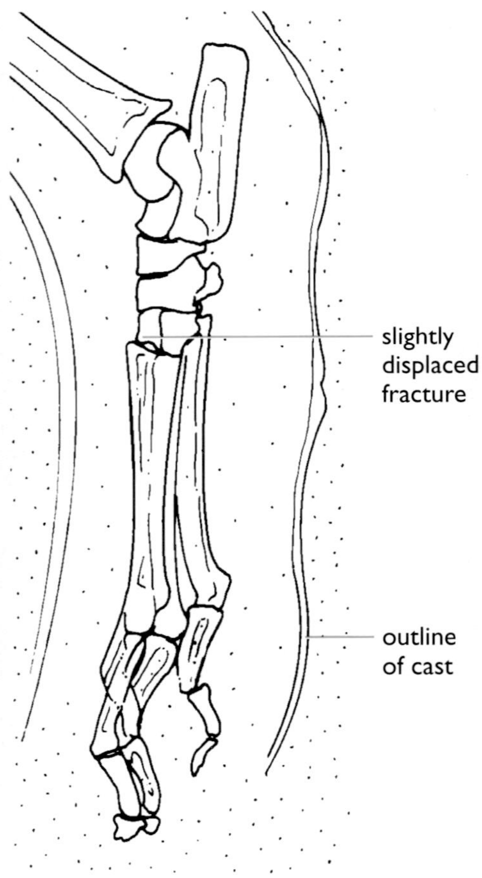

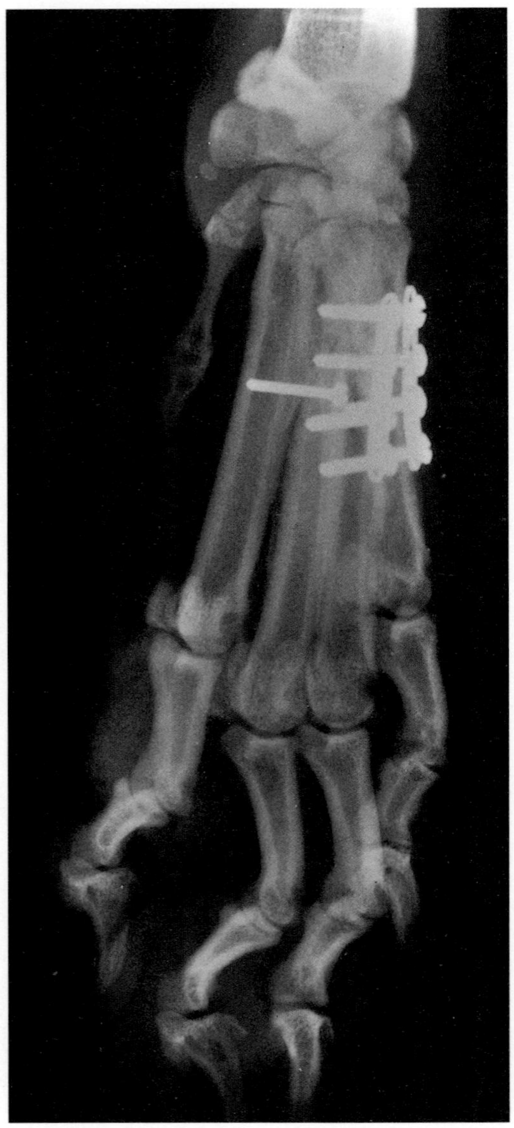

FIGURE 4.5 These fractured metacarpals have been treated with bone plates and a lag screw.

wire or, if the fragment is large enough, one or two small screws (two are preferable) are inserted to lag the fragment in place (Fig. 4.7).

A figure-8 tension band cerclage wire may be placed through a hole drilled through the fragment. Another may be placed through the shaft. With small fragments, a dorsally-located tunnel is drilled across the shaft. The cerclage wire is inserted through the tunnel and over the fragment. It passes under and next to the bone, where the ends are then twisted tightly together, cut off, and bent close to the bone (Fig. 4.8).

Closure is done by suturing the fascia, subcutaneous tissue, and skin. The foot is placed in a cast.

Fractures of the Metacarpal/Metatarsal Shaft

Fractures of the shaft of the metacarpal bones are reduced at open reduction and treated with intramedullary pins or small bone plates.

SURGICAL TECHNIQUE

Exposure for a single bone is made by incising the skin directly over the affected bone. If two adjacent bones are fractured, the incision is made between them. If all of the bones are fractured, a skin flap is raised. The incision begins at the proximal head of metacarpal II, curves distolaterally to the shaft of metacarpal V, and curves distomedially to the distal portion of metacarpal II. The skin is undercut, elevated, and retracted. The heavy subcutaneous fascia is

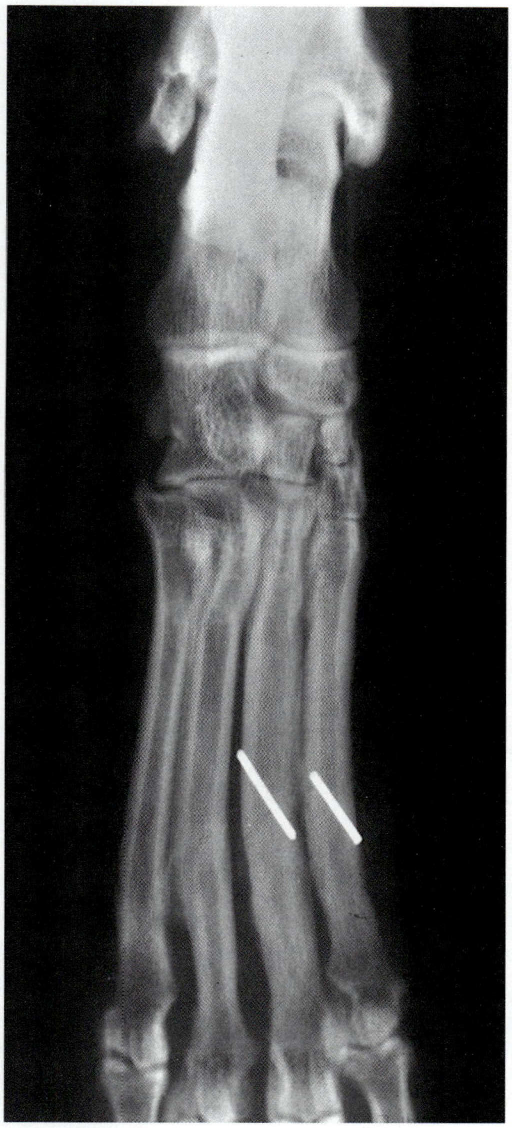

FIGURE 4.6 Excellent healing has been obtained in these metatarsals treated with K-wires across the fractures.

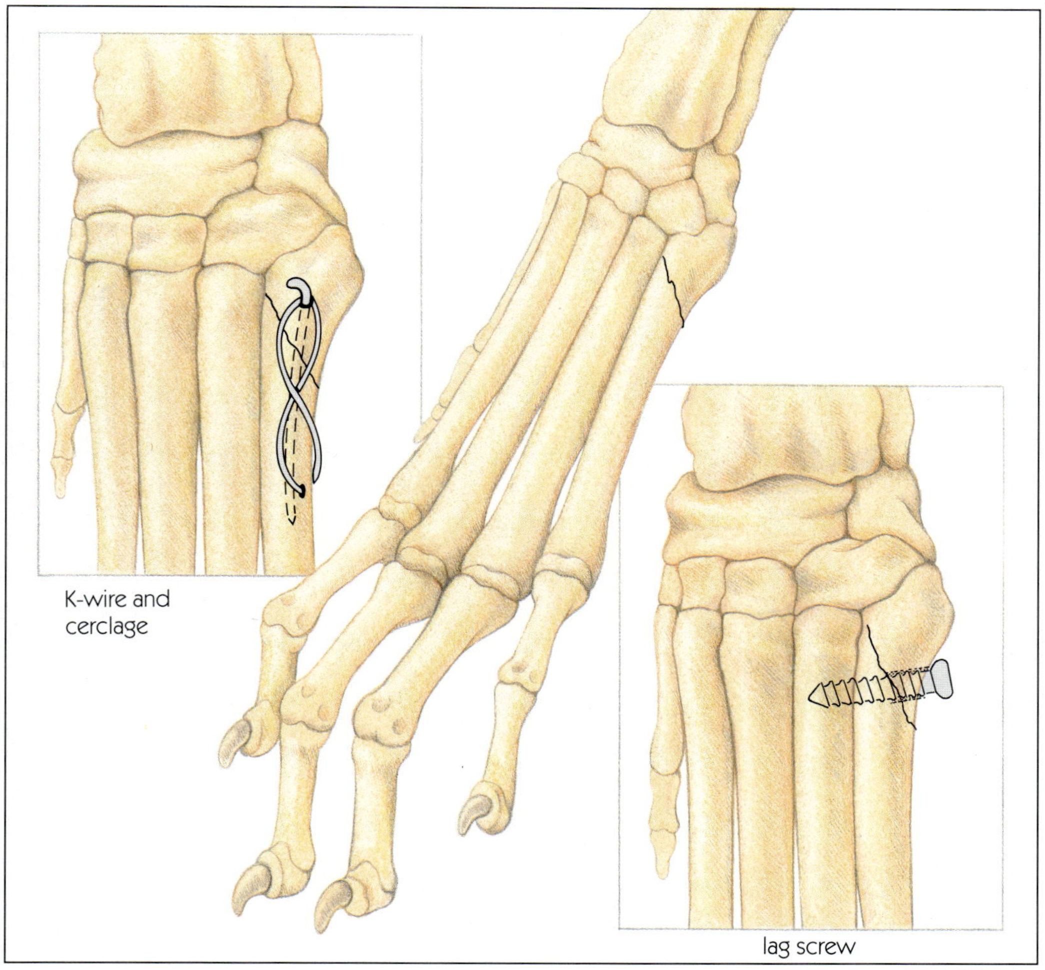

FIGURE 4.7 Repair with a K-wire and cerclage of a proximal metacarpal fracture involving the joint surface. A lag screw can also be used in larger dogs.

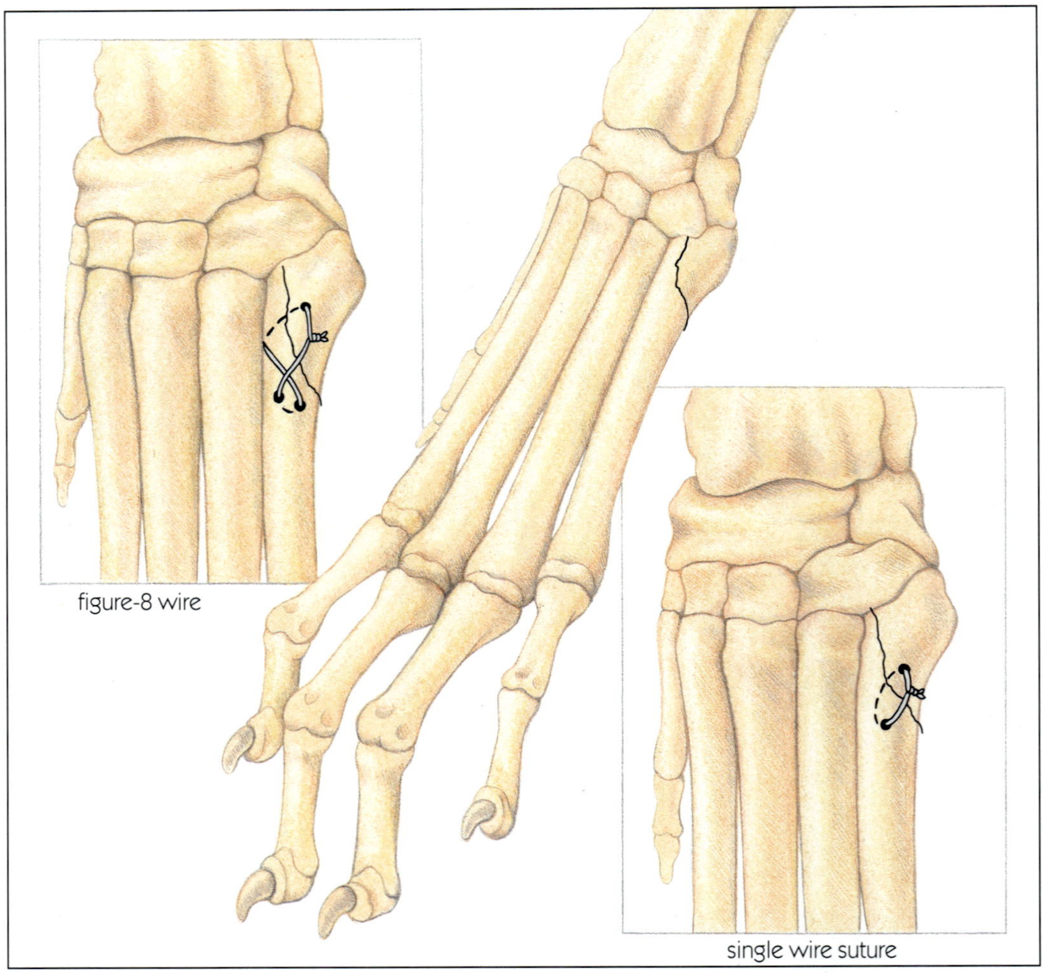

FIGURE 4.8 This proximal metacarpal fracture involving the joint was treated with a figure-8 tension band.

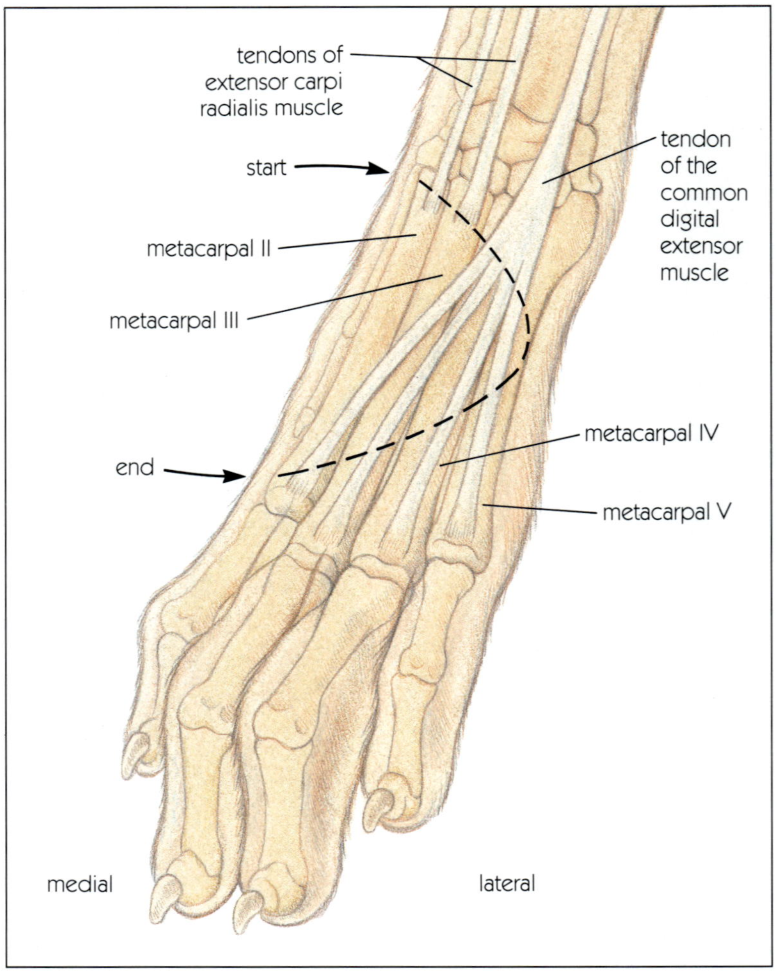

FIGURE 4.9 Surgical exposure of the metacarpals.

incised to expose the several diversions of the common and lateral digital extensors with their fascial supporting structures (Fig. 4.9).

Small intramedullary pins of a diameter that will not completely fill the fractured bone's medullary cavity are selected. With the proximal phalanges firmly flexed, the pin is introduced at the dorsal edge of the distal articular cartilage of the fractured bone. The pin is inserted through the distal fragment into the proximal fragment. Each affected bone is treated similarly. The projecting end of each pin is bent at a right angle and cut off. The pins are now seated firmly into the proximal fragments. The bent ends are directed outwards, allowing the proximal phalanx to assume as natural a position as possible. The bent ends protect the phalanges from injury and provide a grip for pliers when the pins are removed (Fig. 4.10).

Small bone plates in various styles are available. Usually it is difficult to place more than two screws per fragment. The overlying tendons are carefully elevated and gently retracted enough to allow plate insertion after the fracture has been reduced. With nonunions, the fragment ends are curetted to provide fresh bone-to-bone contact (Fig. 4.11).

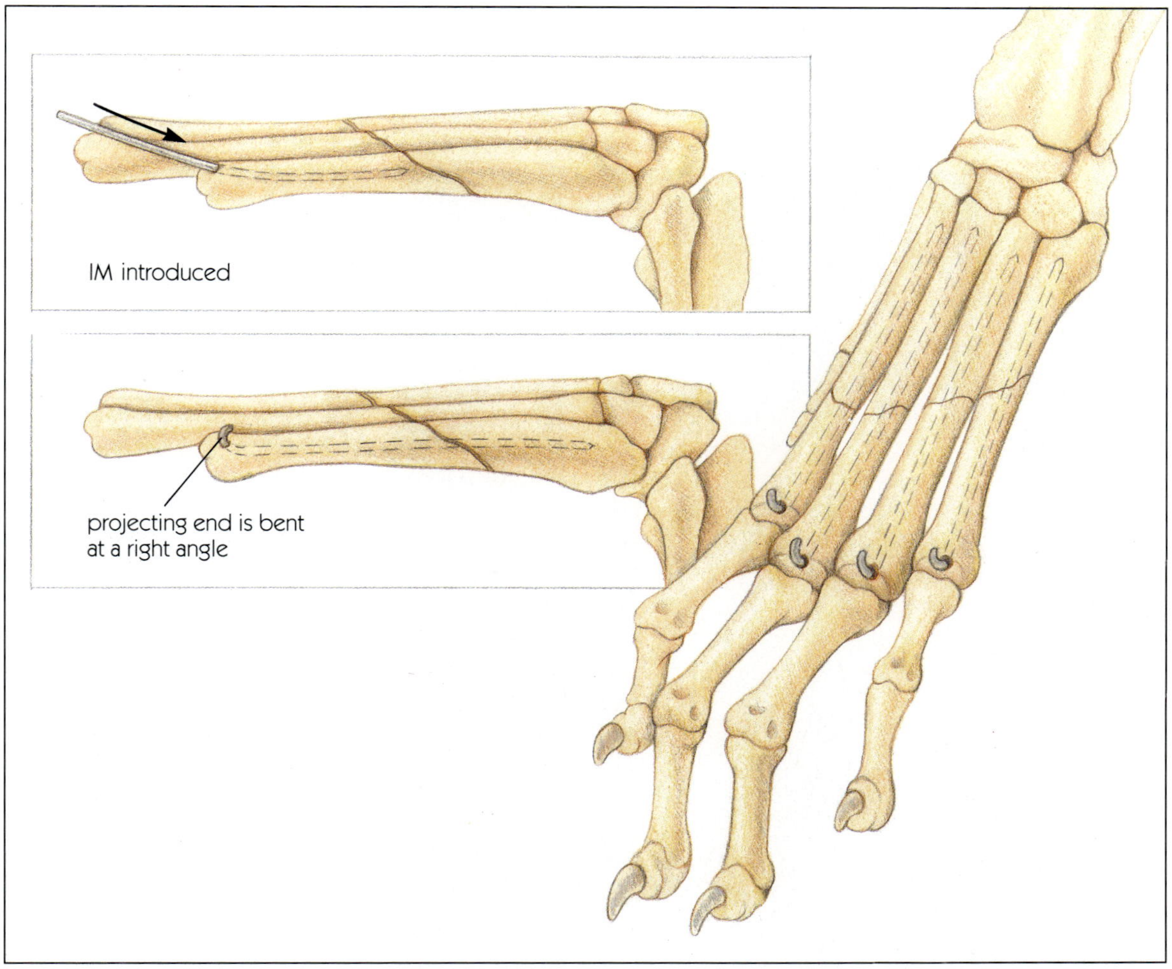

FIGURE 4.10 Placement of IM pins in fractures of the metacarpals.

Closure is done by suturing the incisions in the fascia, subcutaneous tissues, and the skin. Plates are usually removed in 3 months or when healing is complete. The foot is placed in a cast.

The plate's solid support makes it possible to remove the cast in about three weeks. With intramedullary pins, the cast is left on 2 or 3 weeks longer.

FRACTURES OF THE PHALANGES

Fractures of the shaft of the phalanx are usually treated by placing the foot in a cast. In very large, valuable, or show animals, an extremely small plate is used. If the fracture is proximal and involves the metacarpophalangeal joint, open reduction and fixation is required to prevent degenerative joint disease from misaligning the joint surfaces.

SURGICAL TECHNIQUE

The surgical approach is made by incising the skin directly over the affected area.

In very large dogs, the fragment is stabilized by lagging it with a small screw or introducing a small intramedullary pin (Fig. 4.12). Smaller fragments are secured by a hemicerclage wire placed through a hole that is drilled through the bone and the fragment. If the fragment is too small be drilled, the wire is inserted through a tunnel, which has been drilled through the dorsal portion of the proximal end of the proximal phalanx. The wire is placed over the fragment and around the bone, where the ends are tightly twisted together. The wire may pass over the heavy fascia, protecting the flexor tendon.

Wires and screws remain in place permanently. The foot is placed in a cast for 4 weeks. Amputation is a common alternative

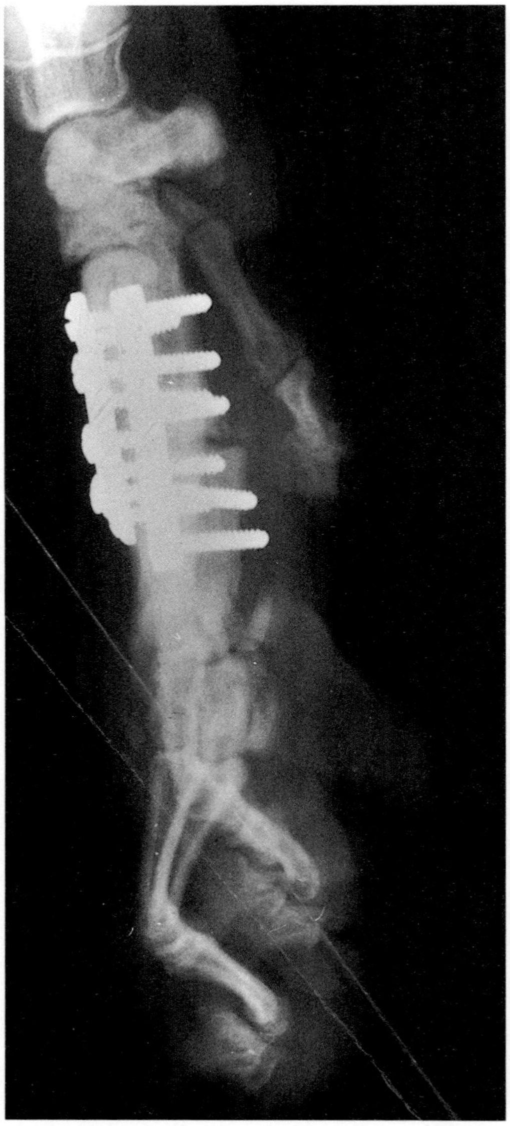

FIGURE 4.11 Fractured metacarpals treated with small bone plates.

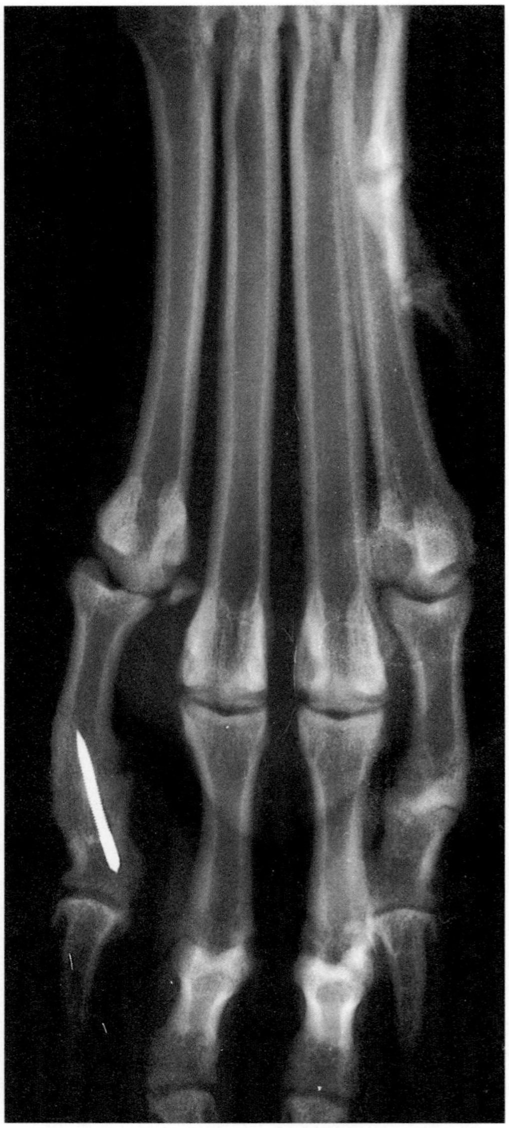

FIGURE 4.12 This phalangeal fracture was treated with a threaded IM pin.

treatment in fractured phalanges of the second and fifth metacarpals. Removal of the center toes will cause almost permanent lameness.

FRACTURES OF THE PROXIMAL SESAMOIDS OF THE METACARPOPHALANGEAL JOINT

These fractures are occasionally seen in large breed dogs and can cause intermittent lameness. Special radiographic techniques may be required to identify the fracture. The sesamoids are paired and numbered 1 to 8, from the second metacarpal to the fifth. The second and seventh are most often affected. Small fragments are extracted. In a central or multiple fracture, the entire sesamoid is removed.

SURGICAL TECHNIQUE

The area is exposed by making an incision through the skin medial or lateral to the large central foot pad. Reflection of the skin exposes the proximal annular ligament and the tendon of the superficial digital flexor. A midline vertical incision is made through these structures directly over the sesamoids. The incision is retracted medially and laterally to expose the deep digital flexor tendon. The sesamoid bones lie on each side of the joint. A small fragment or the entire sesamoid is removed by sharply dissecting the attached ligamentous structures (Fig. 4.13).

The incision is closed by suturing the annular ligament and the superficial digital flexor tendon. The skin is closed. The foot is protected with a padded bandage for a week.

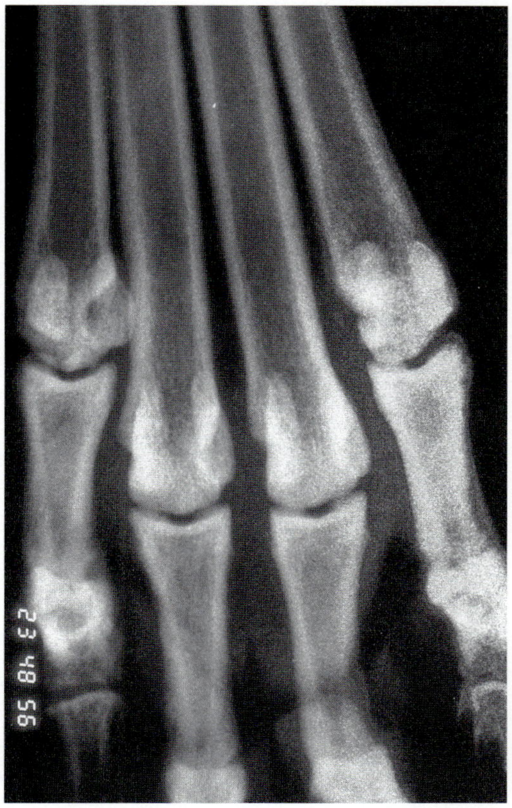

FIGURE 4.13 Fractured sesamoids. The second and seventh sesamoids, seen in this radiograph, are the most commonly injured.

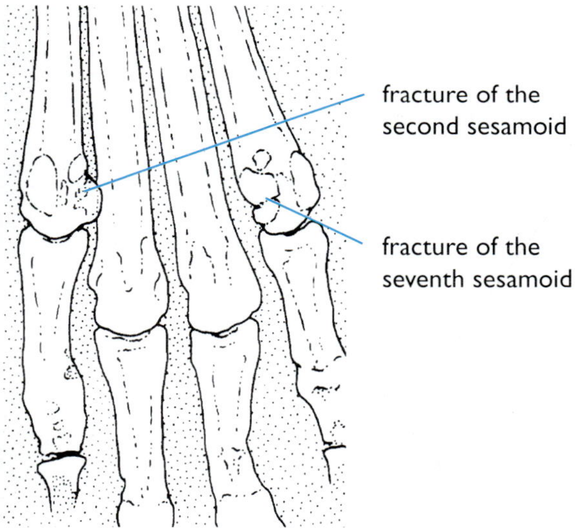

CHAPTER

5

JOINTS

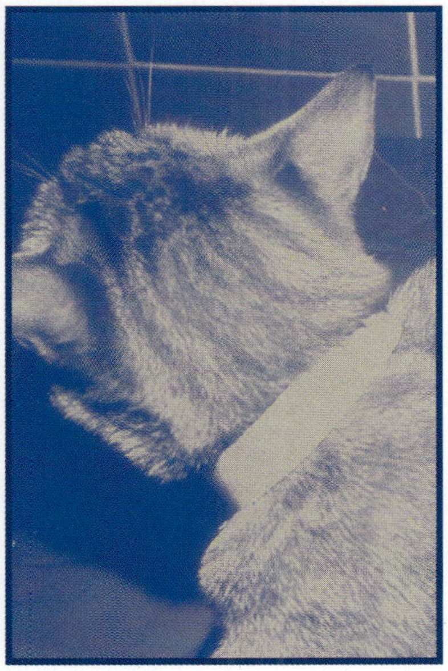
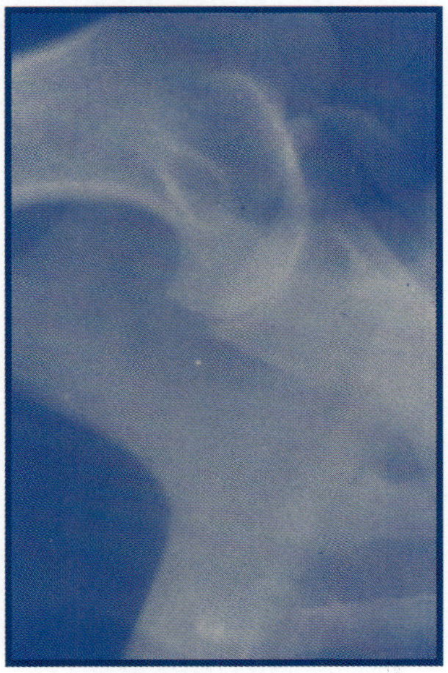
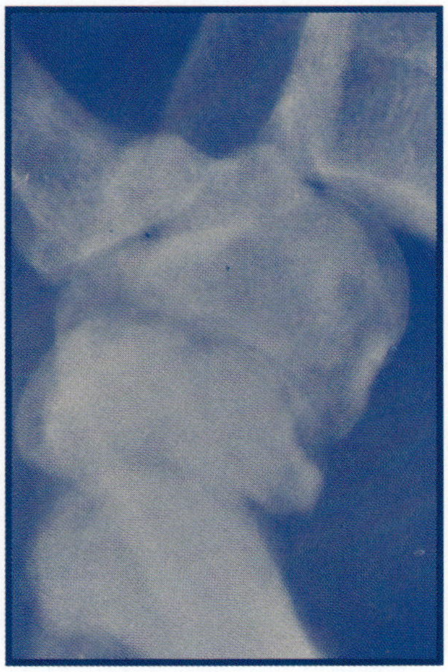
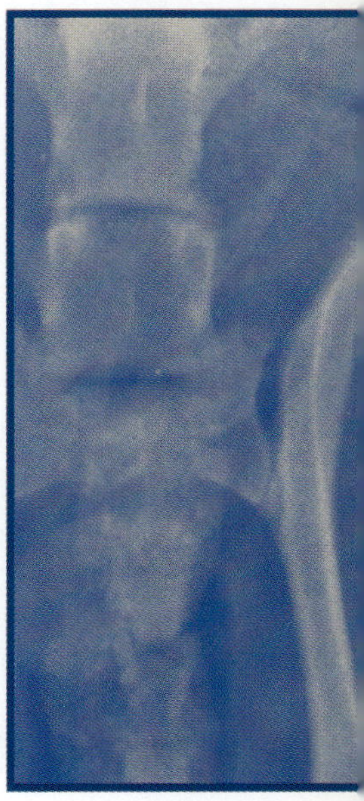

Surgeries of the joints make important demands on the surgeon. Strict asepsis, joint surface congruity, gentle handling of joint cartilage, radiographic and anatomic understanding, and excellent technique are essential for good functional results. Open joints should be debrided and systemic antibiotic therapy begun as soon as possible. Sterile wound dressings should be applied, as should a means of limiting activity, such as a Robert Jones splint.

LUXATIONS

Luxation of the Scapula

Luxation of the scapula is relatively rare and is usually related to trauma. It occurs in both dogs and cats and can be bilateral. The dorsally projecting hypermobile scapula is very noticeable and diagnostic (Fig. 5.1). The attachments of the serratus ventralis, rhomboideus and trapezoideus muscles are torn away, permitting dorsal movement on weightbearing.

Treatment consists of securing the dorsal caudal edge of the scapula to the fifth rib by a strong wire suture (Fig. 5.2). The torn muscles are replaced and sutured where possible.

SURGICAL TECHNIQUE

An incision is made through the skin and subcutaneous tissue along the dorsal caudal edge of the scapula to expose the thoracic portion of the trapezius and the caudal edge of the deltoideus. Some of the muscular attachments to the dorsal edge of the scapula and its undersurface will appear to have been torn loose. A collection of serum is usually found under the scapula. Depending on the time elapsed since the injury, the torn edges will have retracted and healed.

The dorsal caudal edge of the scapula is freed of muscle with a periosteal elevator. The underlying rib, usually the fifth, is exposed by sharp and blunt dissection. Two holes are drilled through the scapula over the exposed area of the rib. The periosteum with the underlying pleura is carefully separated from the rib to allow passage of orthopedic wire under it. The chest cavity should not be penetrated. The wire ends are inserted through the holes in the scapula and are twisted tightly, binding the scapula to the rib. The twisted ends are flattened to the bone. With the scapula stabilized, muscles are reattached using mattress sutures.

Closure is done by suturing the fascial, subcutaneous, and skin layers in the usual manner.

A full foreleg splint is applied for 5 days; activity is restricted for 1 week. Excellent recovery should be expected.

When both legs are affected, they are placed in full-length foreleg coaptation splints with wrappings around the cranial chest. This allows the animal to stand and move on a smooth surface. Extra care is needed to provide soft bedding and to ensure the animal's comfort.

Luxation of the Shoulder

Medial and Lateral Luxation of the Shoulder

Luxation of the shoulder can be acquired or congenital. The latter is usually seen in very small breeds such as toy poodles, Pekingese, and very small terriers. Frequently the joint is so poorly developed that it precludes any form of functional repair (Fig. 5.3). These joints can be fused to provide a more stable front leg.

Acquired luxations are usually the result of severe trauma (Fig. 5.4). Most of them are medial, though a few are lateral. Cranial and caudal locations have also been reported. Early repair is necessary because movement of the joint causes the humeral head to erode the medial or lateral lip of the glenoid. This results in a glenoid that is insufficient to form a stable joint, even with surgical repair. The standard repair is to transpose the biceps brachii's tendon of origin medially for medial luxation and laterally for lateral luxation (Figs. 5.5, 5.6).

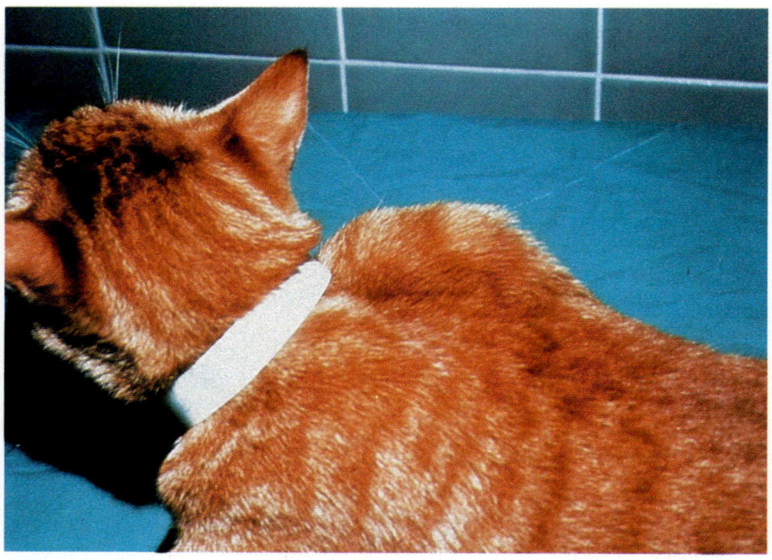

FIGURE 5.1 A dorsally projecting blade of the scapula is diagnostic of luxation.

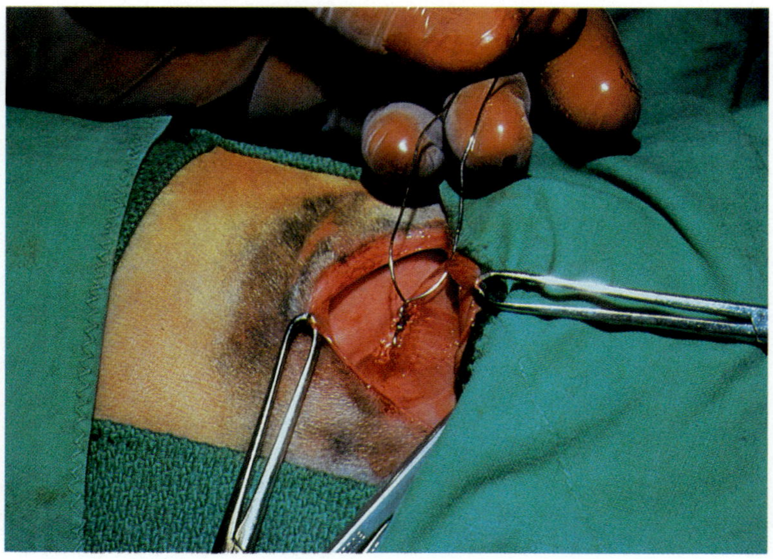

FIGURE 5.2 The dorsal caudal edge of the scapula is wired to the fifth rib.

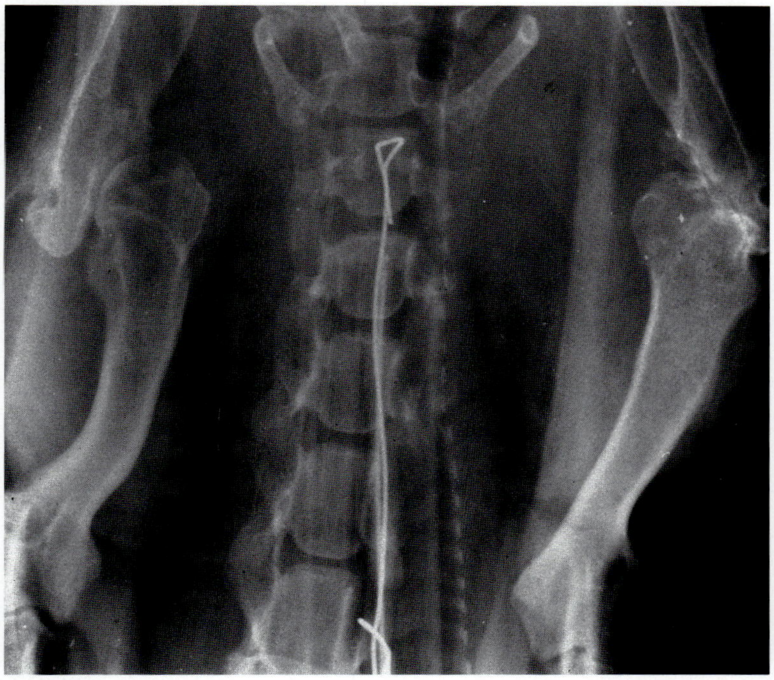

FIGURE 5.3 A congenitally luxated shoulder in a Pekingese.

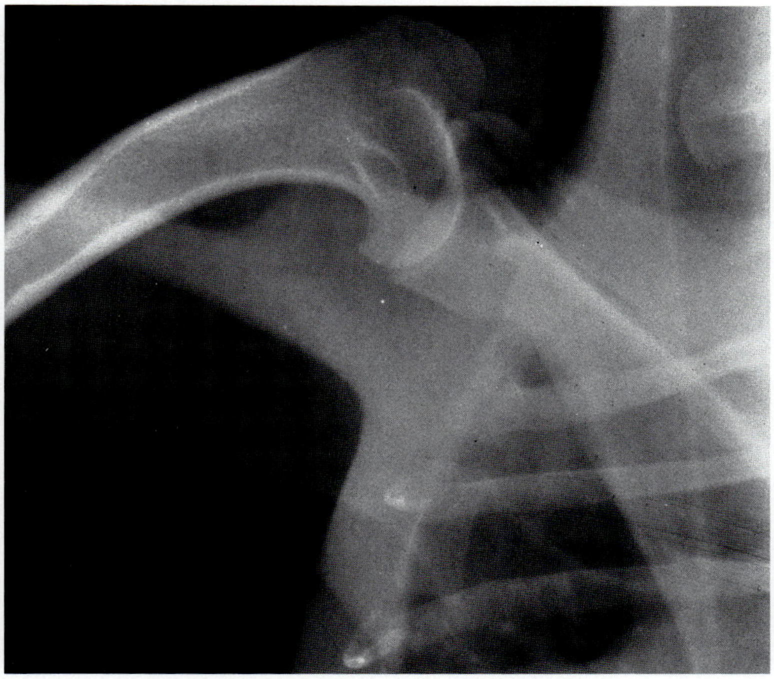

FIGURE 5.4 Radiograph of a traumatically luxated shoulder in a dog.

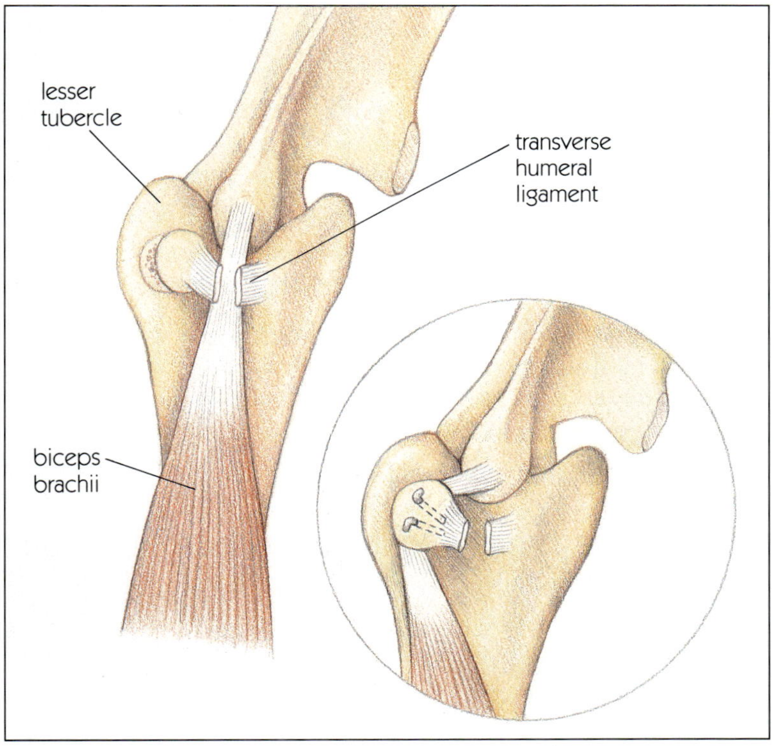

FIGURE 5.5 In the groove of elevated bone in the lesser humeral tubercle, tendon of origin of the biceps brachii is transposed for correction of medial luxation of the shoulder.

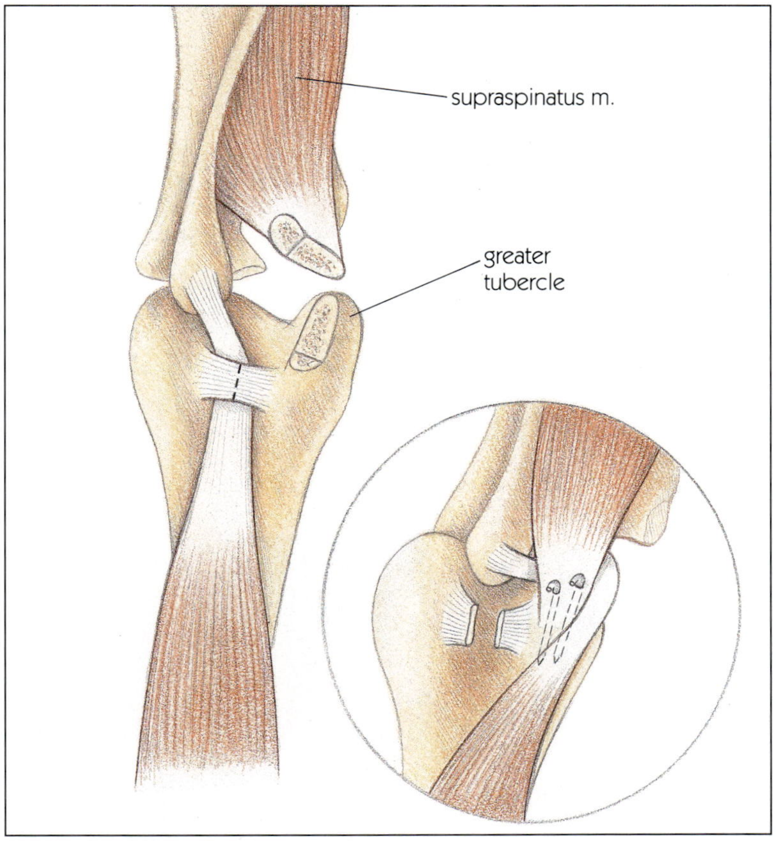

FIGURE 5.6 Transposition of the biceps brachii's tendon of origin to the lateral surface of the greater tubercle for correction of lateral luxation of the shoulder.

Medial Luxation

SURGICAL TECHNIQUE

An incision through the skin and subcutaneous tissues is made along the lower third of the cranial edge of the scapula over the point of the shoulder and along the cranioventral portion of the humerus. The incision is continued through the fascia of the shoulder to permit ventral retraction of the cleidobrachialis and expose the greater tubercle of the humerus. The ventral edge of the omotransversarius is retracted dorsally. The insertion of the deep pectoral is incised and the muscle is retracted medially from its insertion on the greater tubercle of the humerus. The superficial pectoral is incised along its insertion on the shaft of the humerus, then retracted medially. Further blunt dissection exposes the supraglenoid tubercle. The biceps brachii's tendon of origin is isolated and the transverse humeral ligament is incised. The tendon is exposed in its groove.

The lesser humeral tubercle is cleared of fascial and muscular insertions. A cut is made with an osteotome to provide a groove medial and parallel to the original intertubercular groove. An undercut is made to elevate a portion of the bone of the upper aspect of the new groove. The tendon of the biceps brachii is elevated from the intertubercular groove and slipped into the new groove under the elevated piece of bone. Two K-wires are driven into the elevated bone fragment, bent over, and cut off. The wires are driven flat to the bone with a mallet. The tendon now pulls the head laterally, thus preventing luxation (Fig. 5.7).

Lateral Luxation

For repair of lateral luxation of the shoulder, the incisions in the skin, subcutaneous tissues, and fascia are made as for a medial luxation. The cleido-brachialis is retracted ventrally and the omotransversarius dorsally. The area of the insertions of the supraspinatus on the greater tubercle is cleared laterally. The insertion of the deep and superficial pectorals are incised and retracted medially. The fibrous insertion of the supraspinatus is cleared of tissue so that it can be osteotomized. This is done by delineating the area laterally, medially, and ventrally with cuts of the osteotome. The osteotome is then directed from the ventral cut to remove a solid section of the greater tubercle containing the insertion. The supraspinatus is isolated by sharp and blunt dissection, then retracted dorsally.

The biceps brachii's tendon of origin is removed from its normal location after incising the transverse humeral ligament. The tendon is brought to a location lateral to the osteotomy site. The supraspinatus is now replaced and secured by two K-wires or small intramedullary pins that are driven into the humerus. Each pin or wire is bent at a right angle, cut off, and flattened to the bone surface with a mallet. The tension on the tendon of the biceps brachii now prevents lateral luxation of the humeral head (Fig. 5.8).

The closure of both repairs is the same. The deep and superficial pectorals are reattached by suturing them to adjacent fascia. The incision in the fascia of the shoulder is sutured so that the cleidobrachialis and omotransversalis are returned to their former locations. The subcutaneous tissues are closed with 2-0 catgut and the skin is closed with nonabsorbable suture.

Postoperative care consists of confining the dog in a cage and exercising it on a leash for 2 to 3 weeks. Use of the leg may take some time and require some physiotherapy. The end result, though not always perfect, will be an improvement over the dog's initial condition.

Luxation of the Elbow

Elbow luxations usually occur laterally. The large square-ended shape of the medial epicondyle contains the ulna, whereas the rounded shape of the lateral condyle permits the ulna and the anconeal process to move to a lateral and caudal position.

The elbow is painful, especially when it is moved. The foreleg is held abducted and is nonweightbearing in the acute stage.

Acute Luxation of the Elbow

Acute elbow luxation is not common. There is a history of recent trauma, usually of only a few hours' duration. The affected leg is not used, the joint is very painful, and the forelimb is held extended dorsolaterally from the elbow.

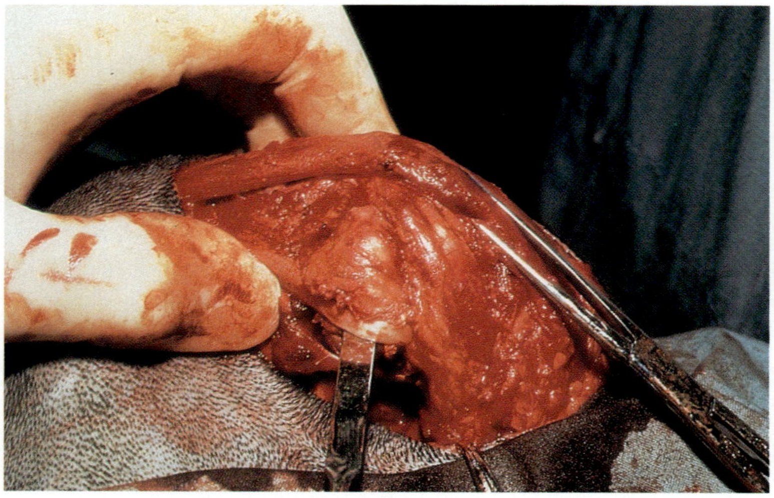

FIGURE 5.7 The biceps brachii's tendon of origin is placed medially on the lesser humeral tubercle for correction of medial luxation of the shoulder.

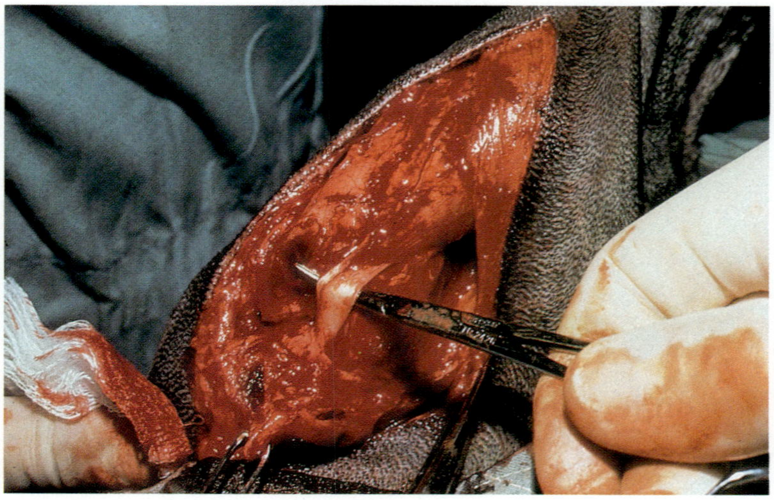

FIGURE 5.8 The tendon of origin of the biceps brachii is placed laterally on the greater humeral tubercle for correction of lateral luxation of the shoulder.

A good radiograph is essential, especially the AP view. It will identify the luxation as well as reveal any fracture that might be present (Fig. 5.9).

The luxation may possibly be reduced manually under deep anesthesia. Enough traction has to be applied to maneuver the anconeus into its original position from its luxated position, lateral and caudal to the lateral humeral condyle.

The distal humerus is grasped firmly in one hand, with the thumb and forefinger holding the distal condyle. The proximal radius and ulna is grasped with the other hand. A combination of firm caudal traction and flexion of the joint will angulate and rotate the olecranon back into place. Once reduced, complete smooth range of motion is achieved. The head of the radius is reduced to its normal position at the same time.

The reduced joint usually will stay in place. If the joint reluxates easily, there is probably some ligamentous damage that will require surgical repair.

In a simple luxation, a Velpeau bandage is applied for 4 days, followed by a week of exercise on a leash. A radiograph is taken for forensic purposes and to show that the luxation has been completely reduced. Return of function is to be expected.

On occasion, it will be difficult to apply enough traction to the radius and ulna to bring about reduction. Under sterile conditions, an intramedullary pin is introduced transversely through the olecranon. It is then cut off, but enough of the pin remains projected to afford a good grip for the fingers. Traction on this pin provides a means of controlling the ulna and overcoming the pull of the triceps muscles. The olecranon is drawn caudally, the joint is flexed, and the anconeus is angulated over the lateral condyle. The proximal radius and the ulna joints will be reduced. The pin is then removed.

In those cases where reduction cannot be obtained because of size, swelling, physical damage, or chronicity, either from the owner's neglect or a veterinarian's misdiagnosis of the condition, open reduction is required.

Chronic Luxation of the Elbow

After the initial injury, the body attempts to stabilize the joint by inflammation and the proliferation of fibrous and cartilaginous tissue and bone deposits. As the pain decreases due to the immobilization of the joint, use of the limb returns but lameness persists. Reduction of the luxation will bring about a return of much of the limb's function and full weightbearing, as well as decreasing the degree of lameness. Open reduction is recommended, even when the luxation is several months old.

SURGICAL TECHNIQUE

A caudally-curving incision is made laterally over the anconeal muscle midway between the olecranon and the lateral epicondyle.

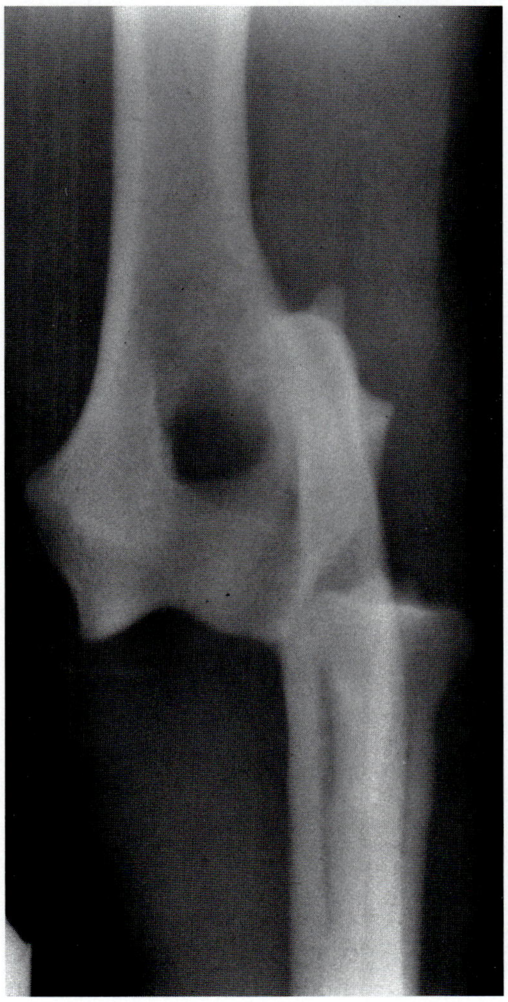

FIGURE 5.9 An AP radiograph of a luxated elbow.

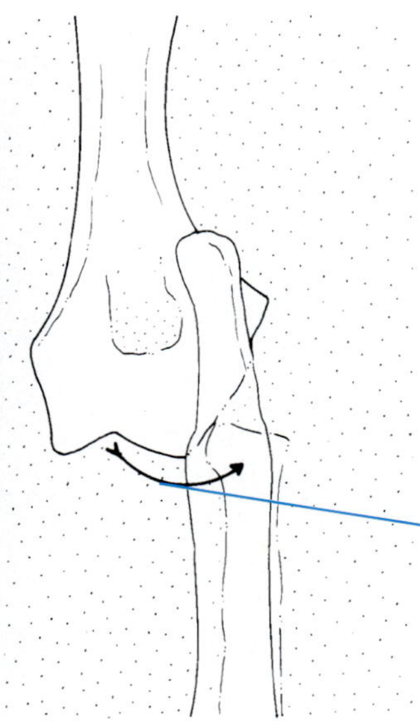

Because of the luxation, these landmarks are less easily identified (Fig. 5.10). The skin and subcutaneous tissues are reflected over the olecranon. Blunt and sharp dissection through the fibrous connective tissue and the adventitious cartilage and bone deposits will identify the caudal edge of the lateral humeral condyle and, caudolateral to it, the anconeal process. An intramedullary pin is driven down the olecranon into the medullary cavity of the ulna. The pin is removed. A Gigli saw is used to transect the olecranon, and the triceps muscle group is reflected craniodorsally. The saw cut must be made at the joining of the anconeus and olecranon. The cut is made straight back (Fig. 5.11). Further sharp and blunt dissection will identify the intercondylar notch. Traction, angulation, and rotation will reduce the luxation, replacing the anconeus in its proper location. Smooth function and a good range of motion will prove that reduction has now been obtained (Fig. 5.12).

The osteotomized fragment is now replaced by driving an intramedullary pin down the previously drilled hole. This will provide accurate realignment. An additional pin is inserted cranially to prevent rotation of the fragment. It must not enter the joint. The pin ends are bent at right angles and cut off.

A transverse hole is drilled lateral to medial through the ulna a few centimeters below the osteotomy site. A figure-8 compression band is made by inserting orthopedic wire through the hole and over the caudal pin in the olecranon. When tightened, it will prevent the pull of the triceps from moving the osteotomized fragment. The pins are tapped close to the bone with a bone hammer (Fig. 5.13).

Closure is done by replacing the reflected skin and subcutaneous tissue after the anconeal fascia or its remnants have been closed.

The leg is placed in a Velpeau sling for 4 days; the dog is exercised 1 week on a leash. Reasonably good function is to be expected.

Congenital Luxation of the Elbow

Congenital luxation of the elbow is rare. When seen, it is often bilateral. The joint is shallow, with little or no trochlear notch and so poorly formed that the ulna merely contacts the humerus in a luxated position (Fig. 5.14).

Depending on the degree of deformity, attempts can be made to provide a functional joint. With marked deformity, the elbow is fused in a natural standing position.

Some of these dogs have borne weight only on their forearms since birth. Once the elbows are fused, the dogs become active and walk well.

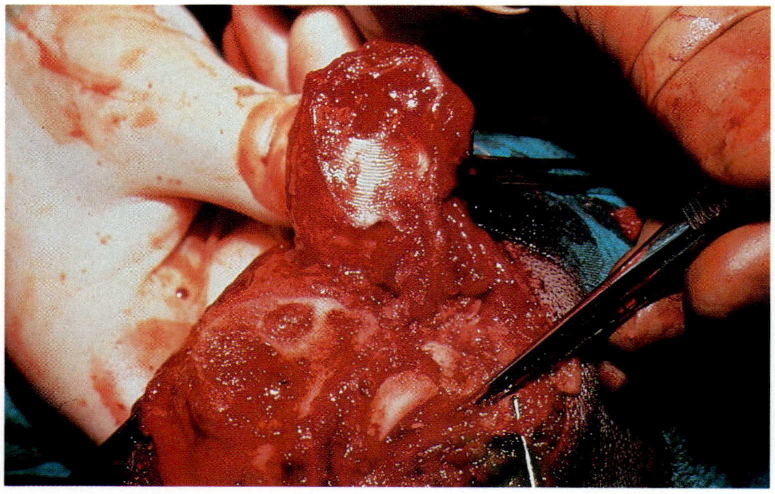

FIGURE 5.10 A luxated elbow at surgery.

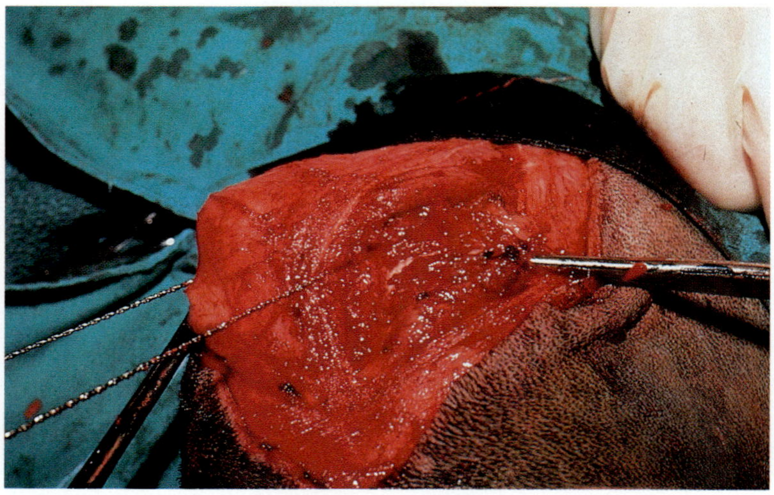

FIGURE 5.11 Osteotomy of the olecranon with a Gigli wire.

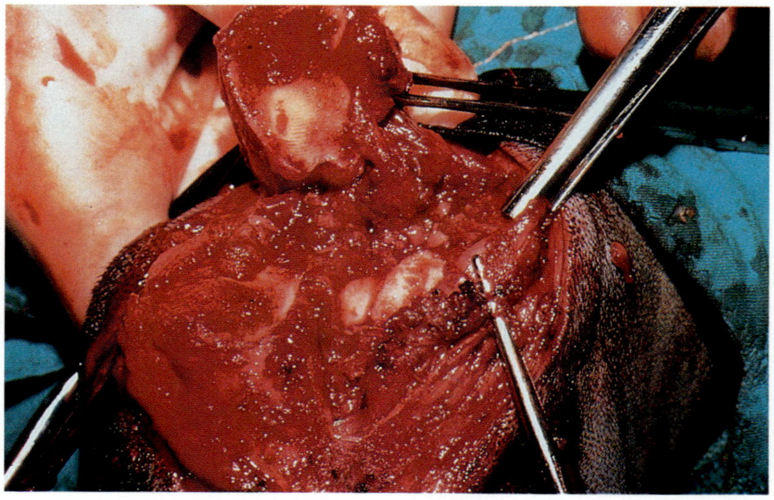

FIGURE 5.12 Reduction of a luxated elbow at surgery.

SURGICAL TECHNIQUE

An incision is made over the elbow joint from the dorsal aspect of the distal humerus to the caudal aspect of the proximal ulna, passing medial to the olecranon, which is located lateromedial to the lateral condyle in its aberrant position. The skin and subcutaneous tissues are undermined and reflected over the olecranon to expose the caudal aspect of the humeral condyle, which is thinly covered with tissue, and the insertion of the triceps on the olecranon. The anconeus is incised to expose the deformed elbow's false joint. The tendon of insertion of the triceps is transected about 1 cm from its insertion. The triceps muscles are reflected to expose the distal humerus. Usually there is a failure of development of the usual features. The false joint surfaces between the olecranon and the humerus are removed with a burr or a high-speed drill.

The head of the radius is also deformed and has no true articulation. The false articular surface of the radial head and its contact with the humerus is removed in the same fashion.

Due to the deformity, the usual location of lag screws and pins for an elbow fusion is not available.

A lag screw, small intramedullary pin, or a K-wire is introduced through the ulna and into the humerus across the former false joint. Depending on the degree of deformity, a small pin is

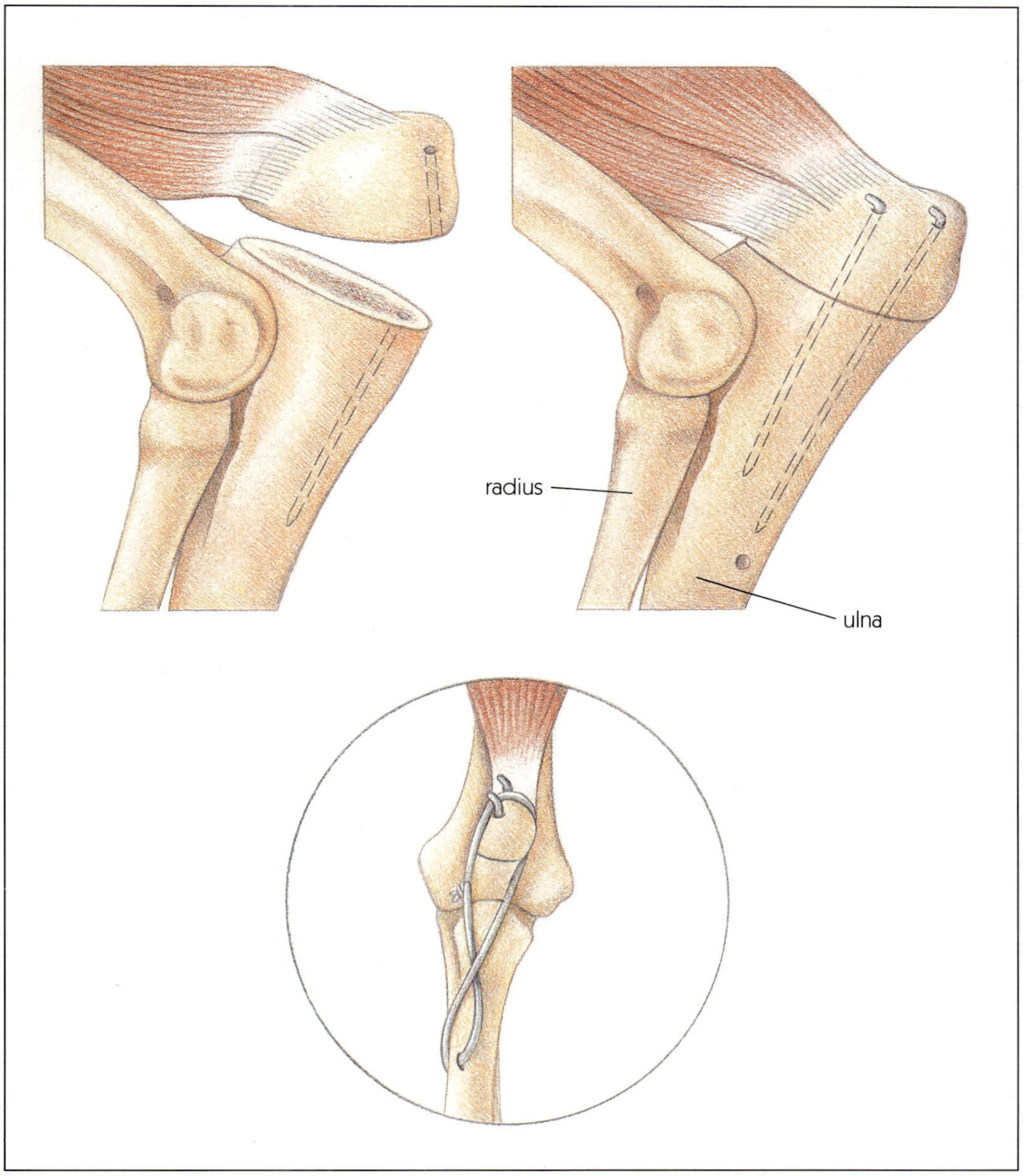

FIGURE 5.13 Compression band figure-8 wire and pins in closure of olecranon osteotomy.

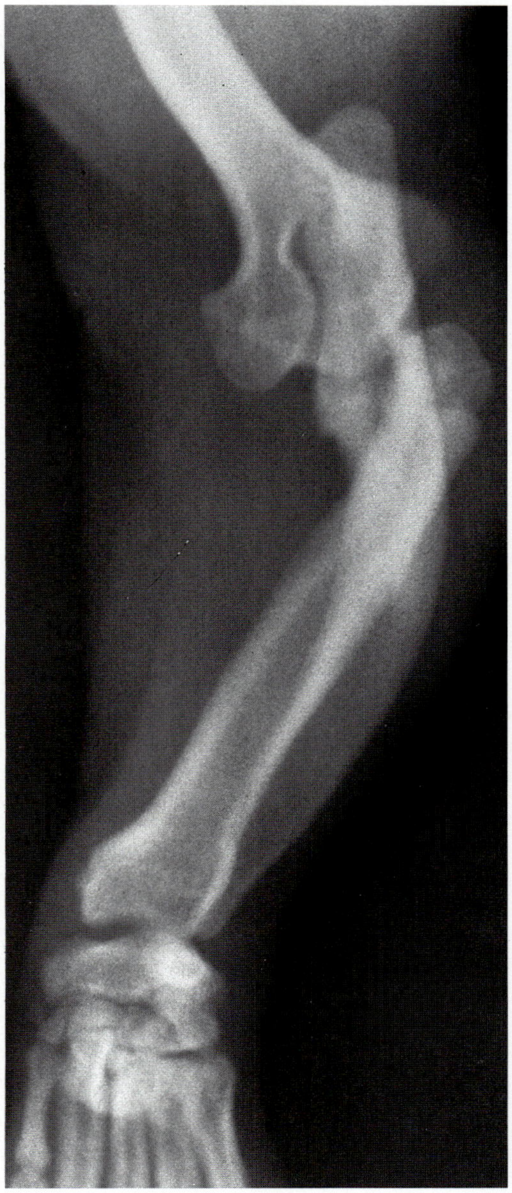

FIGURE 5.14 An AP radiograph of a congenital luxation of the elbow.

driven from the dorsal surface of the humerus into the radial head. Alternatively, a pin is inserted from the lateral surface of the proximal radius across the false joint and into the humerus (Fig. 5.15).

The ends of pins or K-wires are bent at right angles and cut off. They are tapped in close to the bone. A cancellous bone graft is packed at the contact site.

Closure is done by suturing the transected triceps tendon, followed by the usual closure of the skin and subcutaneous tissues.

The leg or legs are placed in full foreleg coaptation splints. Additional care must be given to dogs with bilateral surgeries to prevent pressure sores and soiling.

It takes 4 to 6 weeks to achieve adequate union. The pins and screws are left in place.

Shearing Injuries of the Elbow

Shearing injuries to the elbow occur when a dog is dragged along street pavement by an automobile. The lateral collateral ligaments are destroyed and the joint is unstable, exposed, and contaminated. Repair is by thorough debridement and synthetic replacement of the lateral collateral ligament.

SURGICAL TECHNIQUE

All foreign material as well as dead and useless tissues should be removed completely. A suitable self-tapping bone screw is inserted on the lateral surface of the humeral condyle at the origination of the lateral collateral ligament. A similar screw is inserted on the lateral head of the radius at the insertion of the cranial crus of the lateral collateral ligament. A figure-8 of nonabsorbable suture woven between the two screws replaces the missing ligament (Fig. 5.16).

Usually there is not enough skin and subcutaneous tissue to cover the wound. The area of the wound is covered with sterile antibiotic dressings and allowed to granulate in. The prosthetic ligament provides enough support to allow reasonable joint function. The length of time between the start of healing and complete skin coverage depends on the injury's severity. The prosthetic material remains in situ. Rejection is rare; good results are expected.

Rupture of the medial collateral ligament is rare and is seen in association with fractures and severe luxations.

A medial approach to the area is made through an incision in the skin and subcutaneous tissues directly over the area of the ligament. The origins of the long and lateral digital extensors, if not torn away, are transected and reflected distally. The ligament is inti-

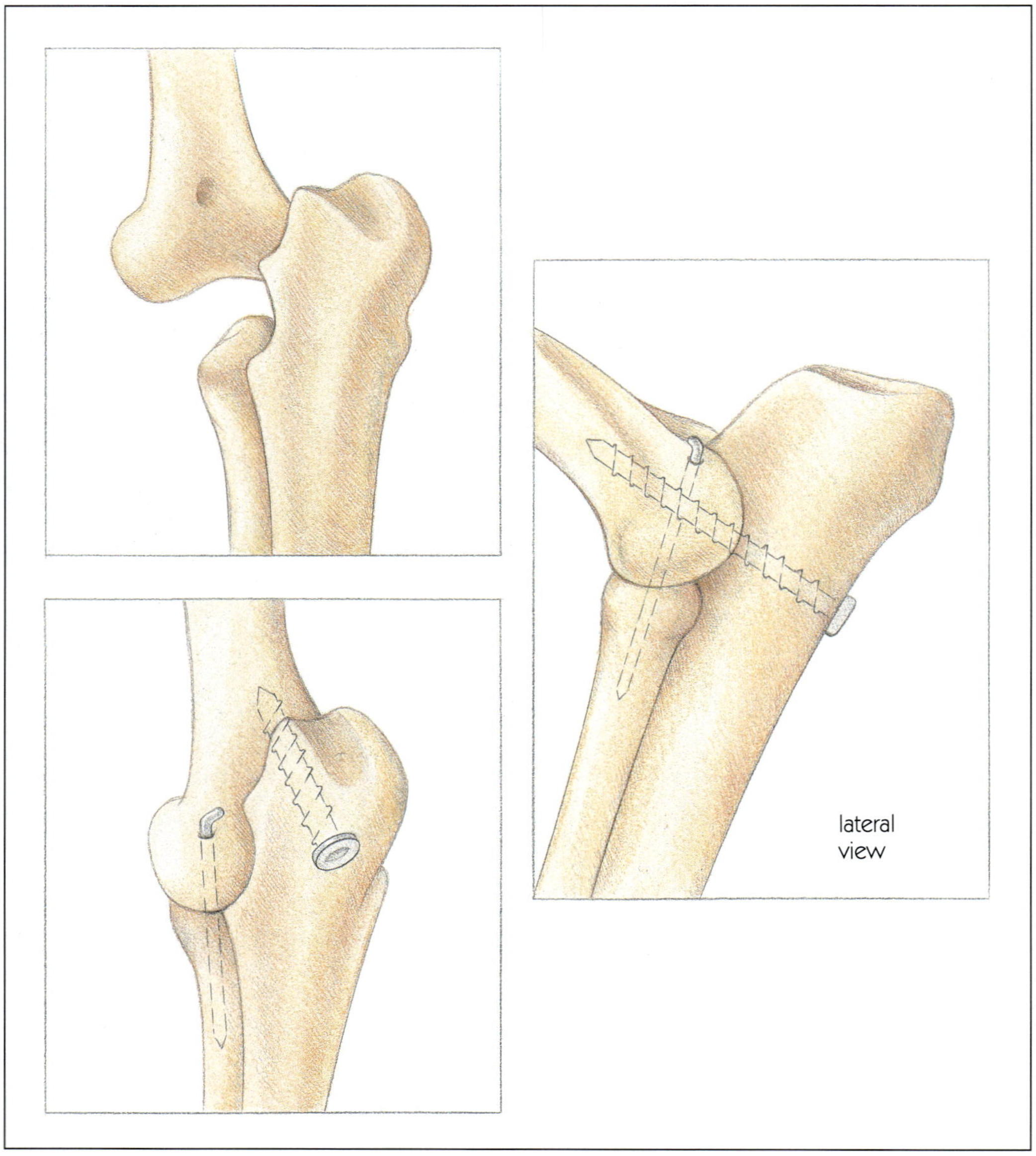

FIGURE 5.15 The fusion of a congenitally luxated elbow.

mately associated with the joint capsule, which may well be partially destroyed. The exception is avulsion of the origin of the ligament from the medial humeral condyle. Here the fragment is replaced and fastened with a small K-wire inserted through it. The wire is bent at a right angle, cut off, and tapped into place with a mallet.

A prosthetic ligament is made by weaving a figure-8 of non-absorbable suture between self-tapping bone screws placed at the ligament's origin on the medial humeral condyle and the most proximal portion of the radius. The transected bellies of the long and lateral digital extensors are sutured back in place. The skin and subcutaneous tissues are closed in the usual manner.

The leg is immobilized in a full foreleg splint for 2 weeks. Good results may be expected, depending on the severity of the concomitant injuries.

Luxation of the Carpus

Luxation (hyperextension) of the carpus is a common, disabling injury (Fig. 5.17). It is seen in either one or both legs and is usually the result of jumping or falling from a height to hard ground.

The palmar ligaments and, in particular, the palmar fibrocartilage are torn, allowing the foot to assume a plantigrade stance. Little pain is involved after recovery from the initial fall, but the dog is quite lame. Some dogs will be completely plantigrade while others may have only exaggerated extension.

The areas affected may be the antebrachiocarpal, middle carpal, or carpometacarpal articulations. Properly taken stress radiographs will be diagnostic (Fig. 5.18). Current treatment is by arthrodesis of the affected carpal articular area. If the antebrachiocarpal articulation is not affected, it is preserved and a partial arthrodesis is performed. If at all possible, this articulation should be preserved. Dogs with a complete arthrodesis of all three levels do quite well, though with some change in gait.

With partial arthrodesis, the flexion of the major carpal joint is preserved. This minimizes the changes in gait and preserves much of the joint's motion.

Partial Carpal Arthrodesis Using Intramedullary Pins

If the hyperextension involves the middle carpal or the carpometacarpal articulations, these may be fused and the antebrachio-

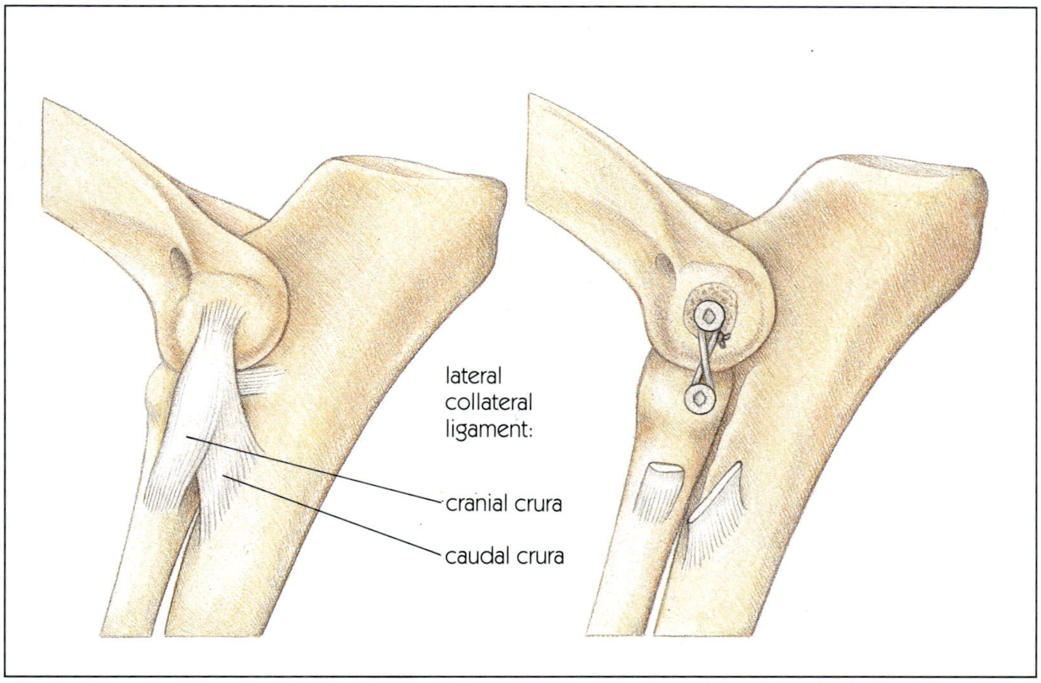

FIGURE 5.16 The placement of screws and sutures for treating a shearing injury to the lateral elbow.

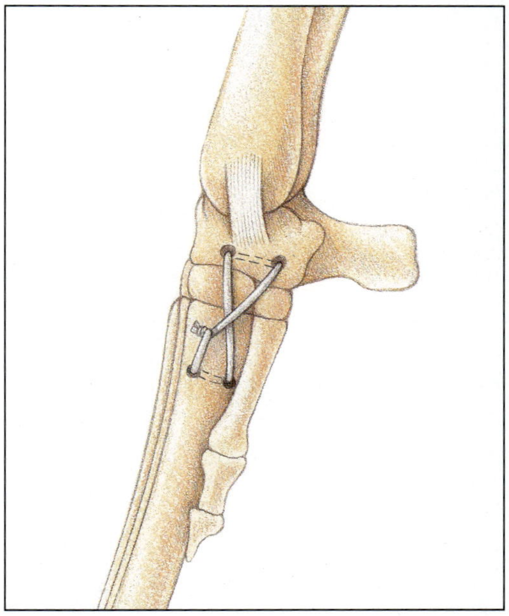

FIGURE 5.17 A middle carpal luxation treated with a figure-8 of wire.

carpal joint preserved. The affected joint articular surfaces are curetted away with a high speed drill and a burr, then packed with cancellous bone grafts from the humerus. Intramedullary pins are introduced up the third and fourth metacarpals to insert into the radial carpal bone (Fig. 5.19).

SURGICAL TECHNIQUE

Just prior to the surgery, a tourniquet is applied over the middle of the forelimb. A dorsal midline incision, through the skin and subcutaneous tissues, is made from the distal radius to the distal ends of the third and fourth metacarpals. Further sharp and blunt dissection over the carpus exposes the tendons of the extensor carpi radialis and distally the tendon of the common digital extensor with all of its branches. The insertion of the tendinous branches of the extensor carpi radialis on metacarpals two and three are preserved.

The articular surfaces of the middle and the carpometacarpal areas and the intercarpal surfaces are removed with the burr of a high-speed drill. These areas will be packed with cancellous bone grafts.

Suitably sized intramedullary pins are driven up the medullary cavities of metacarpals three and four through small holes drilled through the distal dorsal cortex. The carpus is held at a right angle and the pins are driven securely into, but not through, the radial carpal bone. The distal end of each pin is bent at a right angle and cut off.

The tourniquet is removed. The incision is closed by approximating the skin and subcutaneous tissues. The leg is placed in a splint or cast, which should be inspected daily and replaced in 1 week. Fusion is checked by radiographs. The splint or cast is removed in 4 weeks. A modified Robert Jones splint is applied for an additional week.

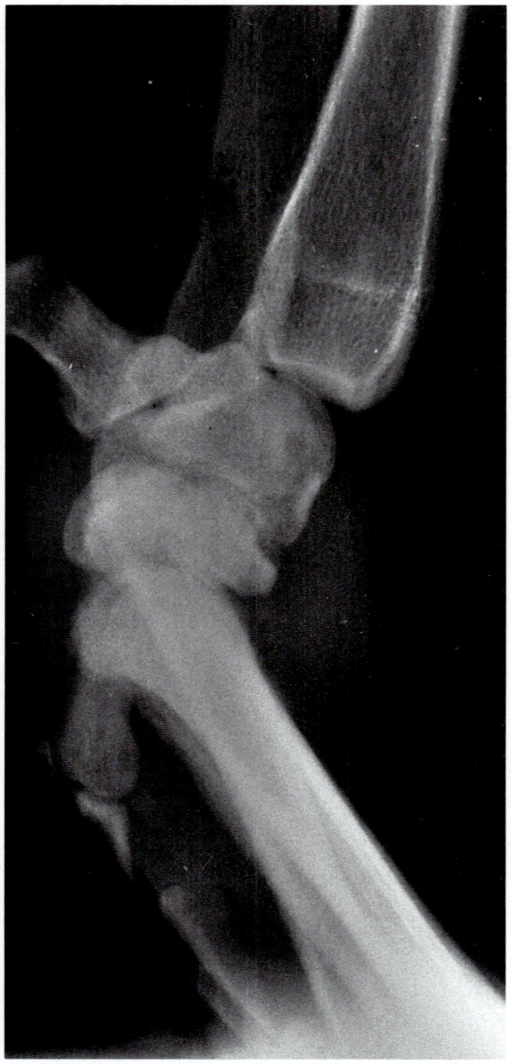

FIGURE 5.18 Radiograph of a carpus under stress, identifying carpal luxation.

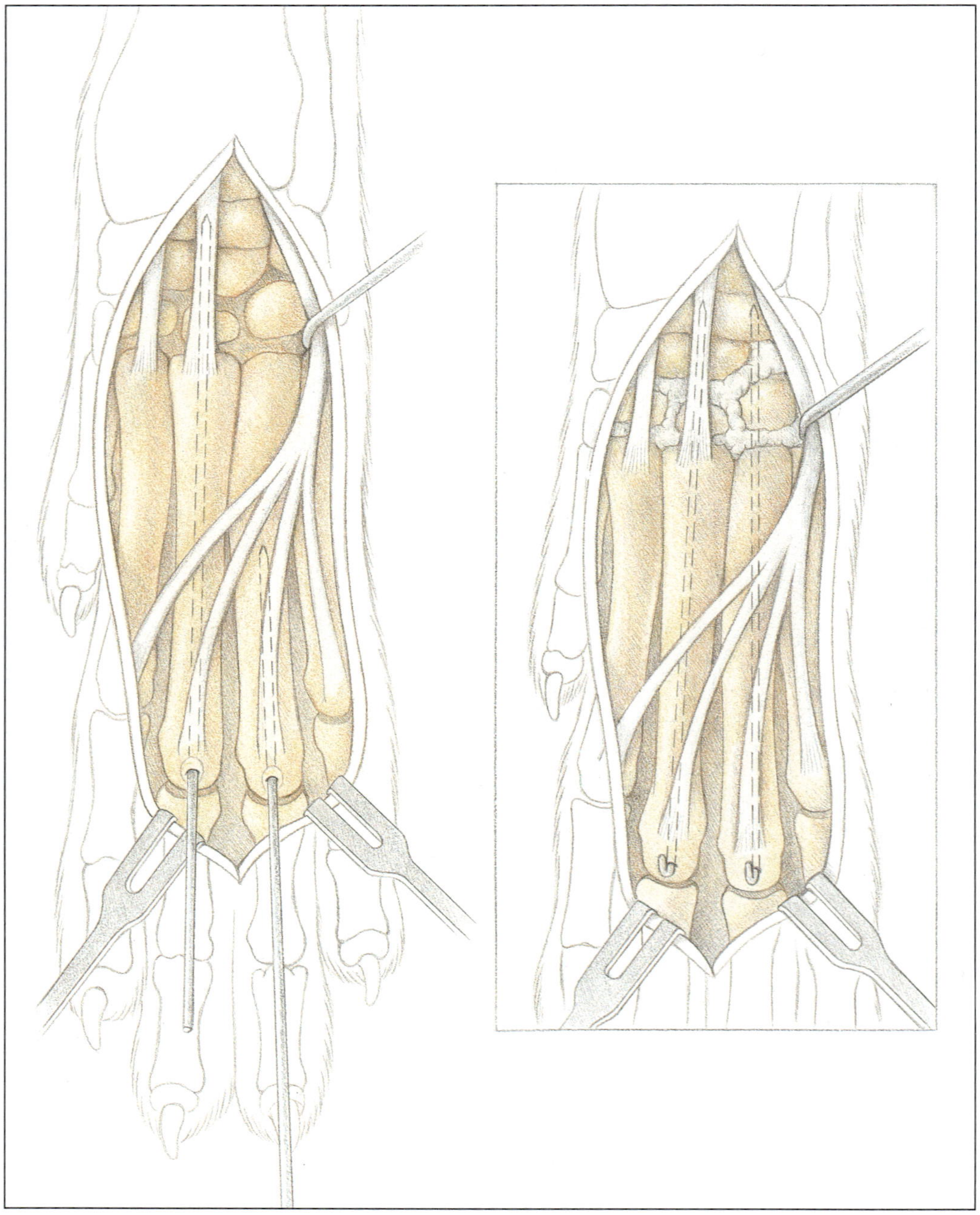

FIGURE 5.19 Partial carpal arthrodesis achieved with intramedullary (IM) pins that were introduced from the metacarpals.

The pins are removed after complete healing. With fusion, the dog will stand in a normal position and have a relatively normal gait.

Partial Arthrodesis Using a Small T-Plate

SURGICAL TECHNIQUE

After surgical exposure, the articular surfaces of the middle, carpometacarpal, and intercarpal areas are removed with a high-speed drill and a burr. These areas are to be packed with cancellous bone graft.

The extensor carpi radialis tendon is severed from its attachment to the third metacarpal bone, elevated and retracted. The small T-plate is contoured to fit the cranial face of the radial carpal bone. It must be located as distally as possible to avoid contact with the radius in full extension. The plate is attached with screws angled proximally to insure solid fixation. The carpus is flexed and the cancellous bone graft material is inserted. The top screw of the center section is inserted into the third carpal bone. If this is not possible, it is inserted in the head of the third metacarpal. The rest of the screws are placed in the shaft of the third metacarpal (Fig. 5.20).

Closure of the skin and subcutaneous tissues is routine. The tourniquet is removed.

The dog is placed in a cast for 4 weeks. When it is removed, a Robert Jones splint is applied for 1 week. With fusion, a satisfactory range of motion and return of function is seen. The plate is not removed.

Complete Carpal Arthrodesis

If the hyperextension is at the antebrachiocarpal level, a complete arthrodesis is done. This involves the placement of a bone plate. All

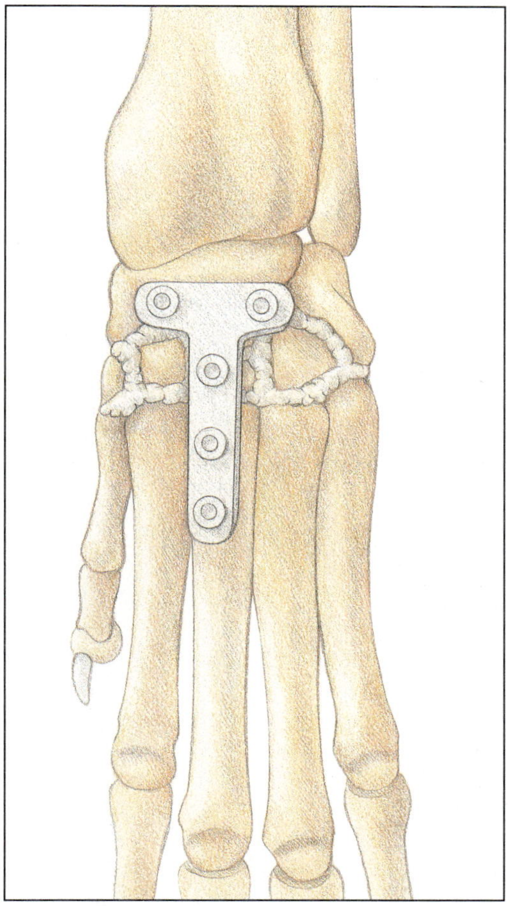

FIGURE 5.20 Placement of a T-plate in a partial carpal arthrodesis.

motion in the carpus is destroyed. A tourniquet is used to control seeping hemorrhage.

SURGICAL TECHNIQUE

A dorsal midline incision is made from the distal third of the radius to the distal third of the third metacarpal. The skin and subcutaneous tissues are reflected and the fascial covering removed to expose the tendon of the extensor carpi radialis, which is retracted medially. Its attachments to the third and fourth metacarpals are cut and the tendon is retracted to expose the groove in which it lies. Further dorsally, the abductor pollicis longus muscle is cut away to provide space for the plate to lie flat to the bone. The joint capsules are cut and the exposed articular surfaces of the antebrachiocarpal, middle carpal, and carpometacarpal articulations are removed with

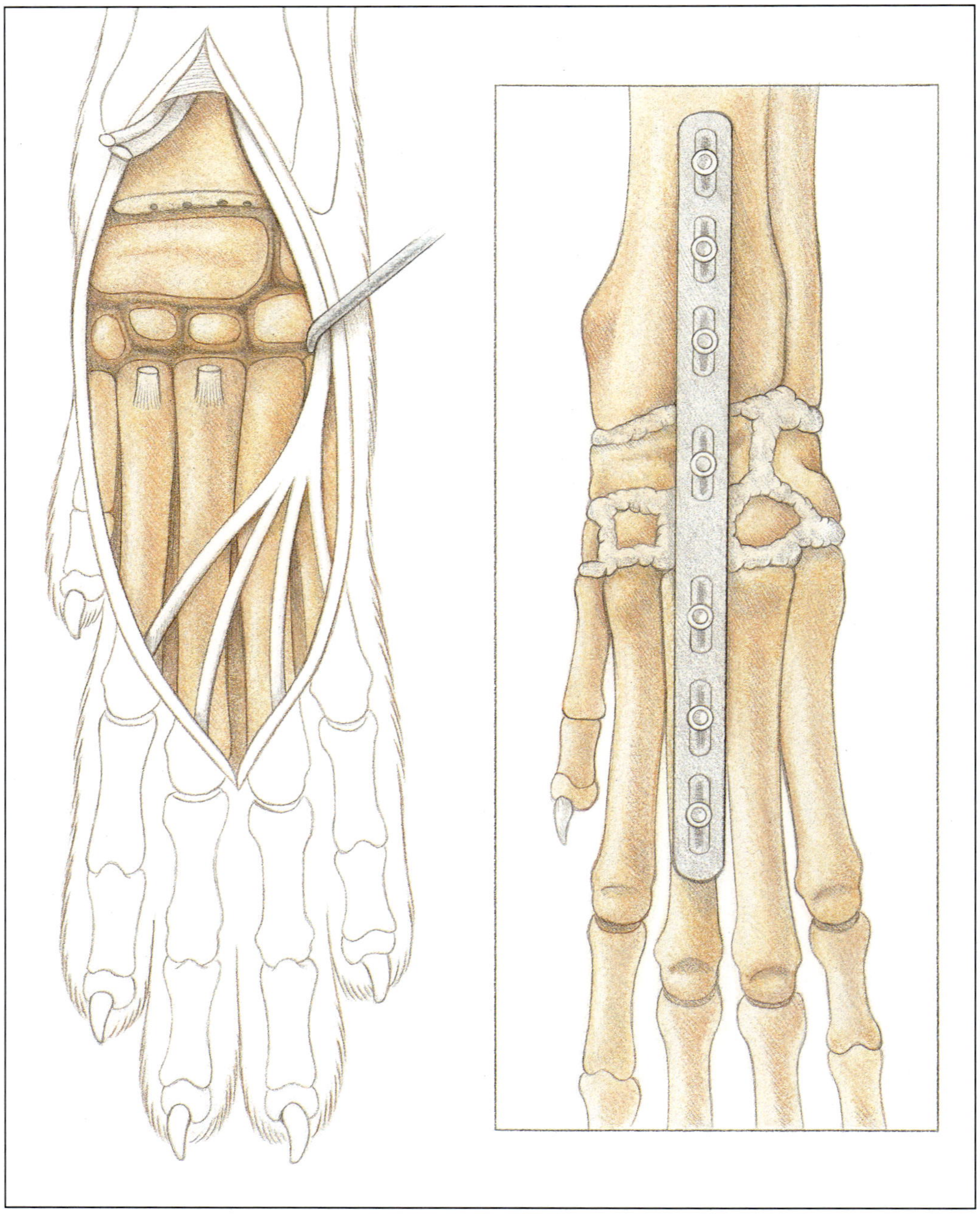

FIGURE 5.21 Placement of a bone plate in a complete carpal arthrodesis.

a high-speed drill and a burr. Small holes are made in the articular surface of the distal radius to contact medullary bone, increasing the opportunity for the ingress of blood vessels.

A suitable seven-hole plate is to be placed with three screws in the radius, one in the radial carpal bone, and three in the third metacarpal. It will be necessary to drill away some of the cranial distal radius to make the plate fit flat to the bone. The plate is bent to allow up to 10 degrees of extension, equal to that of a normal dog.

The debrided articular areas are packed with cancellous bone graft. The plate is placed so that one hole is directly over the radial carpal bone. This screw is placed first. The rest of the screws are placed in the third metacarpal. If a compression plate is used, a hole is drilled so that the screw, when tightened, compresses the antebrachiocarpal space. Cancellous bone is placed under and around the bone plate. The two tendinous branches of the extensor carpi radialis are sutured to the nearby joint capsule fragment. The tendon is replaced over the plate (Fig. 5.21).

A routine closure is performed by suturing the fascia, subcutaneous tissues, and the skin. The leg is placed in a lower leg splint. It is considered good practice to remove plates and screws in 6 to 12 months. A splint is applied for 1 week after the plate is removed. Loose screws cause pain and must be removed or replaced.

The postoperative care is identical to that for partial fusion.

Shearing Injury to the Carpus

This injury is the result of automobile accidents. The lower limb is ground against the pavement, wearing away the skin, muscles, ligaments, and bone. Usually, the medial aspect of the carpus is affected. The radial collateral ligaments are destroyed along with the radial styloid process. The joint surfaces are opened and the area is grossly contaminated. Treatment consists of providing a prosthetic substitute for the collateral ligaments and completely debriding the affected area. Since there is no skin available for coverage, the wound is protected with bandages and treated with antibiotic dressings. The healthy granulation tissue covers the screws and the braided synthetic suture used to replace the ligaments. Draining sinuses rarely occur. Loosening of the screw in the radial carpal bone has been reported. Complete coverage of the denuded area and return of function is to be expected. The area may remain hairless.

SURGICAL TECHNIQUE

The affected area must be thoroughly debrided. The use of a Water-Pic® is recommended. Copious use of physiologic saline or Ringer's solution is needed to ensure good cleaning as well as to remove all dead and severely damaged tissues. Fine thumb forceps are a great aid in picking out bits of gravel, strands of hair, and road debris.

A small, self-tapping bone screw is inserted into the radius at the approximate location of the origin of the collateral ligament. Another screw is placed in the exposed side of the radial carpal bone. A small bone tunnel is drilled craniodorsally at a 45° angle through the craniodistal radius from a position proximal and dorsal to the screw in the radial carpal bone. It exits in normal bone on the dorsal aspect of the distal medial radius.

Heavy braided synthetic suture is placed around the screws and through the bone tunnel to replace the collateral ligament. It is tightened sufficiently to maintain joint stability without interfering with function (Fig. 5.22).

Depending on the severity of the injury, the leg is placed in a splint, which is removed and replaced as the sterile dressings are replaced. If the injury is very severe, stabilization is obtained with a K/E external fixation splint.

About two months or more may be required for granulation tissues to fill the defect and cover the screws and suture material. The K/E apparatus is removed in 3 or 4 weeks, followed by support with a modified Robert Jones splint for 2 more weeks.

What may appear to be an irreparable injury, when treated in this manner, generally results in a satisfactory outcome.

Luxation of the Hip

Acute Luxation

Uncomplicated luxation refers to the condition caused by trauma whereby the femoral head is forced from the acetabulum, usually craniodorsally, with minimal damage to the surrounding structures. Rarely, the femoral head is located caudoventrally.

Replacement should be done as soon as possible, since muscle spasm, scar tissue filling of the acetabulum, adhesion of the ligament of the femoral head, erosion of the femoral head, and false joint formation tend to make replacement and maintenance of the reduction more difficult as time passes.

Good radiographs are essential. Not only do they give information as to the diagnosis and severity of the luxation, but they also offer proof of the diagnosis in case there is litigation (Fig. 5.23).

Closed reduction is effected first, if possible, and the leg is placed in either a flexion maintaining sling (Ehmer) or, preferably, a pelvic limb sling.

SURGICAL TECHNIQUE

The dog is anesthetized and laid on its side with the affected leg uppermost. A soft cotton rope is looped under the groin of the luxated leg and secured firmly opposite the operator. This will restrain the body of the dog while traction is applied to the leg.

The affected leg is grasped around the tibia with the heel of the hand resting near the hock. On the right hind leg, the right-

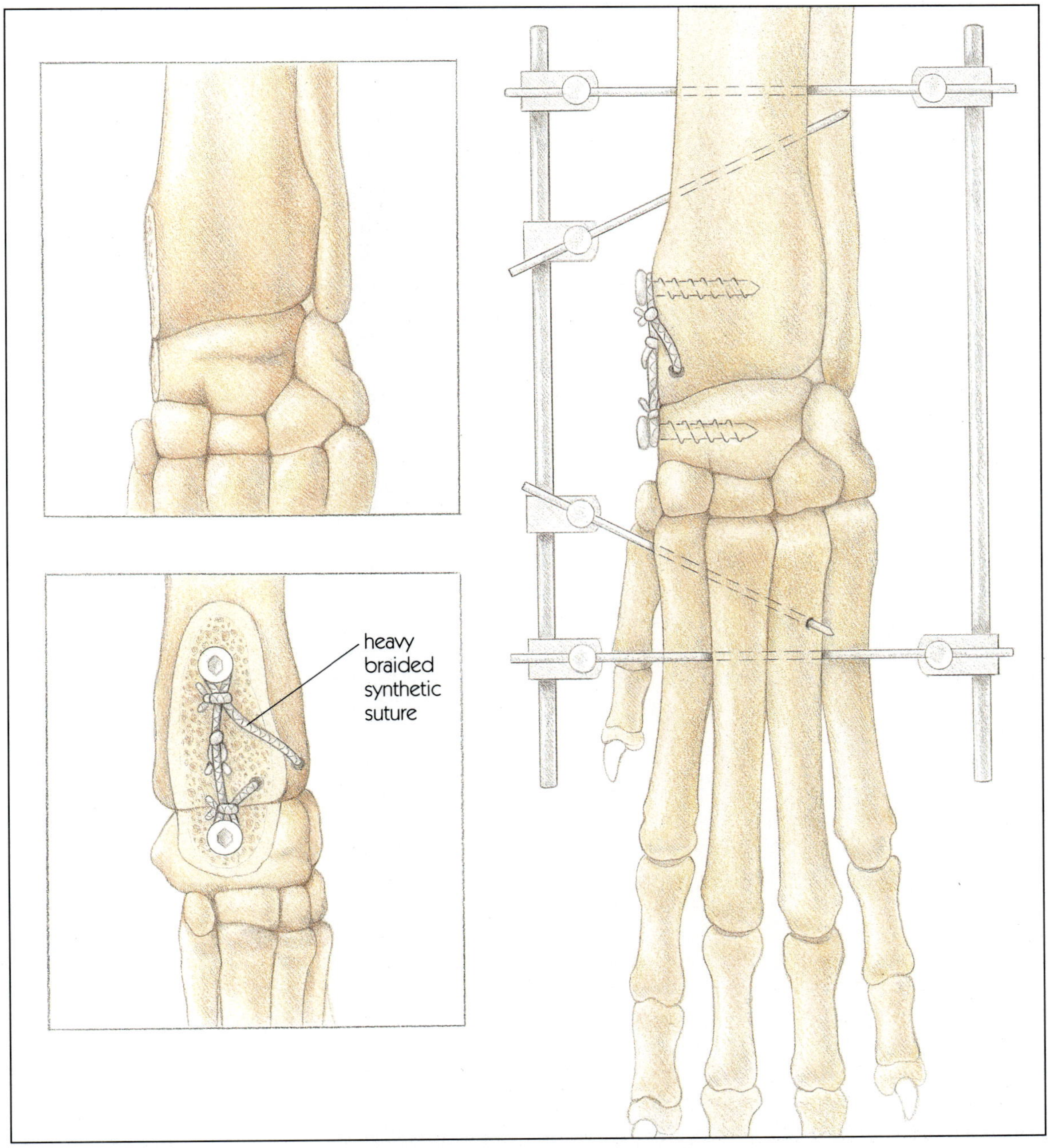

FIGURE 5.22 Placement of screws, bone tunnel, and suture material in treating a shearing injury of the carpus. Additional stability is achieved with an external fixation splint.

handed operator presses with the left hand from the caudal aspect on the trochanter major with the middle finger and against the femur on the medial side with the thumb. This helps to monitor and guide the reduction. The leg is pulled caudally and ventrally as it is held abducted. Firm continued traction will tire the muscles, making it possible for the femoral head to be brought up and over the lip of the acetabulum. The leg is now held flexed and in abduction by an assistant, who keeps pressure on the trochanter and keeps the leg flexed by grasping the hock (Fig. 5.24).

An Ehmer sling may be applied. There are several variations in the application of this sling. A heavy 2-inch or 3-inch adhesive bandage or tape is used. A wrap is made around the metatarsal area with the short end on the lateral side. The tape is brought medially over the cranial femoral region and returned to its origin on the lateral aspect of the metatarsus. The tape is now passed on the medial side of the leg to the dorsocranial femoral region. It is brought high over the thigh and down over the medial hock. The tape is continued ventral and lateral to the metatarsal area and is again passed on to the medial side of the thigh. Additional strips of tape may be applied in the same configuration (Fig. 5.25).

Beginning on the plantar lateral aspect of the hind paw, the gauze roll is unwound so that it progresses up the medial aspect of the thigh over the quadriceps musculature, down the lateral aspect, then medial to the metatarsus. This is repeated to produce a series of figure-8s.

The bandaging may include the paw, using the claws to anchor the bandage. The gauze is covered with adhesive tape.

The metatarsal area is padded with cotton to prevent circulatory obstruction. With the stifle and hock completely flexed, 2-inch or 3-inch adhesive tape is wrapped around the flexed limb from footpad to calcaneus.

A strip of adhesive is now placed from near the calcaneus over the lateral aspect of the limb, over the top of the lumbar spine, where it is held in place by a belly-band of circumferentially applied adhesive tape.

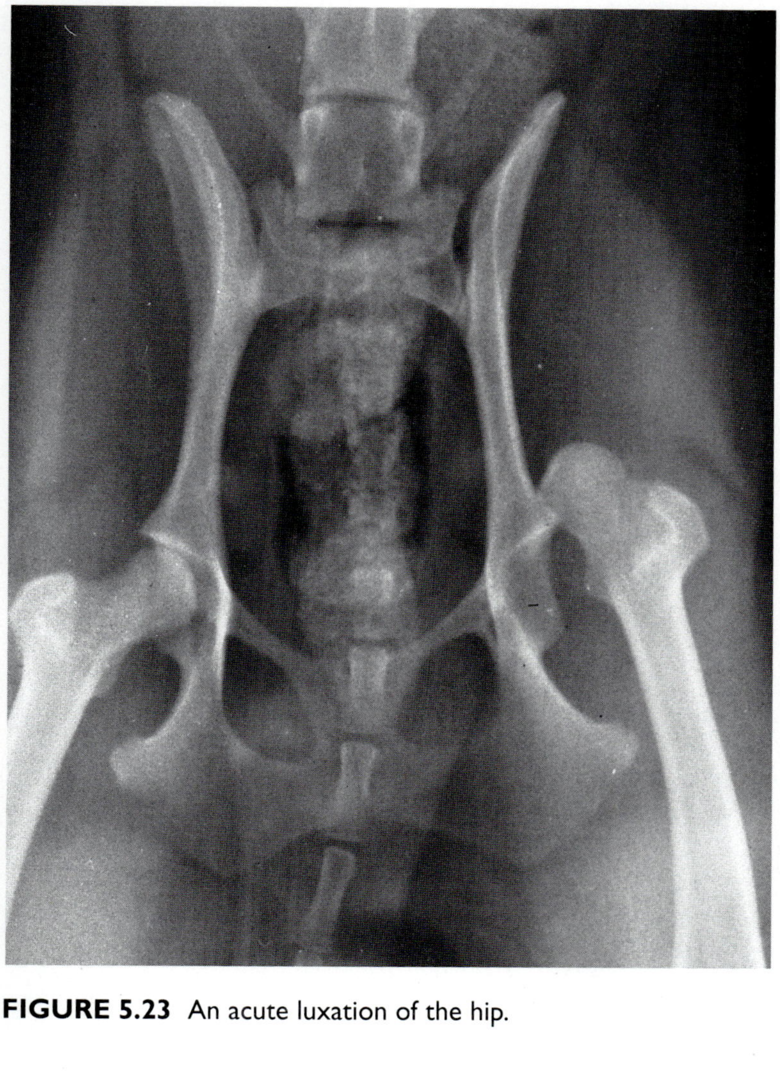

FIGURE 5.23 An acute luxation of the hip.

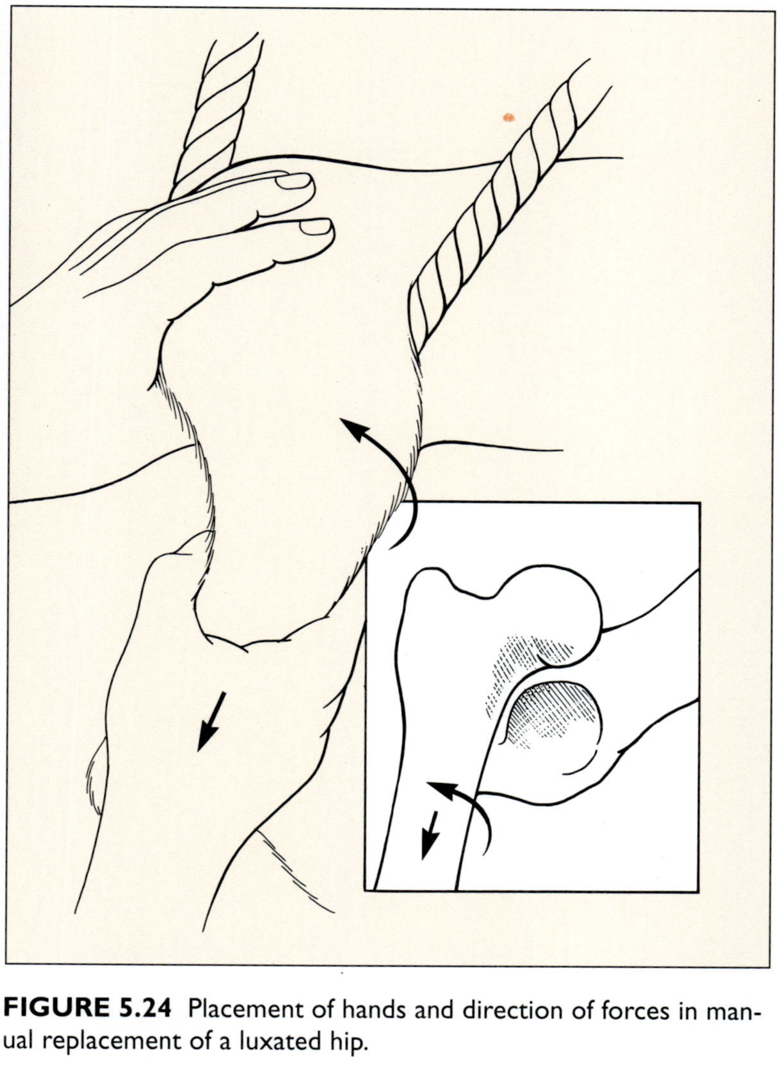

FIGURE 5.24 Placement of hands and direction of forces in manual replacement of a luxated hip.

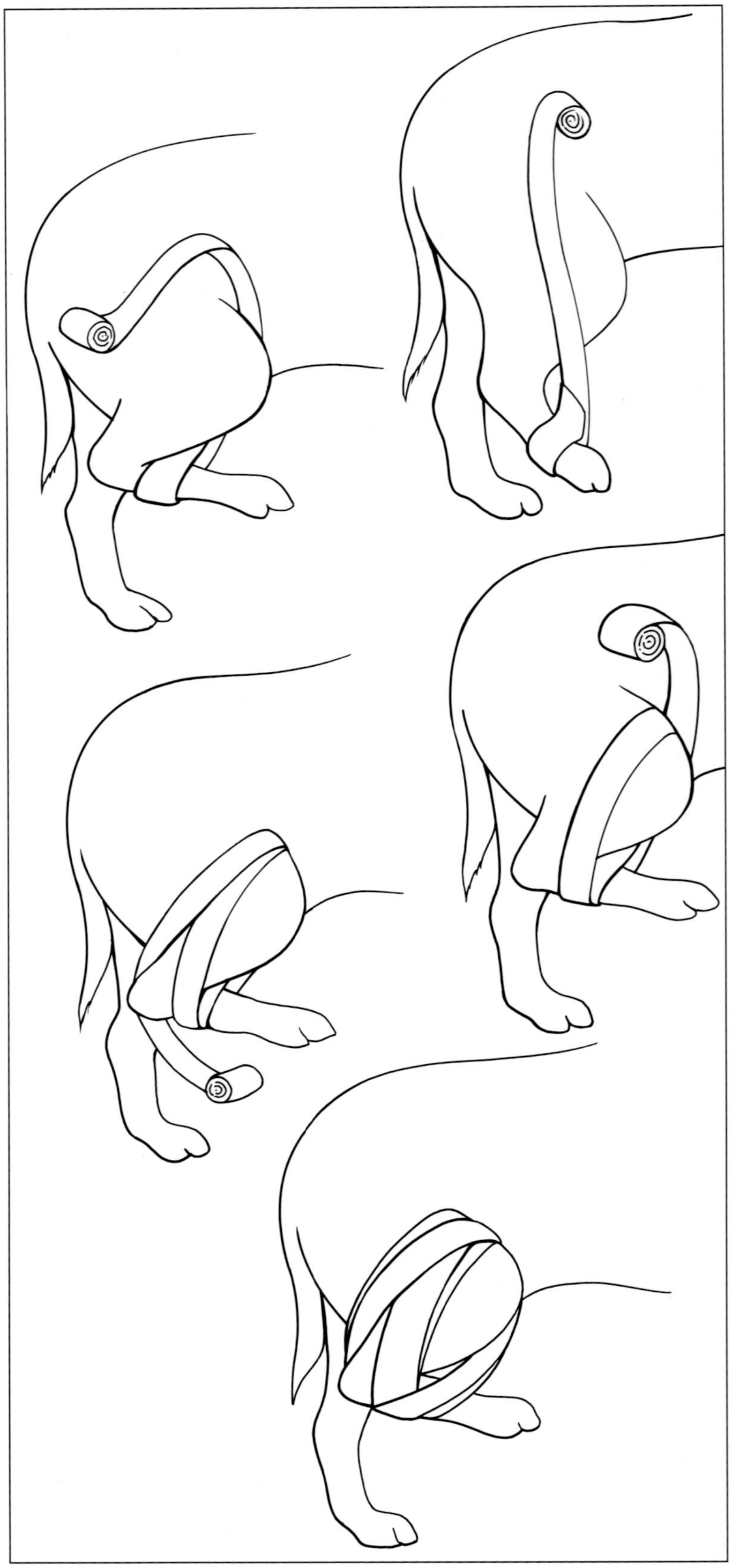

FIGURE 5.25 The application of an Ehmer sling.

The preferred sling is a pelvic limb sling, which will fit all dogs, from the smallest and lightest to the tallest and most obese. It has the advantage of restricting weight-bearing, maintaining some flexion, and minimizing possible circulatory or joint injury and pressure necrosis (Fig. 5.26).

The metatarsus and foot are wrapped in cotton and covered with bandage and adhesive tape. A circumferential adhesive tape bandage is placed around the caudal chest. A heavy band, made of two strips of adhesive pressed together, is placed from the metatarsal area to the dorsum of the spine over the caudal chest and secured to the adhesive tape previously applied. The band from the foot is adjusted to keep the foot forward enough to prevent its use. A restraining loop is made of a doubled strip of adhesive tape and placed from caudal to the head of the tibia to be secured to the long band going from the foot to the spine. This keeps the long strip in place.

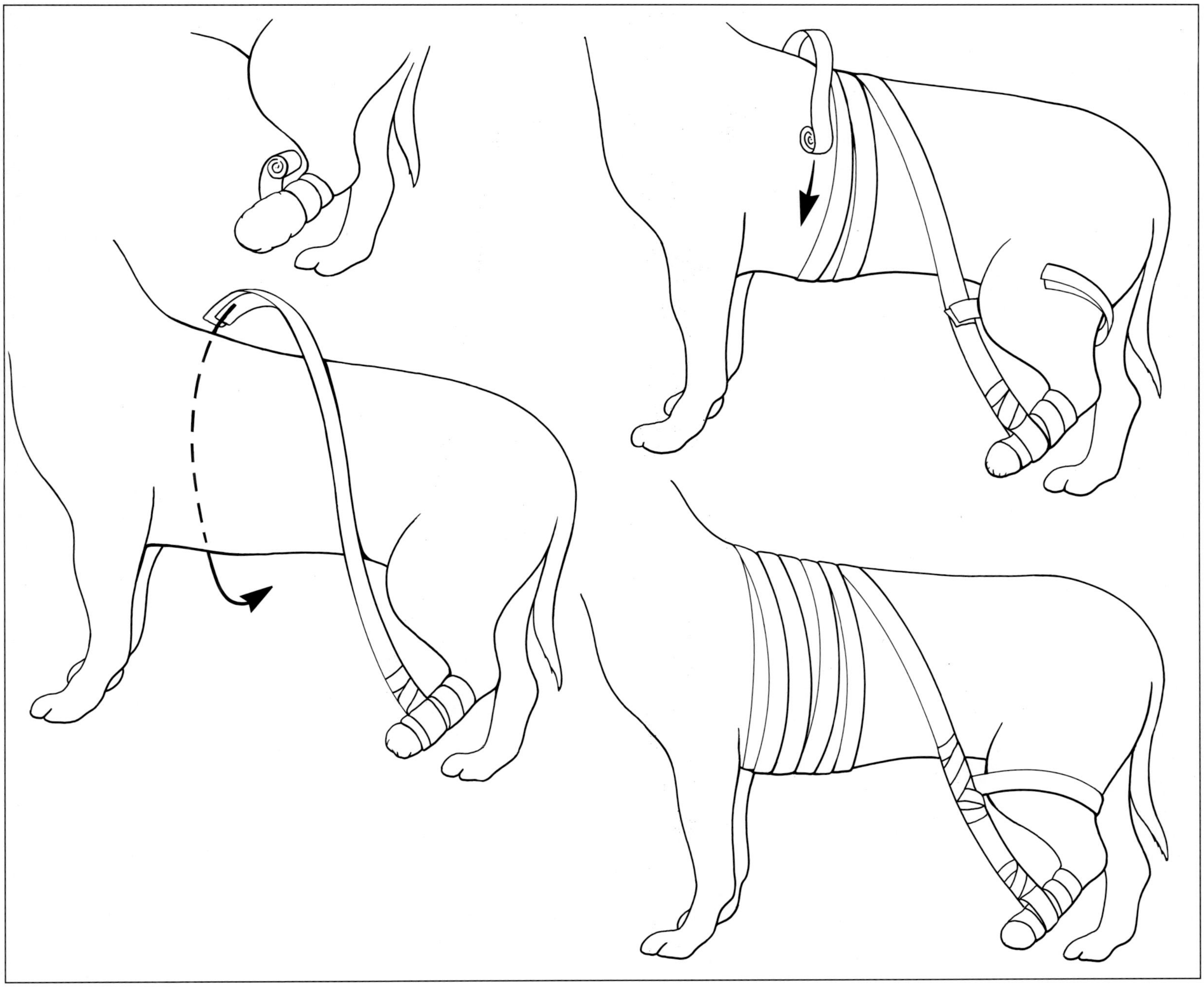

FIGURE 5.26 The application of a pelvic limb sling (Robinson sling).

Slings are kept on for about 10 days. The dog is then caged and not allowed much exercise for another 2 weeks. The leg should be examined daily.

Closed reduction is not always successful. Torn joint capsule, enlarged ligament of the femoral head, scar tissue filling of the acetabulum, and peripheral muscle damage can prevent reduction or its maintenance with a simple sling. These cases will require surgical repair.

Chronic Luxation

Hip dislocations that have been out of the acetabulum for more than a week or two, that have a history of chronic reluxation, or that cannot be reduced manually, often benefit from surgery. Such luxations are common and require good x-rays and physical examination to determine which surgical procedure is the best. Hip dysplasia must be ruled out, since this condition will require a separate mode of treatment. Other conditions such as fracture of the femoral neck, slipped capital epiphysis, fractured acetabulum or other pelvic fractures, well-developed false joints, bone tumors, growth defects, and possible dietary defects complicate the diagnosis. Once the diagnosis is established, an open reduction is performed. The usual approach is craniolateral.

SURGICAL TECHNIQUE

An incision is made through the skin and subcutaneous tissues cranial and parallel to the shaft of the femur from halfway between the trochanter major and the dorsal spine to a point one third the way down the femur. The skin and subcutaneous tissues are retracted cranially and caudally. By sharp and blunt dissection the superficial gluteus is incised and retracted cranially and caudally. The middle gluteus is retracted dorsally. The incision is extended distally to cut through the tensor fascia lata and the fascia lata, exposing the deep gluteus. In most chronic luxations, the femoral head will be located craniodorsal to the acetabulum. Considerable tissue damage may be present. The joint capsule, a portion of the deep gluteus, and the ligament of the femoral head will be torn away. The acetabulum will need to be cleansed of scar tissue and blood clots. Occasionally the ligament of the femoral head will have attached a small amount of bone, which was avulsed from the femoral head. This same ligament can reestablish itself once outside the joint by attaching itself to the pelvis. If more than one third of the femoral head is damaged it cannot remain reduced; a femoral head ostectomy or a prosthetic total hip replacement may be the only surgical choices. If more exposure is needed, the trochanter major may be osteotomized to permit dorsal retraction of the middle gluteus.

SURGICAL TECHNIQUE

A dorsal approach to the hip is obtained by osteotomy of the trochanter major.

The initial approach is identical to the craniolateral approach until the gluteus medius is isolated. Instead of being retracted, its insertion on the trochanter major is osteotomized with a wire saw or an osteotome. The muscle and the attached bone fragment are retracted dorsolaterally, which exposes the dorsal acetabulum. Retraction of the muscle gives a much greater exposure and thus permits removal of tissues from the acetabulum, and makes replacement easier by removing the pull of the middle gluteus. If it is at all possible, the torn joint capsule and damaged deep gluteus are resutured. Replacement of the osteotomized fragment either at the site from which it was cut, or at a new location on the femur prepared slightly more caudal and ventral, is performed. This will increase the inward rotation and compression of the femoral head into the acetabulum. Two K-wires or small intramedullary pins are introduced through the osteotomized fragment, securing it to the femur. Each pin end is bent at a right angle and cut off. A transverse hole is drilled craniocaudally through the proximal femur about 1 cm below the osteotomy line. Orthopedic wire is placed through the drilled hole and over one or both of the K-wires in a figure-8 and twisted tightly to compress the bone fragment into its

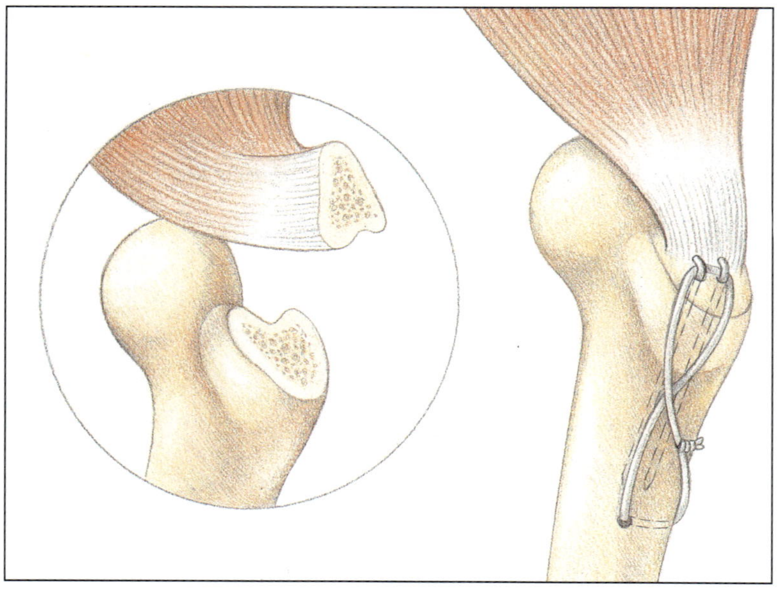

FIGURE 5.27 Figure-8 wiring is shown replacing an osteotomized trochanter.

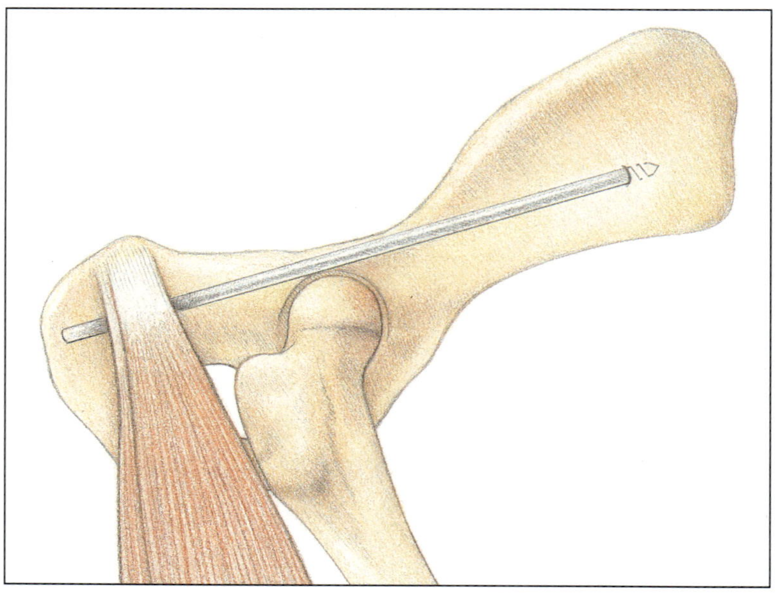

FIGURE 5.28 Placement of a DeVita pin.

bed (Fig. 5.27). Closure is the same as for the craniolateral approach: the incisions in the various layers are closed with 2-0 suture. The skin is closed with nonabsorbable suture.

A variety of modes of restraint have been devised in order to retain the femoral head within the acetabulum. Among these are:

The DeVita Pin

Basically, the DeVita pin consists of a threaded intramedullary pin that is introduced through a small incision in the skin and subcutaneous tissue just ventral to the caudal ischium and driven cranially through the muscle tissue to pass over the area just dorsal to the dorsal rim of the acetabulum. It is aimed slightly upward and outward to insure that it does not injure the ischiatic nerve. The pin is advanced through the muscle tissues to insert in the center of the outwardly flared portion of the illial wing. Once the tip of the pin contacts the bone, the pin is threaded into the ilial wing until it is secure. The pin is cut off under the skin at the ischium and the small incision is closed (Fig. 5.28).

The pin may be removed from 10 days to 1 month later. If the pin becomes loosened from too much activity by the dog, it can migrate into the lumbar area and cause pain.

The advantages of the DeVita are its simplicity, low cost, and ability to give the dog use of the limb. The chief disadvantage is that it is not always effective.

The Transfixion Pin

An open reduction is performed and the femoral head and acetabulum are prepared to be reduced. A small-diameter intramedullary pin is inserted from the fovea capitis through the femoral head and neck and exits laterally on the proximal shaft of the femur. The pin is withdrawn until only the tip of its point is present at the femoral head surface. The hip is reduced and the leg is held in a position similar to a comfortable standing range. The pin is now drilled through the acetabulum until it penetrates the pelvic cavity only a short way. The pin is withdrawn slightly, bent at a right angle, cut off, and tapped back into place with a mallet. This right-angled bend prevents pin migration. The femoral head is maintained in the acetabulum. The amount of activity must be strictly curtailed. The pin must be removed after the repair of tissues surrounding the hip has taken place. This method has the best success in small dogs and cats. Damage to the acetabulum can occur (Fig. 5.29).

The Knowles Toggle Pin

Toggle pinning requires a toggle pin that is made by twisting the smallest diameter intramedullary pin around the next larger sized pin to produce a loop that is then slightly flattened with a pair of pliers. The ends are cut 5 mm away from the central loop. A "button" is also made which consists of two similarly-made consecutive loops. A blunt 15-gauge hypodermic needle is required.

At open reduction a 1/8-inch hole is drilled from the fovea capitis through the femoral head, neck, and proximal femur to exit just below the trochanteric ridge. A special drill guide may be used to insure the proper location of this hole. Heavy #2 nonabsorbable suture is threaded through the loop in the toggle. One end of the toggle is inserted in the tip of the 15-gauge needle, which is then used to push the toggle through the hole in the femoral shaft to exit at the femoral head. The needle is removed. A hole of similar diameter is

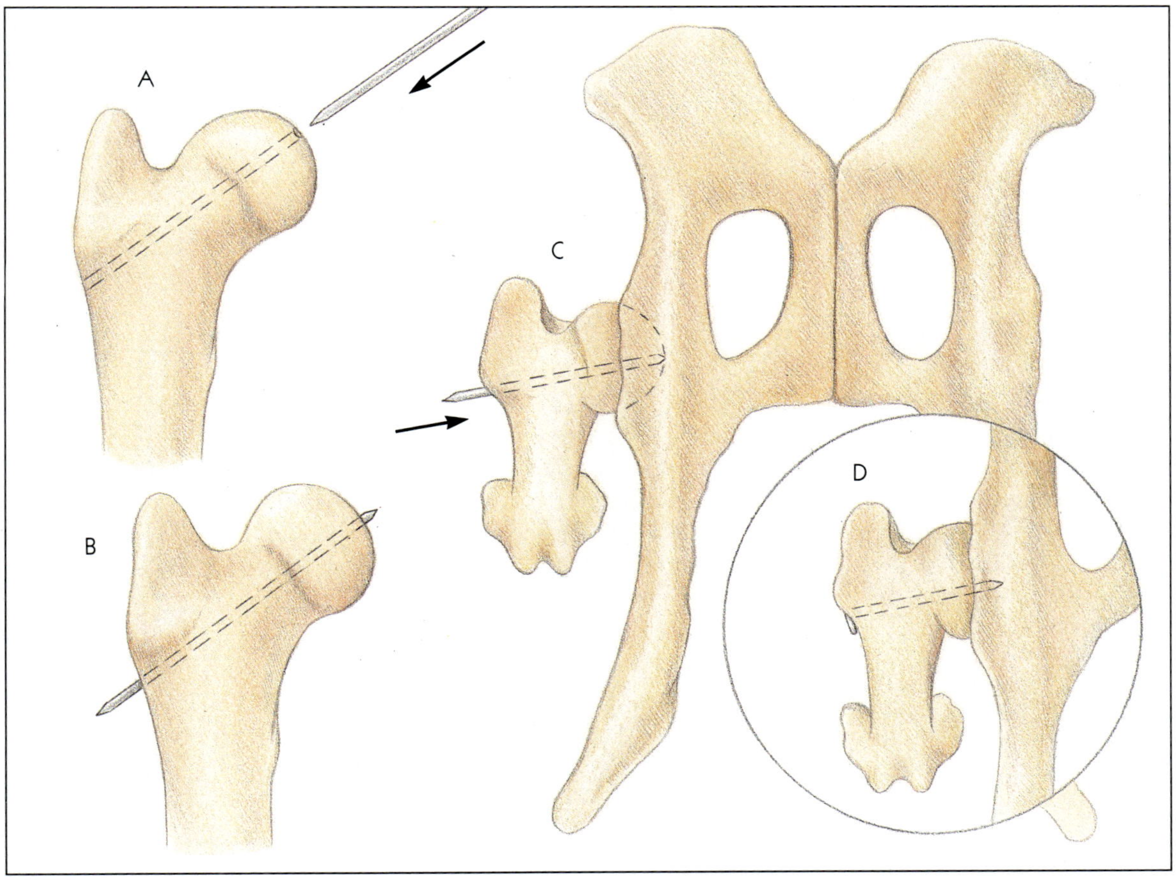

FIGURE 5.29 The placement of a transfixion pin in treating chronic hip luxation. (A) The pin is driven retrograde from the center of the femoral head, through the femoral neck, to exit on the lateral side of the proximal femoral shaft. (B) The pin is withdrawn until its end is flush with the femoral head. (C) The femoral head is replaced. The pin is driven through the acetabulum into the pelvic bone, then bent at a right angle and cut off. (D) It is tapped firmly into place against the femoral shaft's surface.

drilled through the floor of the acetabulum at the point where the ligament of the femoral head had been attached. The toggle pin is pushed through this hole into the pelvic cavity. Here it turns so that it can not be withdrawn, holding the suture in position. The hip is seated in the acetabulum and the two ends of the suture are retracted. Enough slack must be allowed for full range of motion of the hip. The two ends of the suture are passed through the two loops in the "button" and tied securely. The ligament of the femoral head has thus been replaced. This will be quite effective in larger dogs, since there is a size limitation to the hole that can be drilled through the femoral head and neck. Routine muscle and tissue closure is done. The animal must be restrained, using the leg only at a walk for a week or two. Where applicable, this method of prosthetic replacement has proven quite satisfactory, but it is time-consuming and requires ingenuity to correctly prepare the toggle and the "button" (Fig. 5.30).

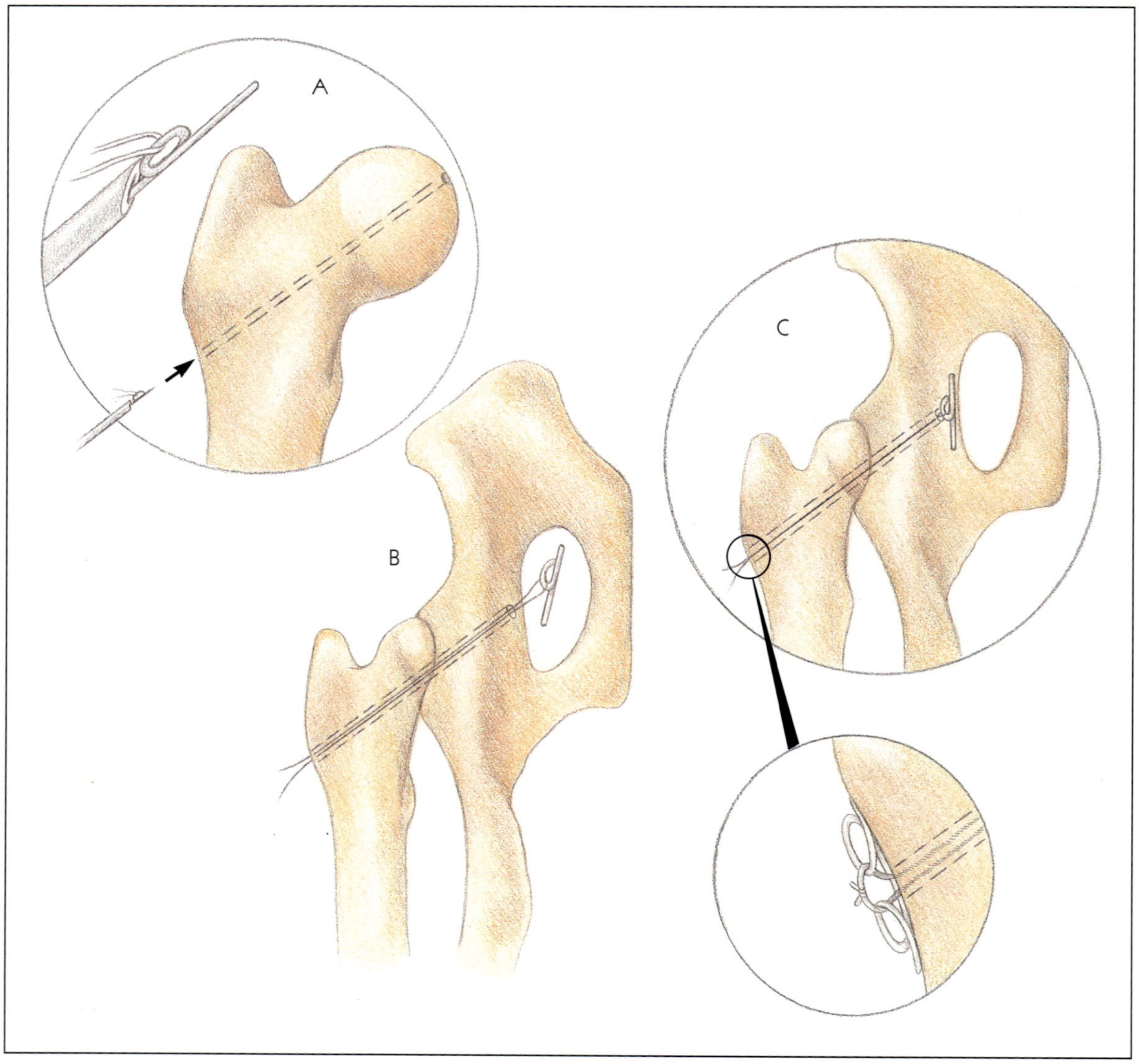

FIGURE 5.30 The placement of a Knowles toggle pin for treatment of a chronic hip luxation. (A) A hole is drilled from the center of the femoral head to the lateral surface of the femoral shaft. The toggle pin with the suture threaded through it is placed in a 15-gauge blunt needle. (B) The pin is inserted through a hole drilled through the acetabulum into the pelvic cavity. (C) The pin is pulled tightly against the pelvic bone, securing the hip, but allowing complete range of motion. The ends of the suture are tied to the double looped pin.

The Synthetic Joint Capsule

A satisfactory method of maintaining the reduction of a luxated hip is to provide a prosthetic joint capsule repair with bone screws and nonabsorbable suture material.

SURGICAL TECHNIQUE

An open reduction is performed and the femoral head is replaced into the cleaned-out acetabulum. The craniolateral area above the acetabular rim is usually free of muscle tissue and joint capsule. A small bone screw is inserted in a dorsal location; care is taken in order to make sure that the screw does not enter into the acetabulum. A similar screw is placed anterodorsally. The tissues at the confluence of the femoral neck on the cranial aspect of the femur are removed with a periosteal elevator. A bone screw is inserted in this location and nonabsorbable suture material is placed in a figure-8 between this screw and each of the acetabular rim screws. The suture should not be tight enough to restrict the hip's full range of motion, but it should have enough strength to restrain any tendency of the hip to luxate. Additional sutures are placed to insure that the figure-8 suture will not slip off. The screws are tightened firmly. Closure is routine. There are many advantages to this procedure. Almost immediate use of the limb is possible. Adverse reaction to the presence of the surgical suture is minimal and results in a stronger joint capsule replacement. Extensive exposure is not required. It is necessary to have some small self-tapping bone screws, a screwdriver and a 1/8-inch bone drill or intramedullary pin with a chuck and a key. This procedure is not applicable to dysplastic hips (Fig. 5.31).

Excision of the Femoral Head

A salvage procedure when all else has failed is to excise the femoral head and neck with a femoral head ostectomy.

SURGICAL TECHNIQUE

A standard craniolateral approach is taken and the tissues surrounding the femoral head and neck are trimmed away so that a good exposure of the neck may be obtained. The hip is usually in a luxated position or is placed in one. It is most important that the femoral neck be completely removed. Any projection that might strike the acetabulum will cause pain to and disuse of the leg. The entire procedure depends on the development of a strong, pain-free, false joint.

A power-driven bone saw, Gigli saw, or osteotome is used to cut the femoral neck. The incision should be parallel to the shaft of the femur. Care must be taken to cut only in the bone since injury to the ischiatic nerve or to nearby blood vessels could occur.

The femoral head is removed and the area of the neck is examined for projections, then smoothed with a small rongeur (Fig. 5.32).

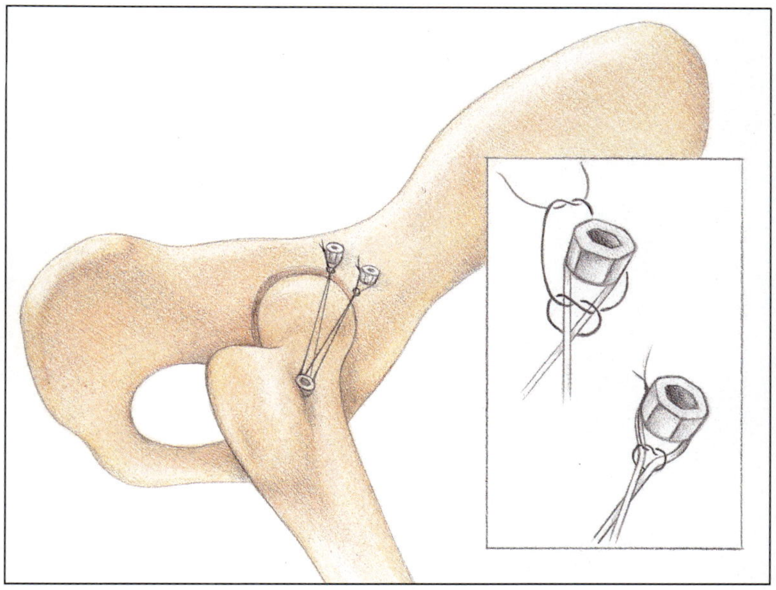

FIGURE 5.31 The placement of screws and sutures for a prosthetic joint capsule in the treatment of chronic hip luxation.

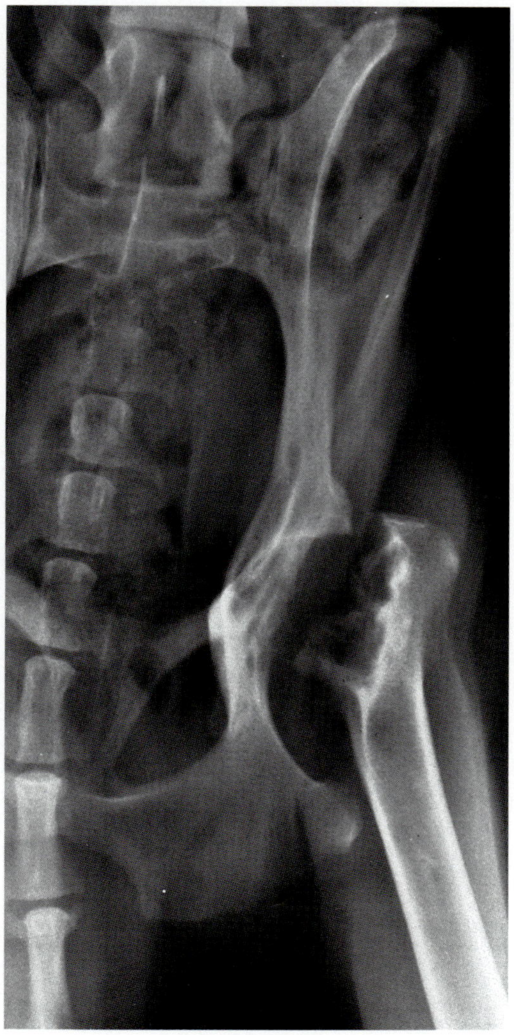

FIGURE 5.32 Radiograph of a femoral head ostectomy.

Although imposition of either a section of biceps or of fascia to provide a gliding surface for the false joint has been recommended, experience has shown that no particular advantage ensues over a simple bone exposure if it has been performed correctly.

Closure of the joint capsule and the deep gluteus cannot be made effectively. The retracted middle gluteus is replaced. It is important that all hemorrhage be controlled, since hematoma formation can lead to the deposit of bone and a painful joint. The rest of the closure is routine.

This procedure and that of total hip replacement are performed more often for hip dysplasia than for chronic hip luxation. It is the treatment of choice in small breeds with Legg-Perthes disease (aseptic femoral head necrosis) (Fig. 5.33).

Femoral head ostectomy is a salvage procedure. It requires a lot of postoperative physiotherapy and is not recommended for large breeds. Postoperative swimming is especially helpful, since it provides a source of nonweight-bearing exercise.

TOTAL HIP REPLACEMENT

Total hip replacement offers repair and return to function of hips suffering from hip dysplasia, degenerative joint disease, malunion or nonunion of the femoral neck, acetabular fractures, irreducible or chronic hip luxations, and avascular necrosis of the femoral head.

The procedure is exacting and requires considerable instrumentation, good assistance, and special surgical training. A competent surgical team must be assembled.

Prolonged exposure of the tissues must be avoided. The highest degree of asepsis must be maintained. The procedure should not be done on animals suffering from infectious processes elsewhere in the body.

Clinical examination must justify the procedure by ruling out conditions confused with hip problems. Not all dogs with hip dysplasia require such surgery. Replacement with a total hip after excision arthroplasty is most difficult. Dogs with degenerative myopathy, disc lesions, nerve root tumors, cauda equina disease and ruptured anterior cruciate ligaments are often mistakenly presented for total hip replacement.

The Biomedtrix® canine modular hip (Biomedtrix® Ltd., Denville, NJ) consists of an acetabular cup of polyethylene and a femoral head of cobalt chrome that fits onto the tapered neck of a titanium femoral stem.

The acetabular and stem components are seated in methylmethacrylate. The femoral head is removed by transecting the neck

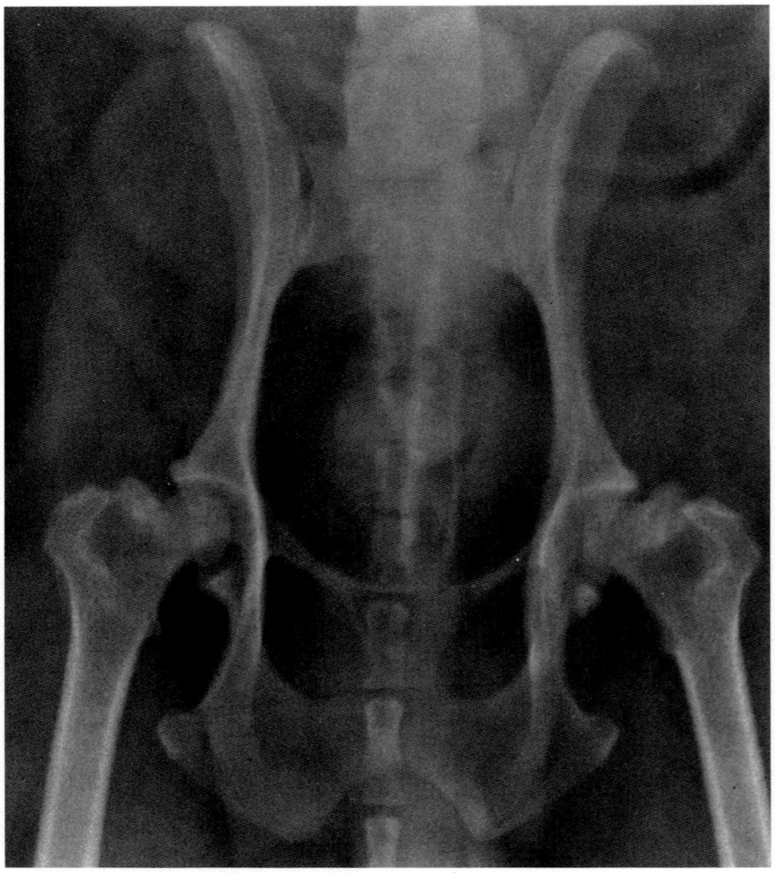

FIGURE 5.33 Bilateral aseptic femoral head necrosis in a small breed dog (Legg-Perthes disease).

to conform exactly to the prosthesis stem. The femoral medullary canal is reamed to accept the stem perfectly. The acetabulum is reamed and prepared to accept the acetabular cup.

A choice of femoral heads fits onto the tapered neck in three positions in order to provide different neck length requirements.

Return of function is seen in about 2 months. Use of the limb is seen within a few days. The dog is restrained in a cage and exercised on a leash for 1 week, then receives restricted exercise for 3 weeks. Good results in the properly operated animal will show full weight-bearing, normal gait, normal range of motion, and no signs of pain.

SURGICAL TECHNIQUE

The approach to the hip is craniolateral with the initial incision made halfway between the trochanter major and the dorsal midline. It is extended cranial and parallel to the proximal half of the shaft of the femur.

The fascia lata and extensor fascia lata are incised at the junction with the biceps femoris. The superficial gluteus is isolated and transected near its insertion on the femur and reflected dorsally. The vastus lateralis is transected near its origin and reflected distally. The middle gluteus is retracted dorsally. A partial tenotomy of this muscle can be done near the trochanter major if more exposure is required. The deep gluteus is elevated and carefully dissected from its insertion and from the underlying joint capsule. It is reflected craniodorsally. A midway radial incision is made in the joint capsule, exposing the hip, which is luxated with a Hatt spoon. The femoral head and neck area is cleared of tissue. Using a neck resection guide, the neck is marked with the electrocautery to identify the line of excision to be followed when the head and neck are removed with an oscillating bone saw. This should be cut so that the femoral component will fit closely against the cut surface (Fig. 5.34A).

The femur is elevated so that the proximal medullary cavity may be drilled. The drill is inserted through a guide to protect the surrounding tissue (Fig. 5.34B). A tapered reamer is used to prepare the femur to receive the femoral component (Fig. 5.34C). A finishing file and a broach complete the preparation. The exactness of the fit is determined with a test component.

The femur is retracted to expose the acetabulum, which is reamed with a special reamer. The joint capsule is retracted with a rake retractor. A 3.5 mm suction hole is drilled from the dorsolateral aspect of the acetabulum just proximal to the origin of the rectus femoris, pointed in a direction that will be

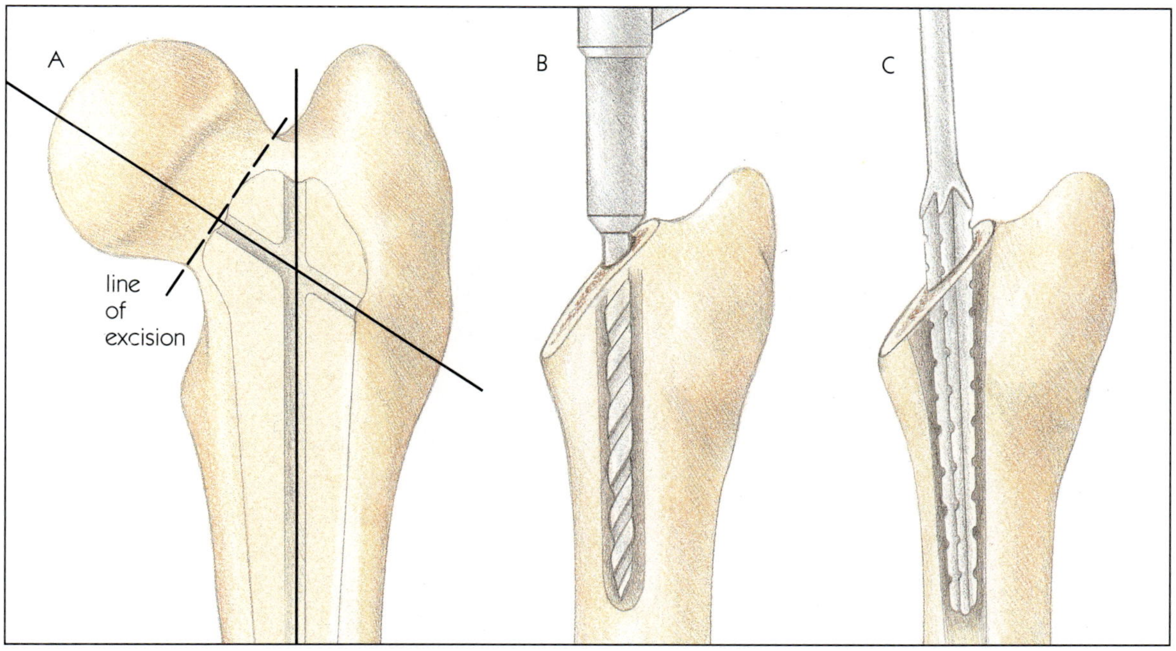

FIGURE 5.34 (A) The use of a guide indicates the exact level of transection of the femoral head for placement of a total hip stem prosthesis. (B) Drill guide and drill. (C) A tapered reamer.

medial to the deepest portion of the reamed area and lateral to the medial cortical pelvic bone (Figs. 5.35, 5.36).

The reamed surface of the acetabulum is further prepared by drilling several 1-mm holes in the trabecular bone to allow for implantation of the methylmethacrylate. Some of these holes will communicate with the suction hole. A 3.5-mm hole is drilled through the lateral cortex of the femur at midshaft for a suction hole.

The acetabulum is flushed, suctioned, and dried with sponges. A disposable suction tip is introduced into the suction hole at the dorsal acetabular area.

A suitable amount of methylmethacrylate mix containing an antibiotic is pressed into the acetabulum. The suction keeps the air and blood from accumulating and ensures good seating of the methylmethacrylate. The acetabular component is placed in a holder and inserted into the acetabulum. The suction is withdrawn. Excess methylmethacrylate is removed. The position of the component is quite critical and its alignment follows the direction indicated by an alignment bar (Fig. 5.37). The holder is removed when the acetabular component is firmly in place, a matter of several minutes until the exothermic reaction is over.

The femur is prepared by flushing, suctioning, and sponging. A disposable suction tip is inserted in the hole in the femoral shaft. This removes blood and clots and keeps the prepared area relatively dry. Methylmethacrylate mix is inserted into the prepared area by hand for small dogs, or by a caulking gun device on a syringe for large dogs. The suction draws the methylmethacrylate deep into the prepared location for the femoral stem. The suction is removed. The stem is inserted so that it is in 15° to 20° of retroversion. Excess methylmethacrylate is removed. When the femoral stem is solidly implanted, a trial head is used to assess the proper neck length required. These trial reductions are aided by use of a bone skid.

The permanent femoral head is selected and tapped onto the cone-shaped neck of the femoral stem with a mallet and a special impactor. A sponge protects the head.

The head is reduced into the acetabulum. Closure is done by suturing as much of the joint capsule and deep gluteus as possible back into its former position. Traction on the gluteus medius is released. The vastus lateralis and superficial gluteus are replaced and sutured. The tensor fascia lata and fascia lata are sutured.

The subcutaneous tissues and skin are closed in the usual manner. A check radiograph is taken (Fig. 5.38).

Intravenous antibiotics are given at the induction of anesthesia and oral antibiotics are given for 5 days after surgery.

Activity is limited for 8 weeks. Exercise is permitted on a leash.

The opposite hip may be replaced in 2 or 3 months.

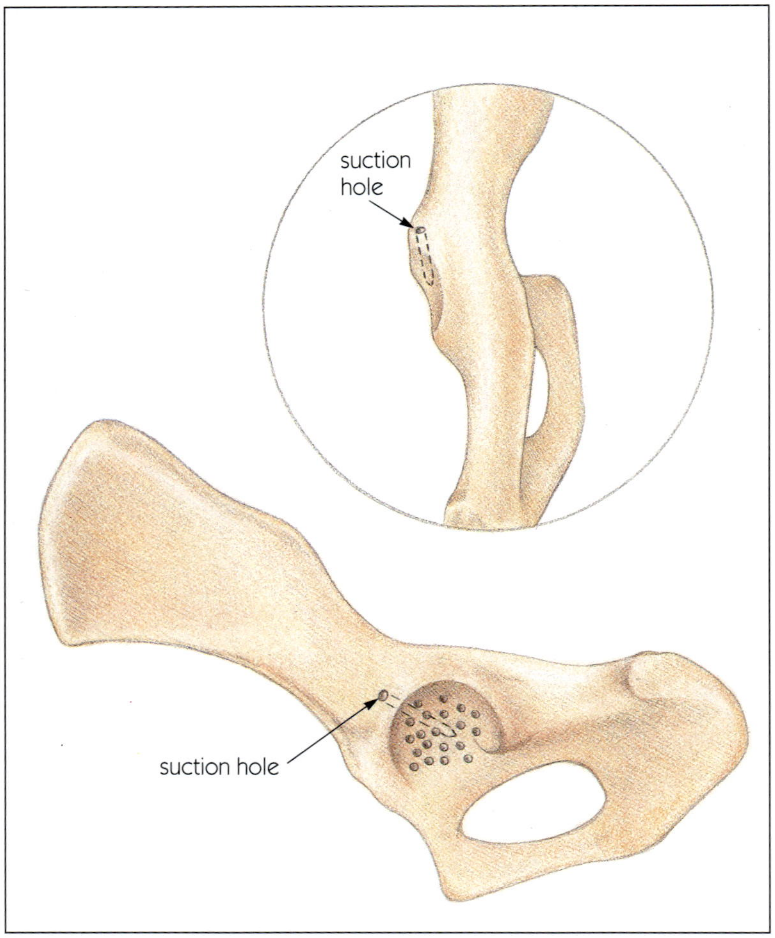

FIGURE 5.35 Placement of a suction hole in the acetabulum. The reamed acetabular surface is drilled with a number of 1-mm holes to establish good bone to methylmethacrylate bonding.

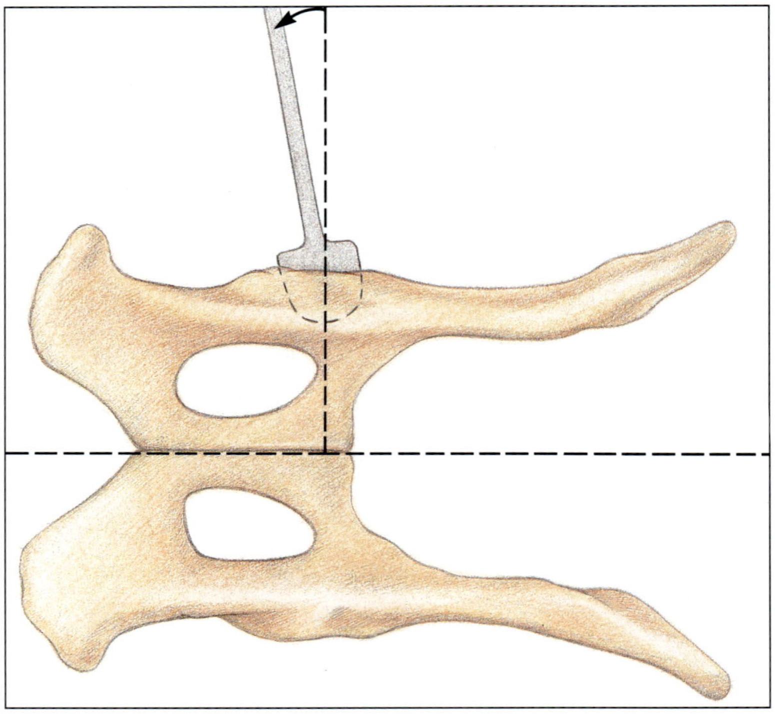

FIGURE 5.36 An acetabular reamer.

LUXATION, INTERNAL LIGAMENT RUPTURE, AND MENISCAL INJURIES OF THE STIFLE

Repair of the Ruptured Anterior Cruciate Ligament

Extraarticular Fixation

Extraarticular fixation for ruptured anterior cruciate ligament depends on the use of a heavy gauge suture to imbricate the joint fascia or to restrain the cranial tibial motion and medial rotation with sutures placed external to the joint. These methods work best with dogs under 30 pounds.

Another method is to advance the head of the fibula. This uses the lateral collateral ligament as the means of restraint of cranial tibial thrust and medial rotation.

The same result is obtained by changing the angle of the tibial plateau. This is done by making a medial to lateral circular cut through the proximal tibia that permits the proximal fragment to rotate, thus tilting the tibial plateau caudally. The transection is secured with a bone plate and screws.

Examination of the joint for meniscal injury and excision of cruciate ligament fragments is done with these repairs.

Extraarticular Stabilization With Nonabsorbable Suture Material

SURGICAL TECHNIQUE

A loop of nonabsorbable suture is placed around the medial fabella and inserted through a hole in the tibial tubercle. A similar loop is placed from around the lateral fabella to the hole in the tibial tubercle. An additional suture is placed from the lateral fabella to the straight patella ligament to aid in control of excess medial rotation.

A medial arthrotomy is done. The remnants of the torn anterior cruciate ligament and damaged menisci are removed. The arthrotomy is closed. The medial fabella is exposed by reflecting the incised fascia of the caudal portion of the sartorius. A large half-round blunt suture needle is used to pass a length of 0 or 1 nonabsorbable suture under the medial fabella. A transverse hole is drilled

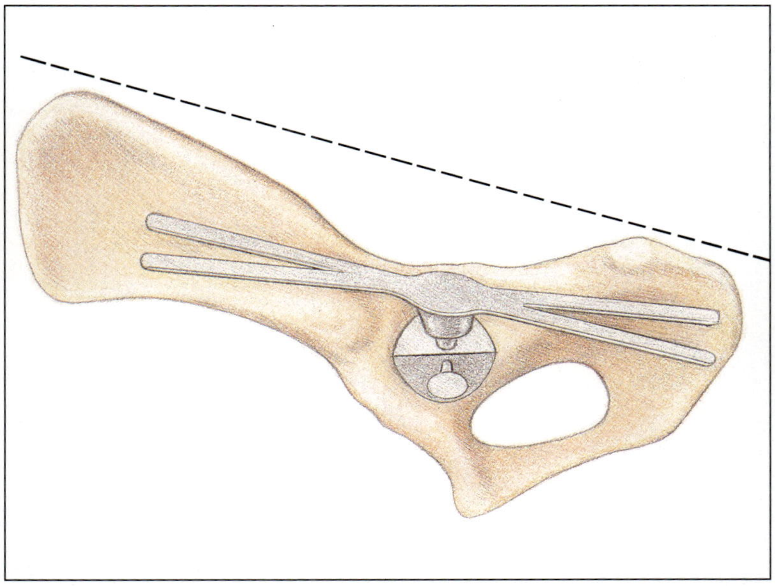

FIGURE 5.37 An alignment bar.

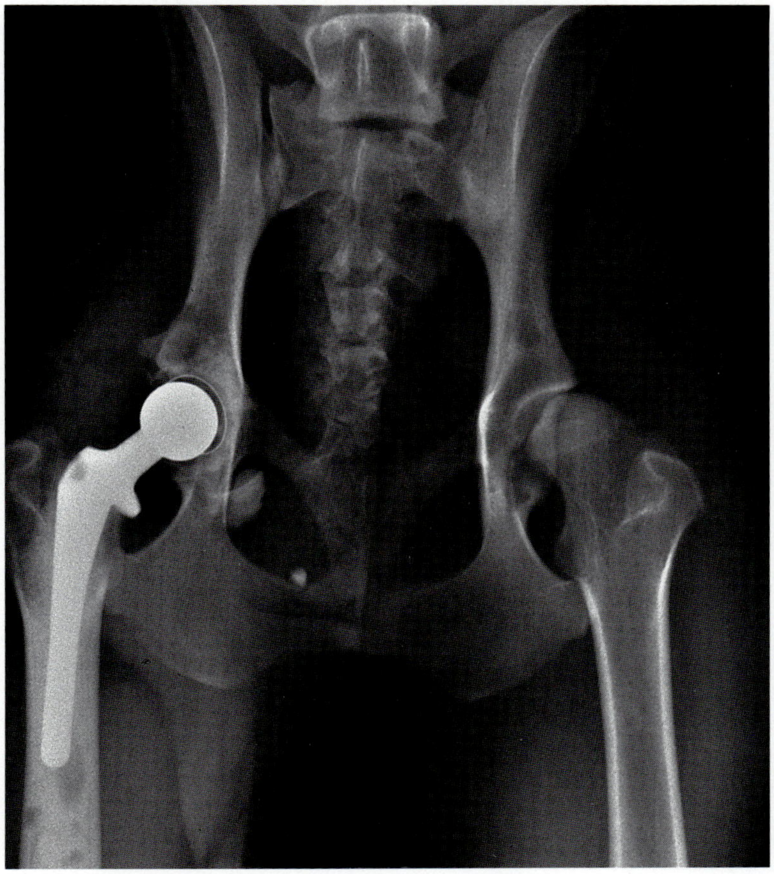

FIGURE 5.38 Radiograph of a total hip.

through the tibial tubercle. The suture is passed through this hole. The lateral fabella is exposed by reflecting the skin and subcutaneous tissues and the fascical insertion of the biceps femoris. A doubled suture is introduced around and under the lateral fabella. The suture is cut at the eye of the needle. One suture is passed through the hole in the tibial tubercle. It is tied with the leg held in normal position. The medial suture is now tied. The second lateral suture is introduced into the straight patellar ligament and tied. This suture will control excess medial luxation (Fig. 5.39).

The fascial edges of the sartorius and the biceps femoris are advanced to the patellar ligament and sutured. This also adds to the control of the cranial tibial movement.

Restricted exercise is maintained for 6 weeks with increased amounts of activity for the following 2 weeks.

Repair of the Ruptured Anterior Cruciate Ligament by Transposition of the Fibular Head

In this surgery, the head of the fibula is freed from its attachment to the tibia and advanced cranially, where it is secured with a K-wire or small intramedullary pin. A tension band wire is inserted between the pin and a hole in the tibial crest.

A routine lateral arthrotomy is done. The joint is inspected for meniscal injury and remnants of the torn cruciate are removed. The fascial insertion of the biceps femoris is incised and reflected to expose the lateral collateral ligament, the fibular head, and the origin of the cranial tibial and peroneus longus muscles.

The fascia between the cranial tibial and peroneus longus muscles is incised. The fascia at the origin of the cranial tibial mus-

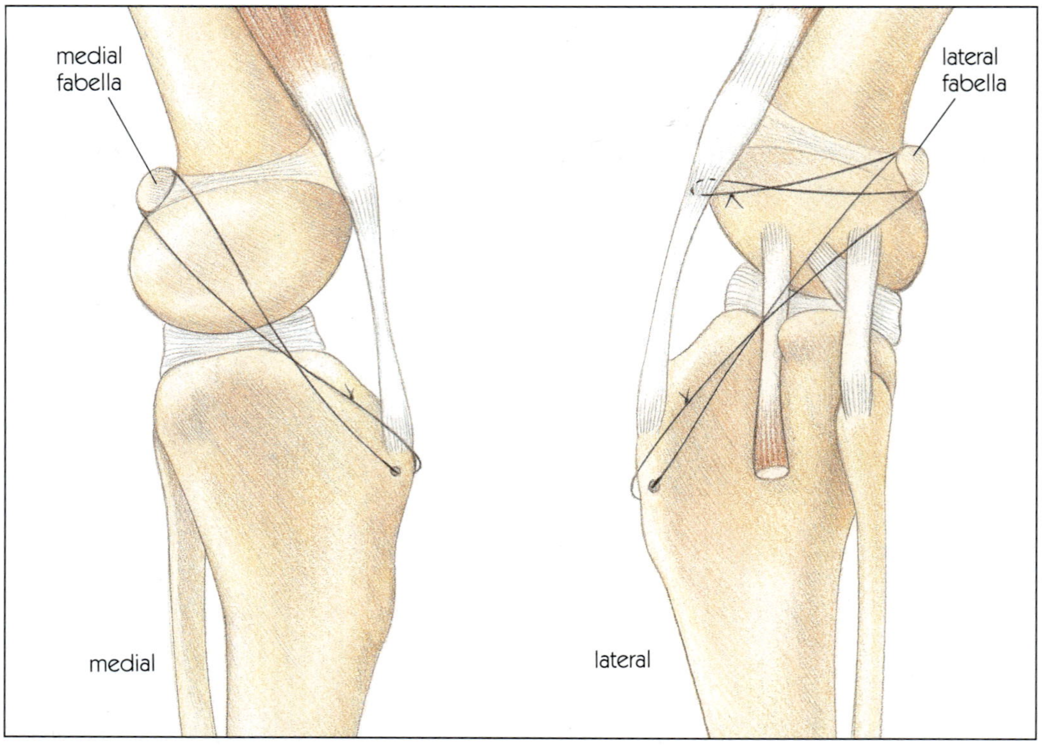

FIGURE 5.39 The placement of sutures in extraarticular repair of an anterior cruciate ligament rupture.

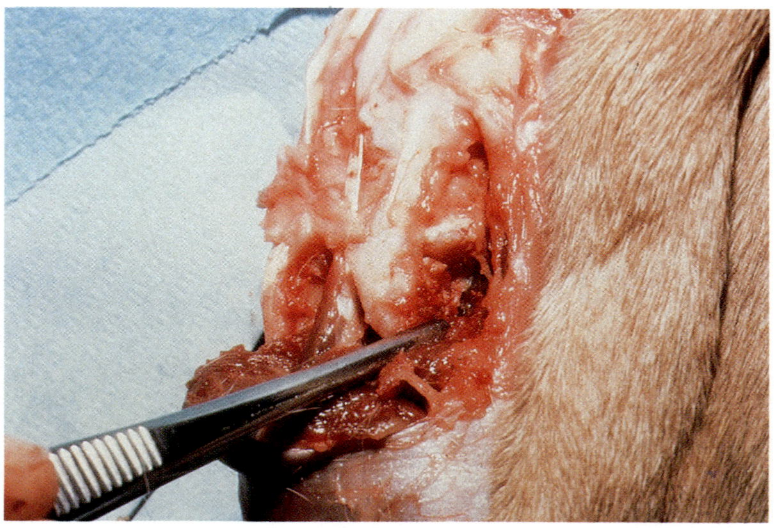

FIGURE 5.40 The fibular head has been moved to a new cranial position.

cle is incised cranially to the tendon of the long digital extensor. The fascia and joint capsule cranial and caudal to the lateral collateral ligament is incised enough to free it. The fibular head is isolated and its attachment to the tibia is sectioned. The dissection plane is at a 45° angle from the saggital plane of the tibia. The fibular nerve lies just caudal and distal to the head and must be protected.

The fibular head is moved cranially. A portion of the intervening edge of the tibia is removed with a rongeur to permit easier transportation (Fig. 5.40).

The stifle joint is held at a normal standing angle. A bone forceps is used to move the fibular head into its new position with one jaw on the tibial crest and the other at the back of the fibular head.

A small intramedullary pin or K-wire is introduced through the fibular head deeply into the tibia. A hole is drilled through the tibial tuberosity. A figure-8 wire is introduced around the intramedullary pin and through the hole. The wire is twisted together tightly. The twisted ends are bent close to the bone. The end of the pin or K-wire is bent at a right angle, cut off, and set firmly against the bone (Fig. 5.41).

The biceps femoris fascia is replaced in a more cranial position.

Closure of the skin and subcutaneous tissue is routine. The anterior drawer sign should now be controlled. Exercise is restricted for 1 month with a gradual return to full activity.

While many surgeons utilize this method, I do not recommend it.

Internal Fixation of Ruptured Anterior Cruciate Ligament

The original internal repair described by Paatsama consisted of a fascial strip introduced through a tunnel drilled into the lateral condyle, which then passed through the joint as a replacement of the torn ligament to exit through a tunnel in the proximal tibia. The fascial strip was secured to the tibia by passing it through a transverse hole in the tibial crest. Unless the holes were drilled so that the fascial strip was placed in the same situation as the ligament, it was easily torn. The strip also could be torn at the sharp right angle at the end of the femoral tunnel.

Substitutes for the fascial strip were developed, such as full thickness skin.

Synthetic ligaments of various suture materials have been advocated.

A sophisticated modification of the repair in humans was described by De Angelis. This consisted of making a strip from the medial third of the straight patellar ligament, a portion of the attached patella and a continuation of fascia lata. This strip was

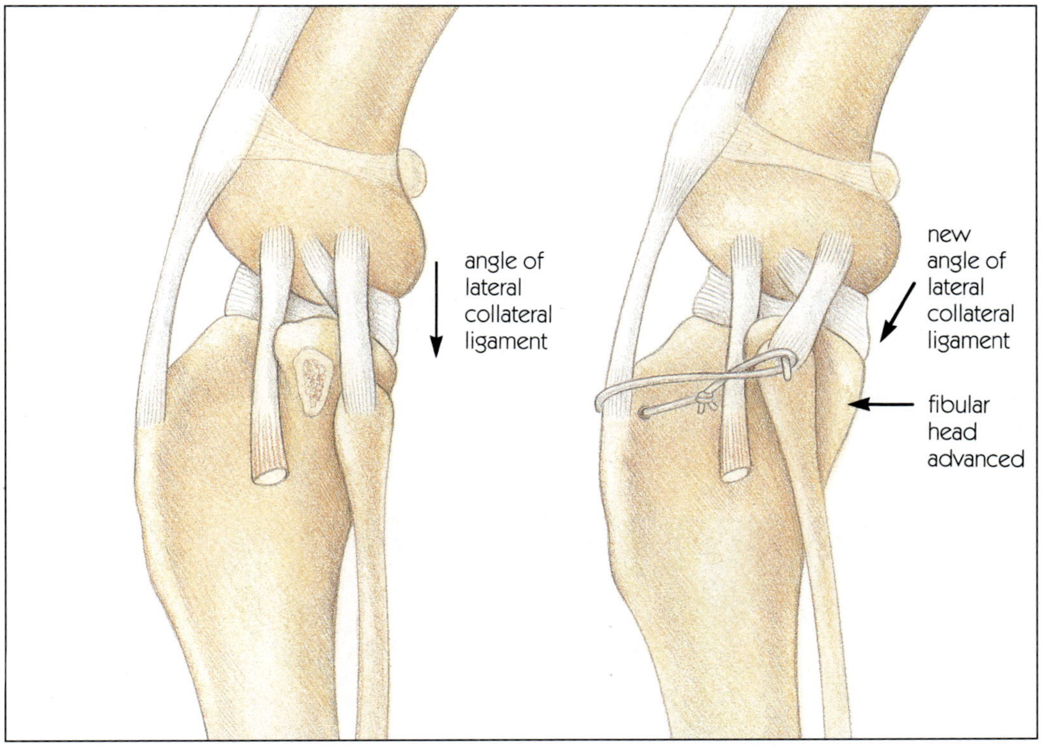

FIGURE 5.41 Advanced position of the fibular head, pin, and figure-8 wire placement and change of angle of the lateral collateral ligament.

brought out over the top of the lateral fabella and secured to the lateral condyle.

A simple but effective repair is to develop a fascial strip as in the original Paatsama repair, pass it cranially to the insertion of the straight patellar ligament, insert it through a slit into the joint in the fascia distally and just medial to the straight patellar ligament, pass it through the joint over the top of the lateral fabella, and secure it back on itself at its origin (Fig. 5.42).

There are several methods of repair, each felt by the particular author to be the best. The over-the-top fascial strip method seems

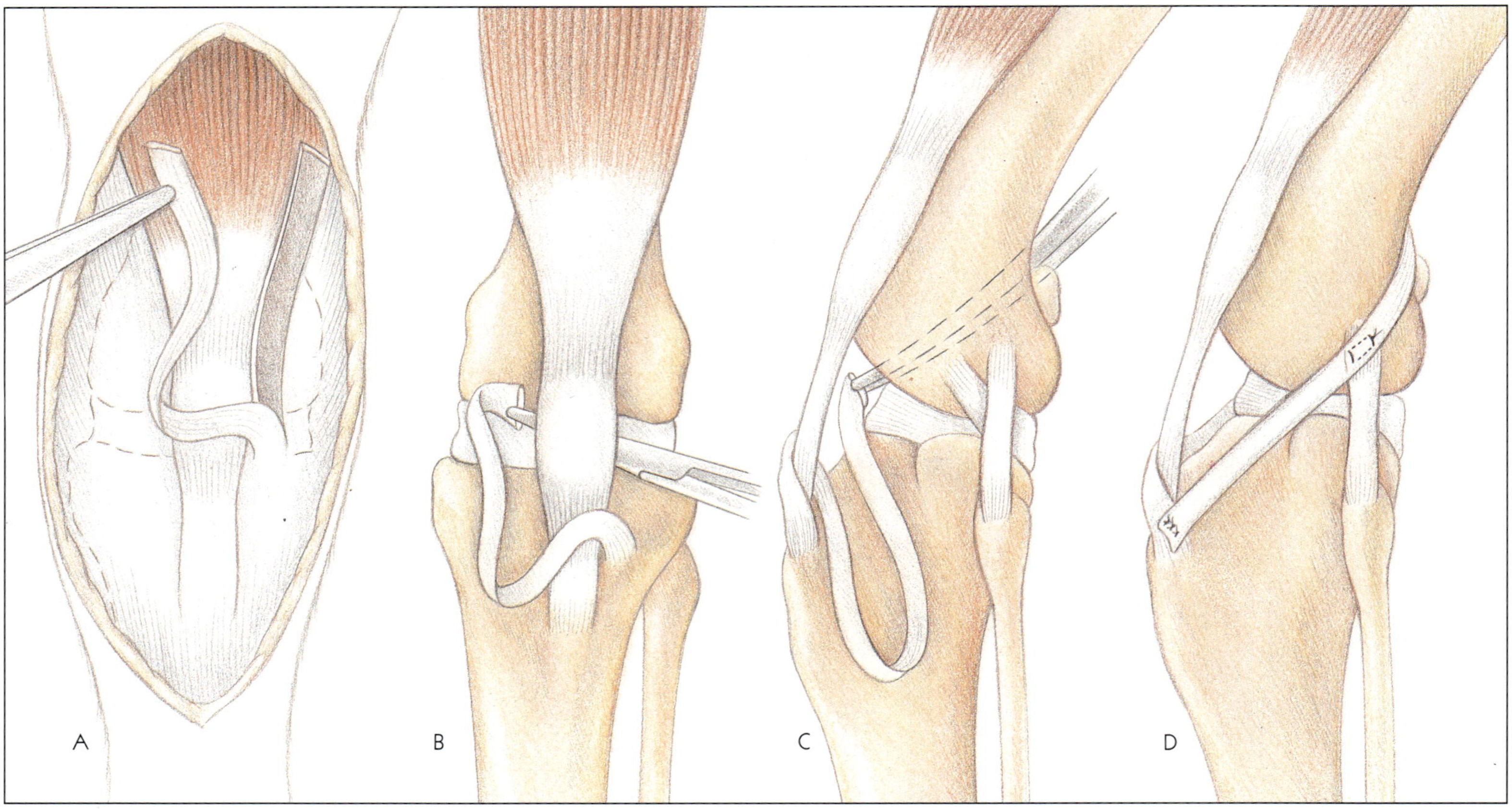

FIGURE 5.42 Repair of a ruptured anterior cruciate ligament with a fascial strip over-the-top method. (A) The fascial strip is obtained beginning at its attachment to the tibia, just lateral to the patellar ligament, extending dorsally through the fascia lata. (B) The strip is drawn over the insertion of the patellar ligament and through a small incision just medial to it. (C) The strip is grasped with a curved hemostat inserted from just medial to the lateral fabella into the joint. (D) The fascial strip is drawn over the top of the lateral fabella to be sutured to its origin. A supporting stitch is placed to secure the strip to the proximal end of the lateral collateral ligament.

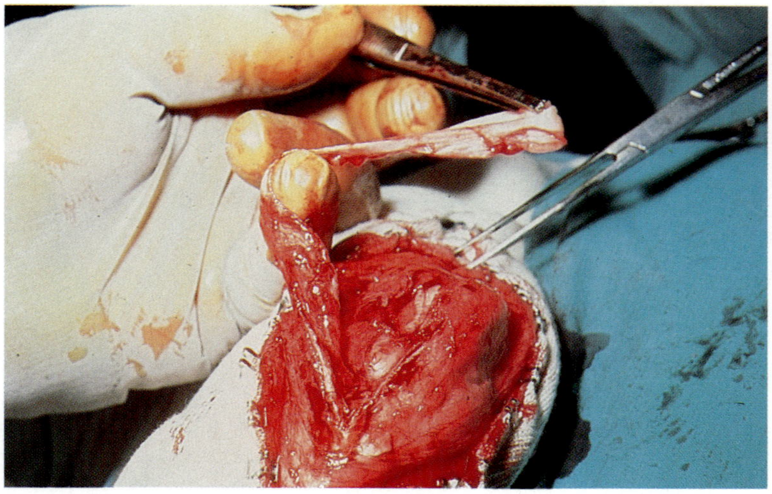

FIGURE 5.43 A fascial strip.

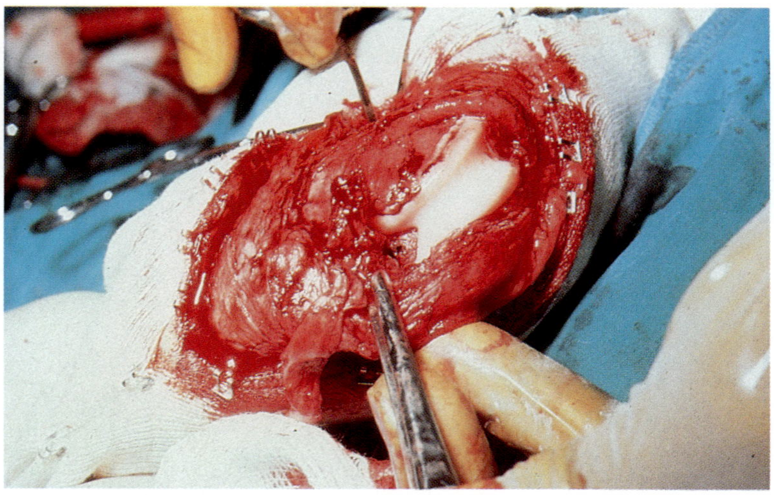

FIGURE 5.44 The tips of this curved hemostat are visible inside the joint preparatory to grasping the fascial strip to draw it out over the top of the lateral fabella.

to be satisfactory. No holes are drilled in the bones and a minimal amount of foreign material is introduced into the joint. The procedure can be done in any size dog and requires no special equipment.

A lateral parapatellar incision is made through the skin and subcutaneous tissues from the head of the tibia to halfway up the thigh. The underlying fascia is exposed and incised. Entry into the joint is made with the scalpel at the soft area nearly opposite the distal end of the patella. Straight scissors are used to enlarge the incision dorsally and ventrally. A small amount of retinacular cartilage should be left attached to the patella for resuturing. The patella is luxated medially. The joint is flexed and the remnants of the torn ligaments are removed. The menisci are inspected. Repair, trimming, or removal of these structures can be done at this time. From the exposed edge of the fascia, the widest possible strip is prepared, extending from the proximal edge of the tibia up to mid-thigh (Fig. 5.43). The strip is now brought around the front of the tibial crest and pulled through a small stab wound made in the distal medial fascia of the knee close to the straight patellar ligament entering the joint.

At this time, the lateral fabella is exposed and the tissues medial and caudal to it are retracted. The caudodistal shaft of the femur is often visible. A curved hemostat inserted through the flexed joint, from just in back of and medial to the lateral fabella, becomes visible in the joint (Fig. 5.44). The free end of the fascial strip is grasped and pulled through the joint and out over the top of the lateral fabella. The leg is extended, the strip pulled taut, and the end sutured to itself and to the surrounding tissues (Fig. 5.45). A stitch is placed from the strip directly into the dorsal portion of the lateral collateral ligament. There should now be no anterior drawer sign. Closure of the joint is performed with nonabsorbable suture material except for the joint capsule, which is closed with 2-0 catgut. Special attention is paid to strong closure of the lateral retinacular structure. The defect from which the strip was taken is closed. The insertion of the biceps femoris is sutured over the fascial strip. Subcutaneous tissues and skin are closed.

A modified Robert Jones splint is applied to the very active dog. Confinement in a run is usually required for only 4 or 5 days. The dog can then be released to the owner to be kept on a leash or housed for about 6 weeks. By that time the dog should be using the leg. At the end of 3 months, light training can begin and regular training at 6 months.

Those dogs requiring meniscal surgery will have an extended recovery. Lighter, smaller dogs will make quicker recoveries, as will those that are operated on early.

Meniscectomy

Meniscal injuries rarely occur singularly. They are frequently a component of other stifle injuries, e.g., ruptures of the anterior cruciate ligament, or of the medial or lateral collateral ligament, or both.

Anterior cruciate rupture with more severe pain and more obvious failure to use the leg gives reason to suspect additional meniscal damage. The injuries seen vary in type and severity. The most common findings are tears, folds, and detachment. The medial meniscus is more liable to be affected.

Diagnostically, a clicking or snapping sensation is felt when the stifle is palpated in the untranquilized animal, but often this is not always present or is hard to elicit.

It is generally believed that the meniscus should be preserved as much as possible. Usually only the portion that is severely damaged is removed. Small tears and folds may be cut away. When this is done, it is recommended that a few radial straight scalpel cuts be made through the meniscus to provide vascular access channels to speed healing. Removal of only the greater part of a meniscus should be avoided; rather, the entire affected meniscus should be removed. As long as the joint instability from the concomitant ligament injury is controlled, a minimal amount of osteoarthritis will occur.

SURGICAL TECHNIQUE

It is essential to use very small No. 11 or No. 15 blades, being very careful not to injure the articular cartilage surfaces.

The ruptured anterior cruciate ligament fragments are trimmed away. A small retractor is used as a pry to bring the caudal aspect of the tibial plateau into view. Although a medial patellar approach is easier for the removal of the medial meniscus, it may not be the desirable approach for repair of the ruptured anterior cruciate.

The intermeniscal and cranial tibial ligaments are cut. The cranial aspect of the meniscus is grasped with a small tenaculum or

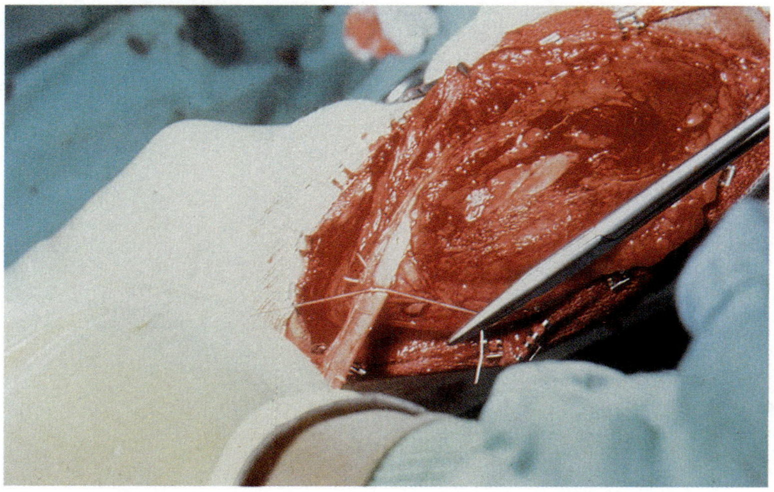

FIGURE 5.45 The fascial strip being sutured in place.

any other toothed clamping forceps. The meniscus is pulled cranially and laterally, then dissected away from its medial contact with the joint capsule. Care must be taken not to cut the medial collateral ligament. Continued dissection and traction draws the meniscus craniolaterally as it is freed from the caudal attachments until the caudal tibial ligament is cut, allowing the meniscus to be pulled free. There are large popliteal blood vessels just caudal to the caudal joint capsule. These must be avoided by very careful dissection (Fig. 5.46).

Repair of the ruptured anterior cruciate ligament or other ligamentous damage is now complete. When the meniscus is damaged, it takes much longer for a normal gait and reasonable use of the leg to return. A rest period of up to 6 months is recommended.

Rupture of the Collateral Ligaments

Rupture of the medial or lateral collateral ligaments of the stifle is not common, but when it occurs it is very debilitating. Direct trauma or ablation by a shearing injury are the most common causes. Associated meniscal and cruciate damage is almost always present and will require repair. The medial collateral is often affected. The

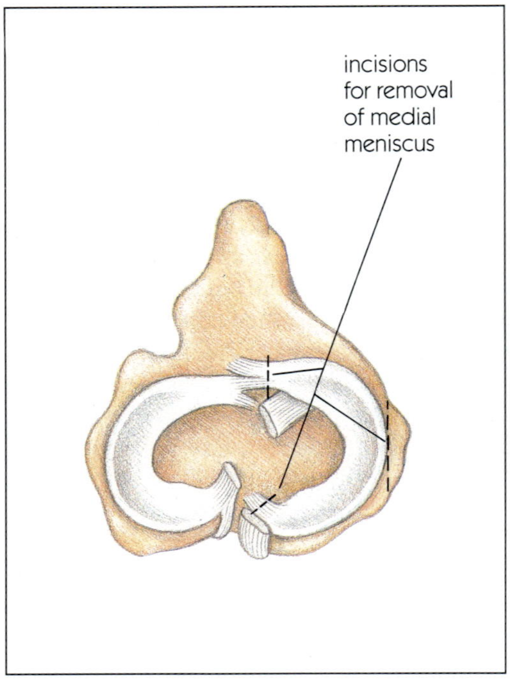

FIGURE 5.46 The location of cuts in removal of the medial meniscus of the stifle of the dog.

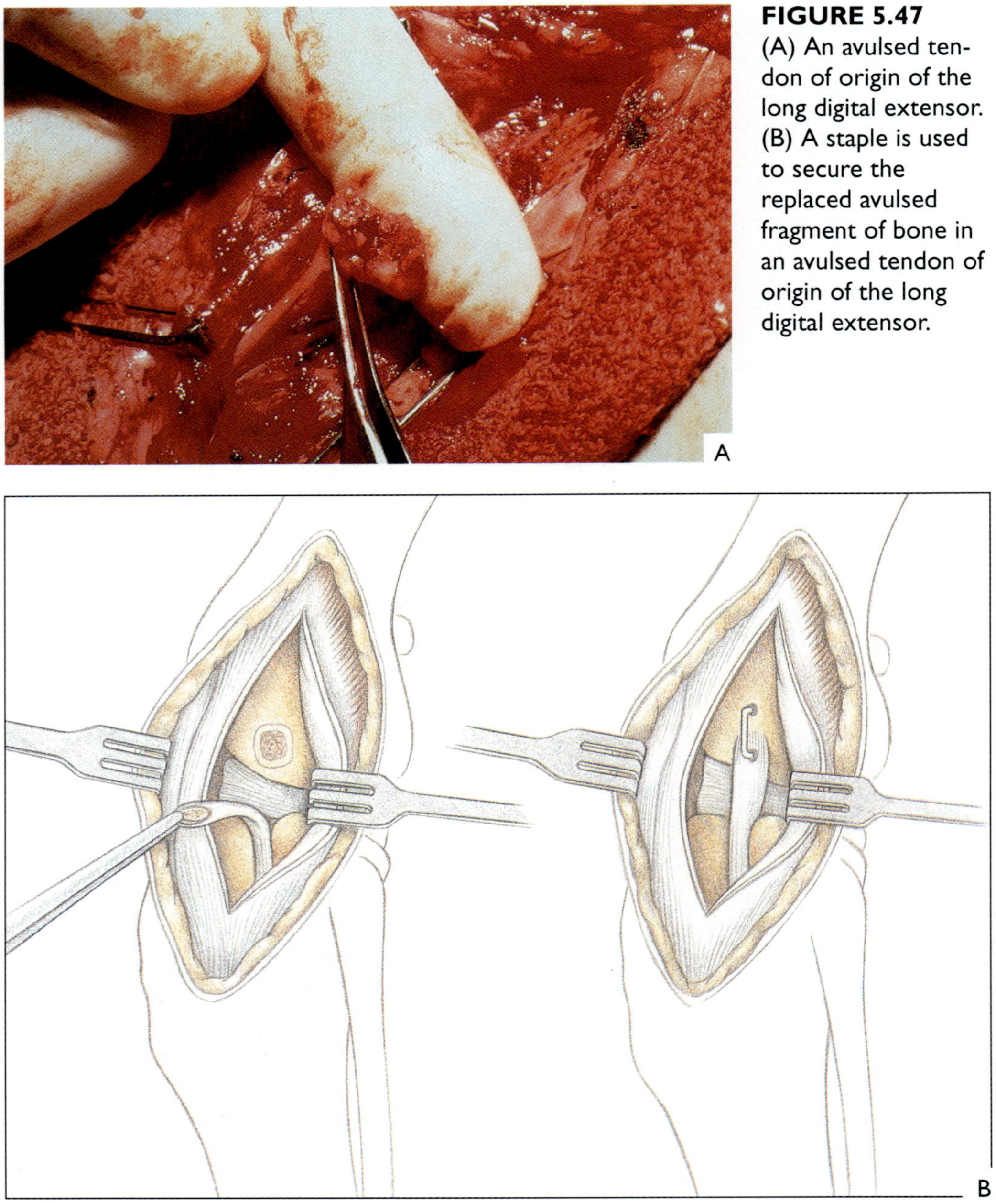

FIGURE 5.47 (A) An avulsed tendon of origin of the long digital extensor. (B) A staple is used to secure the replaced avulsed fragment of bone in an avulsed tendon of origin of the long digital extensor.

collateral ligaments control lateral and medial angulation of the joint, and the medial collateral ligament controls external tibial rotation. Internal rotation is controlled by the lateral collateral and the anterior cruciate ligaments.

The joint will be found to be swollen and nonweight-bearing. Sometimes a joint can be so damaged that the medial, lateral and cruciate structures are torn. Respective repairs of these structures will provide a chance for recovery of a usable knee joint.

Torn collateral ligaments may be able to be replaced, resutured or reattached. Those severely damaged are replaced synthetically.

Repair of Torn Medial Collateral Ligament of the Knee by Synthetic Replacement

SURGICAL TECHNIQUE

An incision is made through the skin and subcutaneous tissues directly over the medial collateral ligament. The medial femoral fascia is transected and retracted. The damaged ligament is obtained by sharp and blunt dissection. The joint is opened by moving the tibia laterally, enabling inspection for damage to the medial meniscus and the anterior cruciate.

The damaged ligament is to be replaced by a figure-8 of nonabsorbable suture material between small bone screws placed at the origin of the ligament in the femur and at the insertion of the ligament in the tibia. The suture is wound around the screws and into a figure-8 to prevent it from slipping off. It is placed with the leg extended to avoid restricting normal joint movement during flexion and extension. The incision in the medial femoral fascia is resutured with 2-0 catgut and a standard closure of the skin and subcutaneous tissues is made.

In a rupture of the lateral collateral ligament, bone screws are placed at the origin of the ligament on the femoral condyle and in the head of the fibula. A figure-8 of nonabsorbable suture material is woven between the two screws with the leg held extended.

Closure is performed by suturing the incision in the fascia of the biceps femoris and closing the subcutaneous tissues and the skin in the usual manner.

The leg is placed in a modified Robert Jones splint for 2 weeks, and the dog is confined for 2 weeks to a run and exercise on a leash. Full activity can resume after 6 to 8 weeks, depending on the amount of damage and the speed of recovery. The screws and sutures remain in place permanently.

AVULSION OF THE ORIGIN OF THE LONG DIGITAL EXTENSOR

Avulsion of the origin of the long digital extensor is uncommon. The lameness that it causes is often difficult to diagnose. Physically there is evidence of minor pain after exercise. Radiographically there is evidence of an inflammatory process occuring at the distal end of the lateral femoral condyle. As with any obscure diagnosis in the knee, an exploratory arthrotomy is warranted. The origin of the tendon will be found to have pulled away a small block of bone from an area of the distal lateral condyle just lateral to the condylar articular surface. Considerable scar tissue production may be present, depending on the duration of the avulsion. Treatment consists of replacing the avulsed fragment.

SURGICAL TECHNIQUE

The knee joint is entered by a lateral parapatellar incision. The patella is luxated medially and the knee is flexed. The area of the avulsion is debrided. The relocation area is deepened with a curette. With the leg extended, the avulsed fragment is replaced. A small bone staple, made from a piece of intramedullary pin, is driven with one prong in the femoral condyle above the fragment and the opposite prong in the bone fragment. The entry holes for the staple ends are predrilled, facilitating placement and entry. The staple is seated with a bone mallet (Fig. 5.47).

The incision is closed by layer suturing. The leg is placed in a modified Robert Jones splint for 1 week.

AVULSION OF THE TIBIAL TUBERCLE

This condition, when seen in young active dogs prior to fusion of the epiphysis, will be a physeal separation. The patella is observed to be located higher than normal. There is considerable pain and lameness. Repair is necessary, but it may bring about premature fusion.

In the mature dog, the fracture is reduced and pinned with K-wires or two small intramedullary pins and a figure-8 tension band wire.

SURGICAL TECHNIQUE

A paramedial incision is made along the tibial crest over the fracture site, which is enlarged to provide adequate exposure. The skin and subcutaneous tissue are retracted with a periosteal elevator to permit reflection of the cranial tibial muscle. The avulsed fragment and the fracture site are cleansed of fibrous tissue. The leg is extended and the two fragments apposed. Two K-wires are inserted through the avulsed fragment and seated deeply into the proximal tibia, but not so deeply that the proximal caudal area is entered. The ends of the K-wires are bent at right angles and cut off. A transverse hole is drilled through the tibial crest about 1 or 2 cm below the fracture site. Orthopedic wire is inserted through the hole and secured around the distal K-wire in a figure-8 tension band. The ends are twisted to tighten the wire, providing compression, immobilization, and resistance to the pull of the quadriceps muscles. The twisted ends should be on the lateral side so that they may be covered by the cranial tibial muscle. The K-wires are seated against the bone with a few taps of a mallet (Fig. 5.48).

Closure is performed by resuturing the muscle fascia, subcutaneous tissue, and skin.

If the dog is young (4–5 months), the tension band should be removed in 3 weeks. This will permit continued growth of the physeal plate. Premature fusion will result in a distorted tibial tubercle.

In mature dogs, the wires are left in place. The leg is placed in a modified Robert Jones splint for about 5 days.

LUXATION OF THE PATELLA

Both medial and lateral luxations of the patella are seen. Medial luxations are much more common, usually occuring as a congenital deformity in small and toy breeds. They occur in larger breeds, usually laterally and in conjunction with other limb deformities, such as hip dysplasia. Traumatic luxation is rare and is usually associated with other severe trauma to the stifle.

Repair of Medial Luxation of the Patella

Medial luxation of the patella, usually a congenital disease, is occasionally caused by trauma. The congenital condition varies from minor to severe, with distortions of the knee joint and compensatory changes in the femur and tibia. In situations where the patella is in place but slips out occasionally and the general architecture of the joint is relatively normal, repair of the ruptured or stretched lateral ligamentous structures of the patella is by prosthetic replacement.

The quadriceps muscle group, the patella, and the tibial crest must be in alignment. An adequate trochlear groove should be present. The radiographic appearance should be relatively normal except in a very chronic situation, when osteophyte overgrowth, wear on the condylar surface, and changes in the patella can be seen. It is usually possible to replace the patella with relative ease.

The more severe cases are those of congenital origin, where changes in the structure of the knee joint are evidenced. The trochlear groove often fails to develop properly. One condylar part of the joint varies in development from the other, causing the planes of the joint surfaces between the femur and the tibia to become divergent instead of parallel, and the tibial crest to be drawn to one side. The patella usually cannot be replaced; if it is, it luxates readily. There is compensatory bowing of the distal femur and proximal tibia. Most important, if the patella is held in the trochlear groove, the alignment between the quadriceps muscle group, the patella, and the tibial crest is changed. The patella is frequently bound down with fibrous tissue and a very short medial ligamentous support. The trochlear groove often fails to develop properly. There is a disturbance in gait commensurate with the degree of deformity.

Surgical repair is obtained by transpositioning the tibial crest and deepening the trochlear groove as needed.

SURGICAL TECHNIQUE

A lateral parapatellar incision is made to enter the joint. The skin and subcutaneous tissues are incised and retracted. The patella is freed of medial attachments (medial patellar desmotomy). The tissues in the area of the lateral fabella are incised and retracted so that the caudal aspect can be seen. A hole is drilled caudomedially

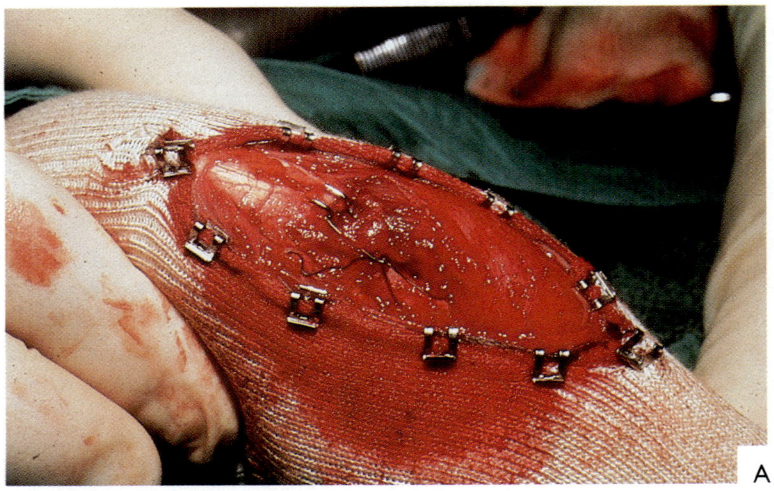

A

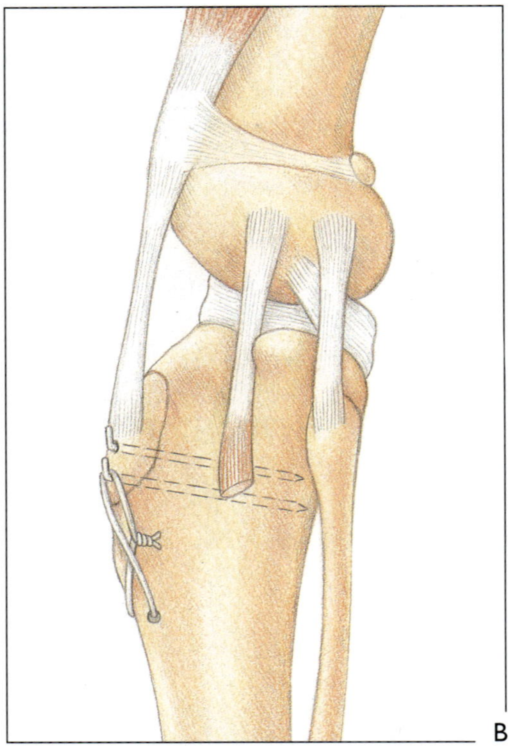

B

FIGURE 5.48 (A) An avulsed tibial tubercle. (B) The repair of an avulsed tibial tubercle with K-wires and a figure-8 wire tension band.

through the lateral condyle, exiting just medial to the inner surface of the lateral fabella. A sharp cutting-edge suture needle may be used for this purpose in toy dogs.

A length of nonabsorbable suture material is threaded through the hole and brought out just caudal to the lateral fabella. A large noncutting curved needle is used. It is inserted through the hole in the bone and through the muscles caudal to the knee. The suture is picked up from the eye of the needle just as it passes caudal to the fabella. The needle is withdrawn from the muscular tissue and the suture is cut at its eye. One end of the suture, which has been placed under and around the fabella, is grasped with a hemostat. The other end is inserted through a hole drilled transversely through the center of the patella. This suture is brought over the top and tied in a knot to its opposite end, which has been held in the hemostat. The suture, which goes from the lateral surface of the condyle under and around the lateral fabella and through and over the top of the patella, is adjusted to permit a full range of knee motion but not luxation of the patella. No repair of the medial desmotomy is done (Fig. 5.49).

Closure of subcutaneous tissues and skin is normal. Use of the limb is permitted. Improved function should be seen in a few days.

TRANSPOSITION OF THE TIBIAL CREST

This surgery is performed when the tibial crest has been pulled medially during the growth of the dog. The tibial tuberosity with the attached straight patellar ligament is isolated and cut free of the tibial crest. It is then moved laterally to a new location, where a straight alignment of the quadriceps and patella can be obtained. The bone fragment is secured with a wire stitch or a K-wire, depending on the size of the dog. If inadequate development of the trochlear groove is present, surgery to deepen or provide a new groove is performed.

SURGICAL TECHNIQUE

To enter the joint, a lateral parapatellar incision is made through the skin, subcutaneous tissue, fascia of the knee, and the joint capsule. The patella is usually held in a medial position, requiring the surgeon to positively identify its location. The patella is freed of its medial attachments. A wire saw or osteotome cuts away a good-sized section of the tibial tuberosity and the attached insertion of the straight patellar ligament. When freed of all attachments, the ligament and bone fragment is retracted (Fig. 5.50). If the trochlear groove is inadequate, it is deepened with rongeurs, osteotome, or scalpel. A nice technique in larger dogs is to make two parallel longitudinal cuts to remove a wedge of bone where the new groove is to be located, the outer section of the wedge being the articular surface. A portion of the inner section of the wedge is cut off so that the wedge can be replaced with its articular surface settled deeper. A new groove has thus been established, with preservation of the cartilaginous articular surface. The wedge does not need to be further secured in position.

The tibial crest fragment is located on the lateral face of the crest after the cranial tibial muscle has been reflected from it. The bone fragment is secured to the tibial crest by transfixing it with a small K-wire in larger dogs or orthopedic wire in small ones. Two small holes are drilled through the fragment front to back and a small piece of orthopedic wire is inserted as through a button. Two correspondingly spaced

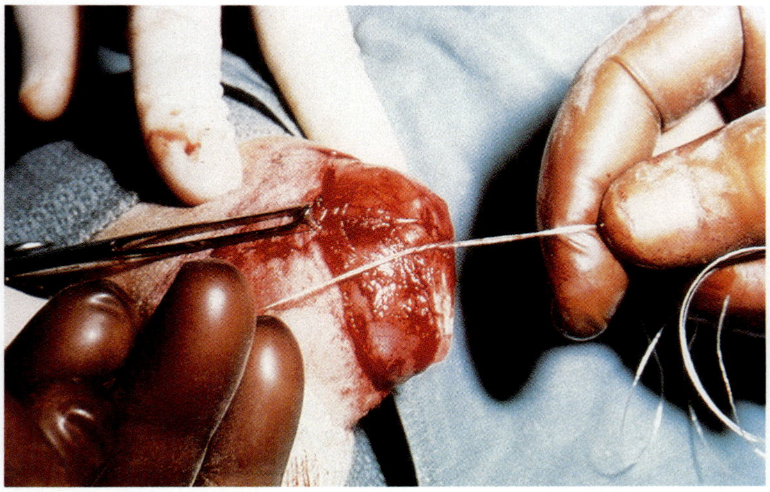

FIGURE 5.49 The tying of a suture that runs from the fabella to the patella in the treatment of minor patellar luxation.

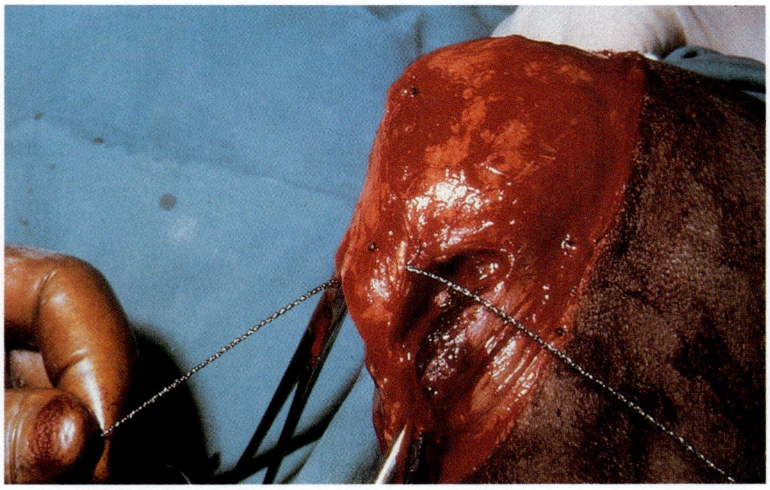

FIGURE 5.50 The tibial crest being cut with a Gigli wire saw.

holes are drilled from lateral to medial at the selected location on the tibial crest. The orthopedic wire ends are inserted through the holes and twisted tightly on the medial side to hold the crest fragment in place. The reflected cranial tibial muscle is replaced. Any redundant lateral knee fascia is trimmed to allow exact replacement of the patella and patellar ligament. No medial closure is possible since these tissues have not developed. The knee joint should function through an almost complete range of motion with the patella staying firmly in place. Closure of the joint is normal.

A modified Robert Jones splint will control pull on the newly-seated crest fragment and is left in for 4 or 5 days. Function will be improved depending on the severity of the previous deformity.

LUXATION OF THE HOCK

Tibiotarsal Luxation with Malleolar Fracture

This is one of the more common hock injuries. The radiographic appearance and degree of physical deformity make the condition appear much worse than it really is. Usually the lateral malleolus is avulsed from the distal tibial area, although the medial one or both can be involved.

An open reduction is performed; the affected malleolus is replaced and secured with a lag screw in large dogs and, in smaller breeds, one or two K-wires with a figure-8 tension band of orthopedic wire or nonabsorbable suture. The tension band material is threaded through a horizontal hole drilled through the tibial cortex about 1 cm above the fracture line. The leg is placed in a coaptation or modified Robert Jones splint for 3 or 4 weeks until healing takes place. Return of good function is to be expected. The pin and wires or screws are left in permanently.

SURGICAL TECHNIQUE

An incision is made through the skin and subcutaneous tissues directly over the malleolar area. Enlargement of the exposure with Metzenbaum scissors isolates the collateral ligament and the bone fragment to which it is attached. The joint is inspected and flushed clean of any blood clots or other tissue remnants.

The luxation is reduced and the malleolar fragment is secured in its proper position with a K-wire. If a lag screw is to be used, a hole is drilled through the fragment into its seat in the tibia. The malleolar portion is overdrilled. After the tibial portion of the hole has been tapped, an appropriately sized bone screw is inserted and the malleolar fragment is lagged to the underlying bone.

In smaller dogs, one or preferably two K-wires are inserted to anchor the malleolar fragment in place. A small hole is drilled through the tibial cortex about 1 cm above and horizontal to the fragment. This hole will provide support for a figure-8 tension band of orthopedic wire or nonabsorbable suture, which is also looped around the projecting ends of the K-wire. After the tension band is in place, the K-wire ends are bent and flattened against the bone (Fig. 5.51).

The incision is closed with 2-0 catgut and nonabsorbable sutures in the skin.

The hock is supported with a light cast or a modified Robert Jones splint until healing takes place–usually within 4 to 5 weeks.

Shearing Injuries to the Medial or Lateral Aspects of the Hock

Massive abrasive injuries to the hock, most frequently on the medial aspect, are the result of auto accidents. The leg is dragged against the highway, grinding off the tissues, ligaments, and bones, leaving

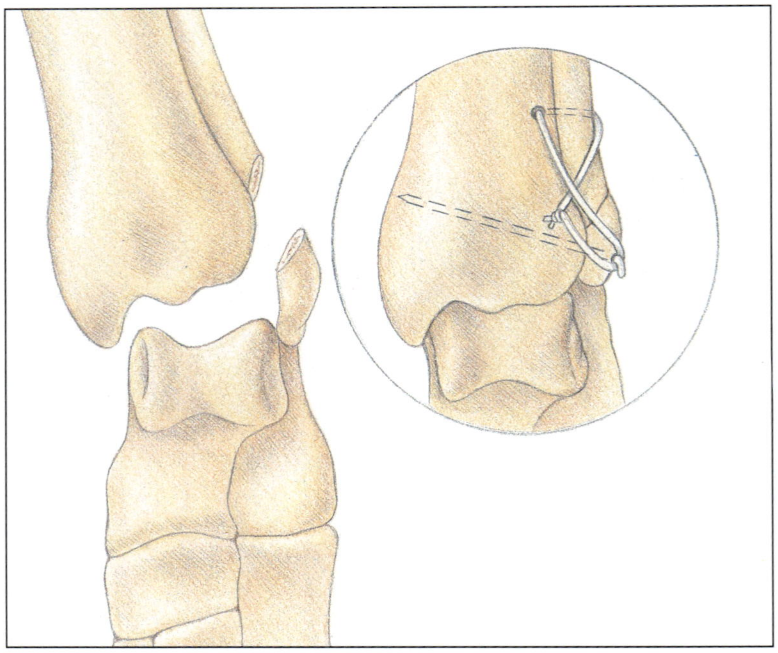

FIGURE 5.51 The repair of a lateral malleolar fracture and tibiotarsal luxation with a K-wire and figure-8 tension band wire.

the joints exposed and without support. There is great instability. Replacement of the key supportive ligaments with nonabsorbable suture material is essential. These will provide support and permit healing to take place. The wound itself must be debrided and is treated as an open wound with surgical dressing, antibiotics, and gentle cleansing.

SURGICAL TECHNIQUE

After debridement of the injured area, a bone screw is placed as distally in the tibia as possible without the screw entering the joint. With a medial shear, two bone screws are placed in the talus: one in the head of the talus to simulate the insertion of the long ligament, the other in the body of the talus to simulate the insertion of the short ligament. Nonabsorbable suture is placed in a figure-8 between the tibial screw and the screws in the talus. The short portion is tied so that it is tight during flexion. The long portion should be tight during extension.

In a lateral shear, the long ligament is replaced between the distal tibial screw and a bone screw in the body of the calcaneus. Additional support is provided by a suture between the tibial screw and is placed in the coracoid process of the calcaneus. The same type of sutures are tied in the same way as for the medial injury (Fig. 5.52).

Remarkably enough, these injuries tend to heal well. Development of a draining sinus is relatively rare; should such a complication arise, the suture or loose screw is removed. Scar tissue is followed by new skin and the eventual return of reasonable function.

The lower leg is protected by a modified Robert Jones splint, which can be easily removed and replaced to allow dressing changes and wound inspections. It may take 2 to 3 months for clinical healing. The general prognosis is very good.

Severe injuries may require external fixation for support or even a joint fusion to preserve the foot.

FRACTURE OF THE CALCANEUS (FIBULAR TARSAL BONE)

This fracture and avulsion of the insertion of the gastrocnemius tendon and slipped tendon of the superficial digital flexor, while not common, are extremely disabling and cannot be treated by simple splints or casts. The affected animal walks with the foot in plantigrade fashion or doesn't use the leg at all. The distraction of the fracture by the pull of the gastrocnemius prevents bone contact, which interferes with healing. The pull of the muscles and the constant movement from walking will tend to bend or break a pin or screw inserted down the bone across the fracture. A repair with two K-wires and a tension band wire stabilizes the fracture satisfactorily.

SURGICAL TECHNIQUE

A lateral incision along the caudal border of the calcaneus is made through the skin and subcutaneous tissue to expose the area of fracture. The superficial digital flexor is freed from the tuber calcanei by incising the lateral fascial supports (retinaculum) and luxating it medially. This allows the fracture to be reduced and two K-wires to be placed. (In larger dogs, a single intramedullary pin through the fragment into the body of the calcaneus suffices.) A hole is drilled transversely through the end fragment below the placement of the K-wires or the pins. A hole is also drilled transversely through the body of the calcaneus. A figure-8 of orthopedic wire is inserted through the holes. The wire is tightened, the ends twisted and cut off, and the remaining twist is flattened to the bone. The two K-wires or the pin are countersunk to keep the projecting ends from

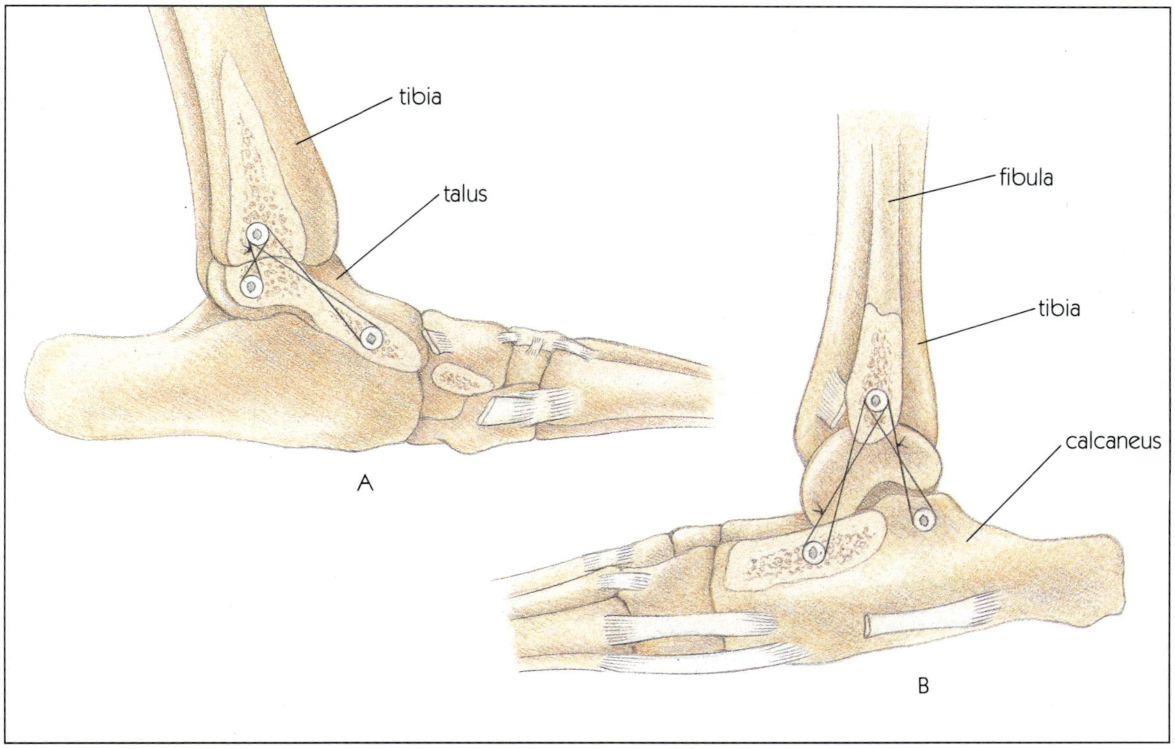

FIGURE 5.52 (A) The repair of a medial hock shear injury with screws and a suture. (B) The repair of a lateral hock shear injury with screws and sutures.

injuring the gliding surface of the superficial digital flexor. The pins will maintain alignment while the tension band will maintain fragment apposition (Fig. 5.53).

The superficial digital flexor is replaced and the lateral fascial support (retinaculum) is sutured with nonabsorbable sutures. The subcutaneous tissues and skin are sutured in place.

If the fracture is close to the end of the calcaneus or there is an avulsion of the insertion of the gastrocnemius tendon, the wire is placed over the ends of the two K-wires. These wires are placed as medially and laterally as possible and the ends are bent over to minimize injury to the superficial digital flexor as it slides over them. The pins and wire may have to be removed at a later date if lameness is observed.

On occasion, the medial or lateral support to the superficial digital flexor (retinaculum) is torn and the tendon slips off the end of the tuber calcis. This causes a lameness that may be somewhat difficult to diagnose because it comes and goes. The tendon may be luxated at palpation, sometimes with a definite snapping sensation.

The approach is made through the skin and subcutaneous tissues on the calcaneus on the side of the fascial support rupture, that is, opposite the side to which the tendon slips. Nonabsorbable sutures are used to repair the damaged fascia that supports the replaced tendon. The subcutaneous tissue and skin closure is then made.

Some additional support is usually provided for calcaneal fractures, such as a modified Robert Jones splint, but not for more than 7 to 10 days.

SUBLUXATION OF THE PROXIMAL INTERTARSAL JOINT

This is a common injury in dogs, especially in the Shetland sheep dog and collie. The injury occurs when the plantar ligament between the fourth tarsal and the calcaneus (fibular tarsal bone) is ruptured and the foot from this area is hyperflexed. The dog will walk almost plantigrade in this position.

SURGICAL TECHNIQUE

The affected joint area is approached by a plantarolateral incision through the skin and subcutaneous tissue. The superficial digital flexor tendon is freed from its fascial covering and retracted medially. The area is debrided, the articular surfaces are curetted and flushed clear. A hole is drilled through the midportion of the calcaneus (fibular tarsal bone). Another hole is drilled through the plantar portion of the fourth tarsal bone. Heavy orthopedic wire is placed through the holes in a figure-8 pattern, but not tightened.

The superficial digital flexor is moved medially from the tuber calcanei by incising the lateral retinacular supports. A hole is drilled down the length of the calcaneus. The bone is very hard and a hand or mechanical drill is useful. An intramedullary pin is inserted down the calcaneus to the fracture/luxation site. This area and the curetted joint surfaces are packed with cancellous bone that can be easily obtained beforehand from the proximal tibia.

The luxation is reduced and the pin is seated firmly into the fourth tarsal. It is cut off close to the bone and countersunk into the tuber calcanei. The tension-band wire is now tightened and the twisted wire ends are cut and pressed flat to the bone. The superficial digital flexor is replaced and the lateral retinacular tissues are sutured with nonabsorbable sutures. The fascia on the plantar surface of the calcaneus and the fourth tarsal is sutured. The tendon of the superficial digital flexor is replaced. The subcutaneous and skin tissues are sutured. The lower leg is placed in a modified Robert Jones splint for 7 days. The pin and wires are left in place (Fig. 5.54).

Subluxation of the Distal Intertarsal Joints

There is a valgus deformity (i.e., the distal part of the foot is spread away from the body). This may be associated with other injuries, which should be looked for.

SURGICAL TECHNIQUE

This injury is repaired by curetting the joint surfaces exposed by an incision over the medial aspect of the affected area, from the central tarsal bone to the head of the second metatarsal. The foot is forced laterally to allow curettage of the area. One bone screw is inserted in the central tarsal and another through the second and third distal tarsals and into the fourth. A figure-8 of orthopedic wire is twisted around the screws and tightened. The twisted ends are cut short, then bent flat to the bone. The subcutaneous and skin incisions are closed. Protection from stress and injury is provided by placing the

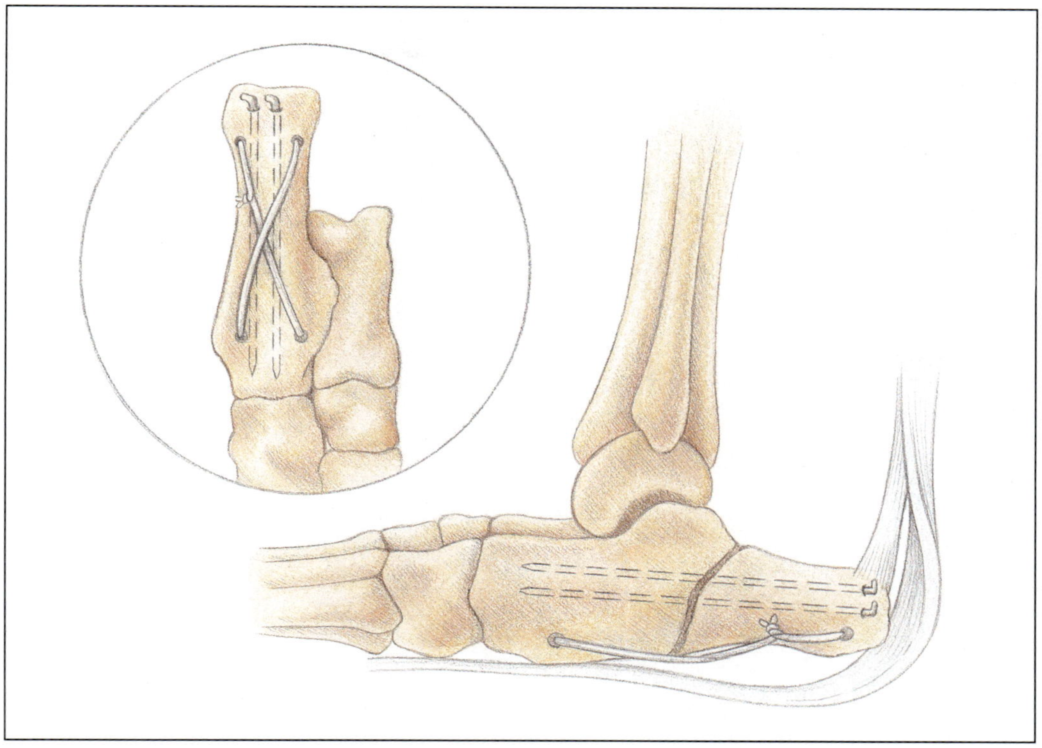

FIGURE 5.53 The repair of a fracture of the calcaneus with K-wires and a figure-8 tension band wire.

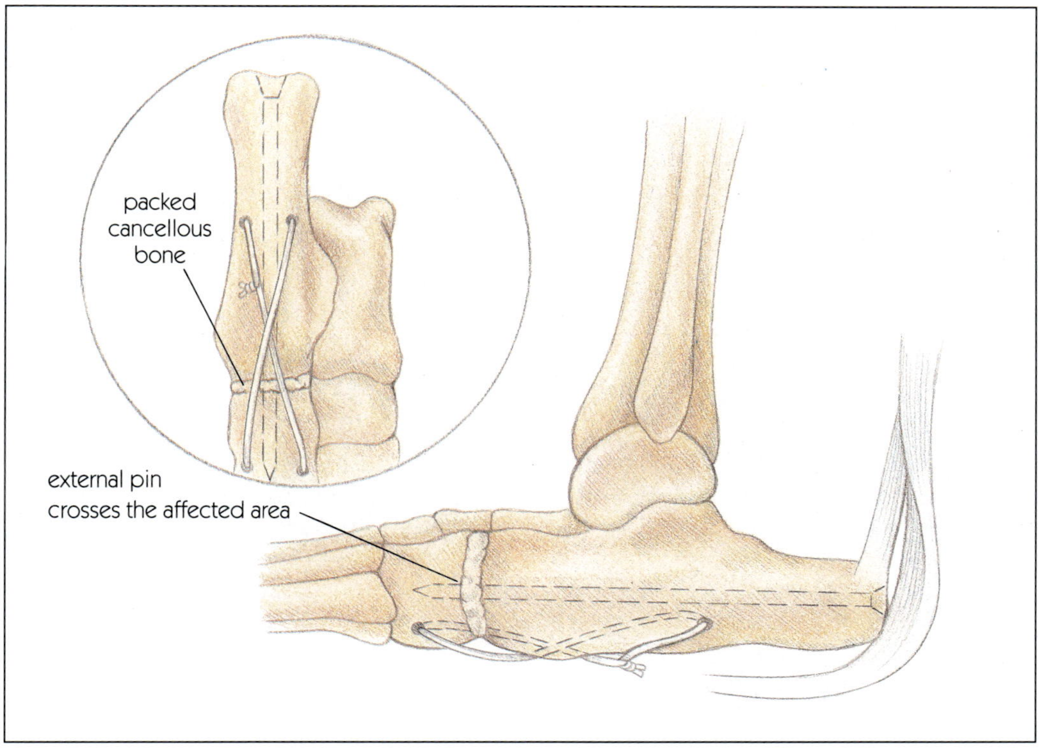

FIGURE 5.54 The repair of a subluxation of the proximal intertarsal joint with an intramedullary pin and tension-band wire.

lower leg in a padded splint or a modified Robert Jones splint for 2 to 3 weeks (Fig. 5.55).

Tarso-Metatarsal Subluxation

This is a common injury, and the results of surgical intervention are far superior to splinting or casting.

The heads of metatarsals V, IV, and III may be found to be torn away from the distal row of tarsal bones (Fig. 5.56).

SURGICAL TECHNIQUE

The approach is over the lateral aspect of the fourth tarsal and metatarsal. The joint surfaces are curetted. A bone screw is placed in the lateral aspect of the fourth tarsal and the lateral aspect of the proximal portion of the head of metatarsal V. A figure-8 of orthopedic wire is placed around the screw and tightened. The twisted ends are cut short and flattened to the bone. The subcutaneous tissue and skin are sutured. The lower leg is placed in a padded splint or modified Robert Jones splint for about 3 weeks.

In larger dogs it may be advantageous to insert a strong intramedullary pin through the length of the calcaneus and the fourth tarsal into the head of metatarsal IV. This pin is countersunk so that it will not interfere with the function of the superficial digital flexor as it glides over the tuber calcanei.

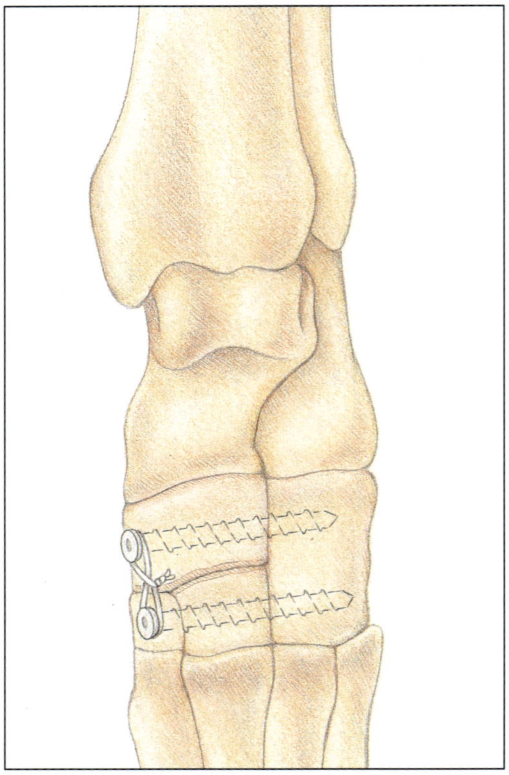

FIGURE 5.55 The repair of a subluxation of the distal intertarsal joint using screws and a figure-8 of wire.

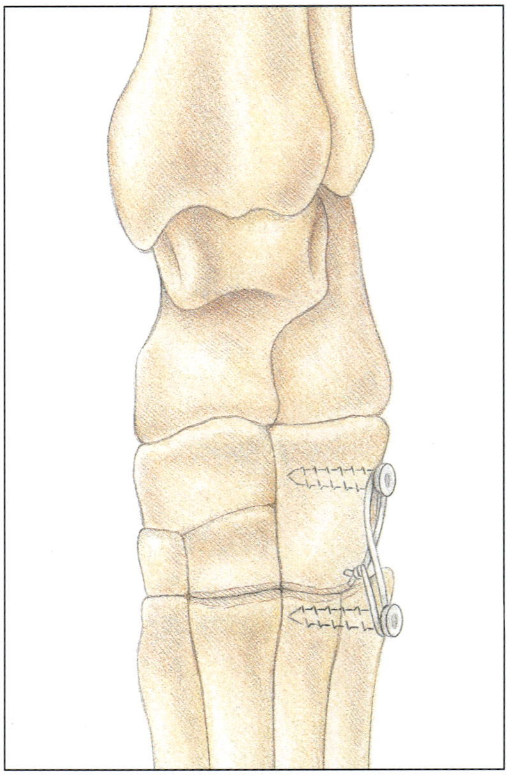

FIGURE 5.56 The repair of a tarsometatarsal subluxation with screws and a figure-8 of wire.

CHAPTER 6

VERTEBRAL COLUMN

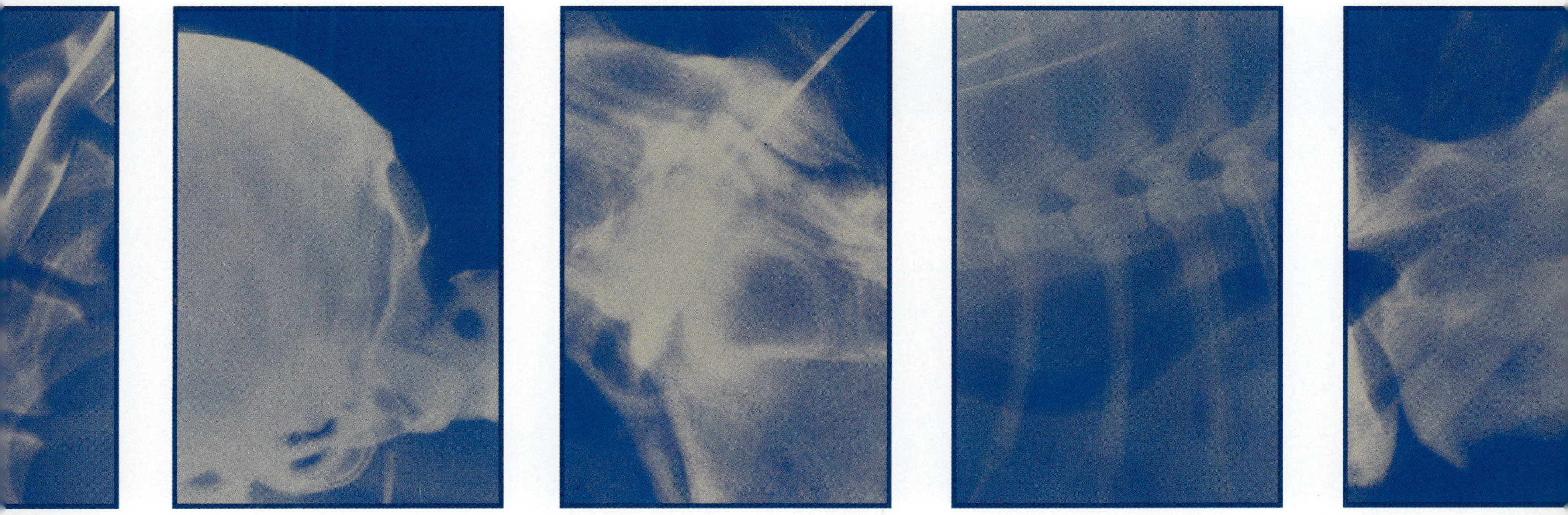

The diagnostic workup is an essential preliminary for any surgery and is especially important for delineating the neurologic component of injuries to the vertebral column. Because determining the prognosis is difficult at best, the client must be informed and must understand the risks. Furthermore, the potential quality of life for the animal must be considered. Delay is often critical for a good outcome. The patient must be handled carefully to avoid further and possibly irreparable damage.

ATLANTO–AXIAL SUBLUXATION

This condition is seen as a congenital defect in dogs of certain young toy and small breeds. It causes compression of the spinal cord at the C1–2 level. Diagnosis is based on neurologic signs and radiography. Extreme care in manipulation of these patients must be observed.

On a lateral radiograph of the flexed neck, the cranial edge of the spine of the axis will be separated from its normal relationship with the atlas and cranium (Fig. 6.1). The abnormal increase in dorsal angulation permits the ventral edge of the axis to impinge on the spinal cord. Surgical correction of the subluxation is obtained by securing the spine of the axis into a proper relationship to the atlas with a nonabsorbable suture sling (Fig. 6.2).

SURGICAL TECHNIQUE

The dog is placed in sternal recumbency with the head in extension and the neck supported on a firm sponge or sandbag. A dorsal midline incision is made through the skin and subcutaneous tissues from the caudal aspect of the occiput to the midcervical area. The underlying fascia is cleared to expose the median raphe. Careful sharp dissection is done to separate the paired neck muscles and retract them laterally away from the dorsal arch of the atlas and the dorsal spine of the axis. Care must be taken to avoid the vertebral arteries when the dissection is deepened and extended laterally. A Gelpi retractor is placed to hold the neck muscles laterally. The periosteum is reflected from the arch of the atlas. The dissection is carried into the spinal canal at the craniocaudal margins of the arch of the atlas. The surgeon must avoid entering the subarachnoid space. The dura may be adherent to the cranial edge of the atlas and must be teased free. If the atlanto–occipital space is too small, a cut is made with rongeurs in either the atlas or the occipital bone.

The dorsal atlanto–axial membrane is isolated and incised to reveal the underlying spinal cord. A small portion of the ligament is removed cranially. A small piece of the caudal edge of the atlas or the cranial edge of the axis may have to be removed with a rongeur to permit passage of a looped piece of 2-0 monofilament wire through the dorsal canal space just under the arch of the atlas. Gentle reduction of the subluxation by an assistant, depressing the axis ventrally by means of a bone forceps grasping the spine, will permit passage of the wire without injury to the cord.

A doubled length of 2-0 Polydek suture is inserted through the looped wire and drawn through the dorsal canal of the atlas. Two holes are drilled transversely through the spine of the axis, one caudal to the other. The looped end of the suture is cut. One piece

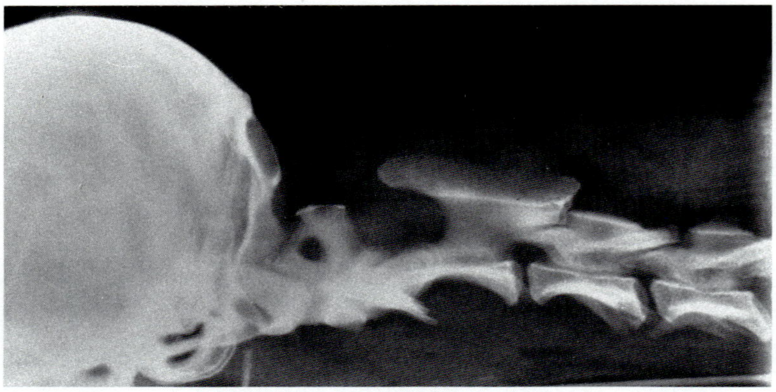

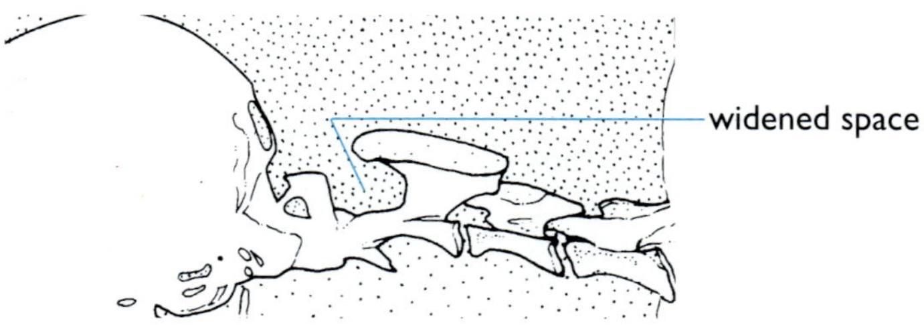

FIGURE 6.1 Atlanto–axial subluxation.

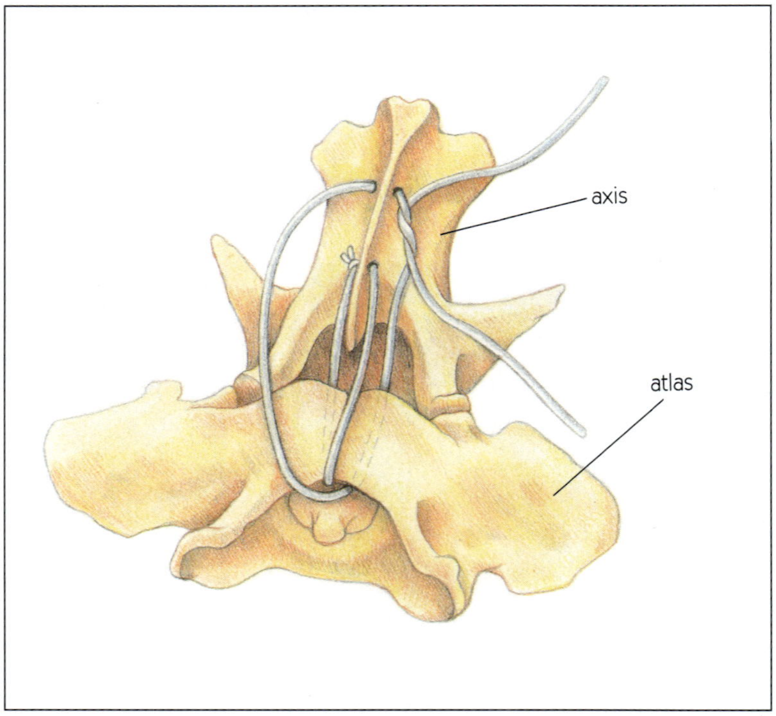

FIGURE 6.2 Suture placement for control of atlanto–axial subluxation.

is inserted through the cranial hole and tied to its end on one side and the other suture is inserted through the caudal hole and tied on the opposite side. The two sutures will form a "harness" over the top of the atlas. The sutures are tied tightly enough to hold the axis in normal position. Not all dogs have a normal-sized axial spine. Such cases require inventiveness on the part of the surgeon to find an area in which to secure the sutures.

Closure is performed by replacing the muscles of the neck and suturing the fascia and subcutaneous tissue. Nonabsorbable suture is used in the skin.

The neck and head are supported by padding and bandages for several days. Improvement will be indicated by relief from pain and improved control of the limbs.

INTERVERTEBRAL DISC FENESTRATION

Cervical Disc

Disc protrusion into the cervical area often causes severe pain by compression of the nerve roots. Knuckling over of the forelimbs and hindlimbs is common. Radiography often demonstrates several discs with various degrees of calcification and narrowing of the disc spaces (Fig. 6.3). When the disc material has not entered the spinal canal, relief is obtained by fenestrating the affected discs.

SURGICAL TECHNIQUE

The dog is positioned in dorsal recumbency, with a pad beneath the neck to arch it towards the surgeon. The incision is made on the ventral midline from caudal to the larynx to the sternum. The subcutaneous tissues are cleared to expose the underlying fascia. This is incised to expose the median raphe between the paired sternohyoid muscles. Incision of the median raphe exposes the trachea, which is then freed by blunt dissection with the finger and retracted to the left to expose the ventral cervical muscles. Care must be taken to avoid damage to the carotid sheath, esophagus, and the right recurrent laryngeal nerve, which lies on the dorsolateral aspect of the trachea.

The vertebrae are identified by using the wings of the atlas and the large transverse processes of C-6 as landmarks. The forefinger is used to palpate on the midline for the ventral vertebral tubercle. A midline incision with a scalpel is made caudal to this structure. Blunt dissection will reveal a pair of yellow fibrous muscle insertions attaching centrally on the ventral tubercle and forming a "V" pointing cranially. These identify the proper location, and are incised with careful blunt dissection to expose the disc's surface. Too wide a dissection will cause severe hemorrhage. A block of the ventral portion of the disc is cut away with a small scalpel. A disc fenestration knife is then used to incise the disc and a fenestration excavator is used to remove as much of the disc material as possible. Calcified material may ooze from the disc, providing evidence of the pressure it has been under.

The disc material must not be forced into the spinal canal. Surgery usually involves C2–3 to C5–6. C-7 can be included when necessary (Fig. 6.4).

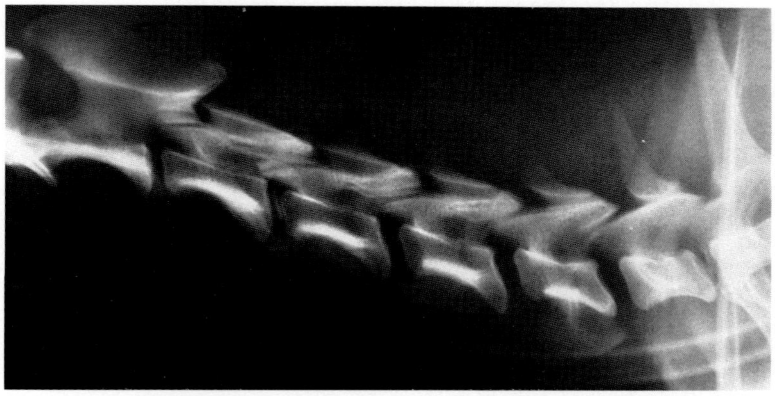

FIGURE 6.3 Cervical disc fenestration. Radiography often demonstrates several discs with various degrees of disc calcification and narrowing of the disc spaces.

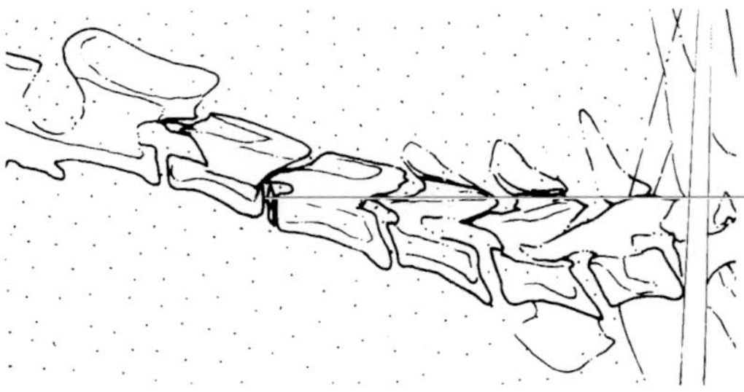

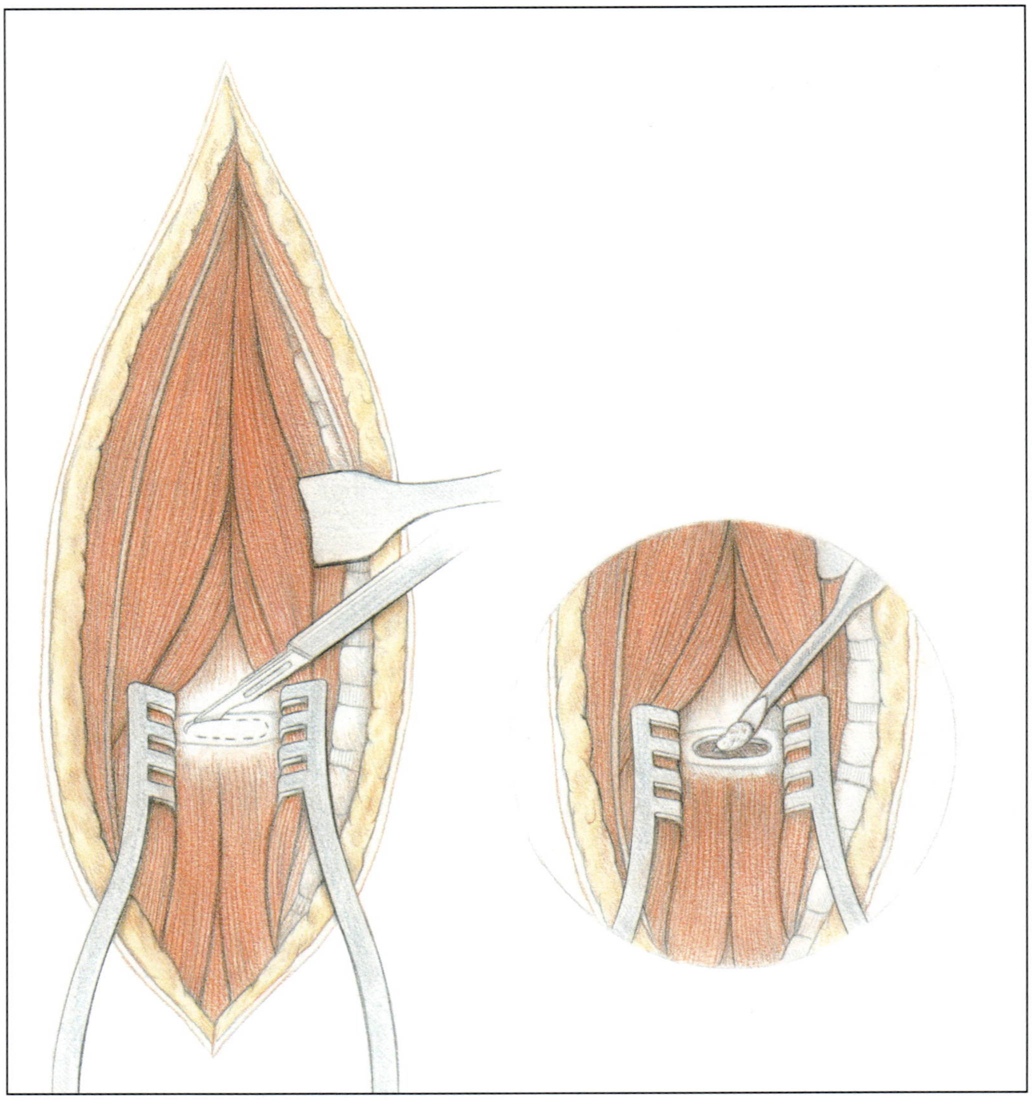

FIGURE 6.4 Disc fenestration.

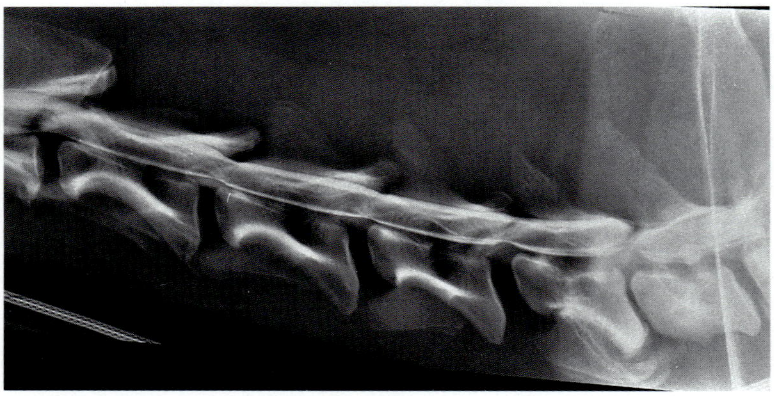

FIGURE 6.5 Ventral cervical disc decompression. Although the affected disc can be located by a plain radiograph, the definitive diagnosis is by myelography, as is shown here.

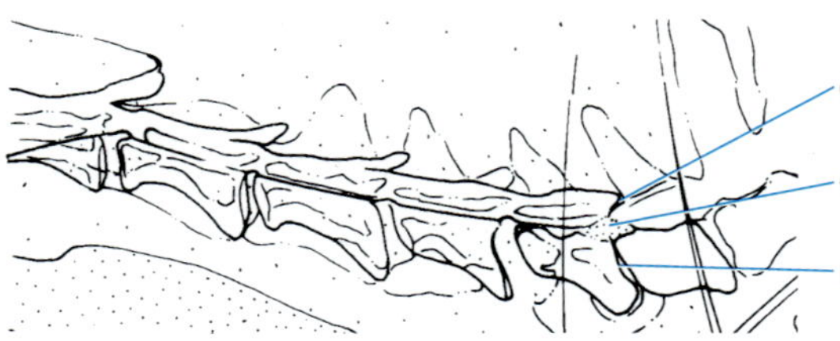

The trachea is released, and closure is performed by suturing the separation between the sternohyoid muscles. Subcutaneous tissue and skin are closed in the routine manner.

Sutures are removed after 7 to 10 days. The response is often dramatic. Some cases, however, require a longer period of time for recovery.

Ventral Cervical Disc

Disc protrusion, ligamentous hypertrophy, and rupture of disc material into the spinal canal require relief from cord and nerve root compression by removal of as much of the offending disc material as possible. Although the affected disc can be located by a plain radiograph, the definitive diagnosis is by myelography (Fig. 6.5). A ventral slotting technique is used to achieve decompression.

SURGICAL TECHNIQUE

The dog is placed in dorsal recumbency, with the neck held gently arched upward with a sandbag. The incision is made on the ventral midline from caudal to the larynx to the sternum. The subcutaneous tissue is cleared to expose the underlying fascia. This is incised to expose the median raphe between the paired sternohyoid muscles. The median raphe is incised and the trachea is isolated by blunt dissection with the finger. The trachea is retracted to the left and the neck muscles spread apart with a retractor. The ventral cervical muscles (longus colli) are exposed. Care must be taken to avoid the carotid sheath, the esophagus, and the recurrent laryngeal nerve lying alongside the trachea. The vertebrae are identified by using the wing of the atlas and the expanded transverse processes of C-6 as landmarks.

The ventral vertebral tubercle is identified, and a midline incision is made caudal and cranial to this structure. The covering muscles are gently dissected laterally to isolate the ventral surface of the disc. Too wide a dissection will lead to excessive hemorrhage from branches of the vertebral arteries. The ventral surfaces of the vertebral bodies above and below the affected disc are exposed. The disc is cut away ventrally with a small scalpel, and any remaining disc material is removed.

The ventral vertebral tubercle is excised with a small rongeur. The exposed flattened area of cancellous bone is first cut with the burr of a high-speed air drill. A ventral slot is made by gently cutting away the underlying cortical and cancellous bone and any intervening disc material from the center of one vertebral body to the other. The sides of the slot are cut downward perpendicularly, with both ends tapered inward (Fig. 6.6). The slot must be vertical, symmetrical, and on the midline. The cut is frequently irrigated with saline and dried with suction. Contact with dense cortical bone indicates that the canal will soon be entered. Once the canal is entered and the cord exposed, the disc material is carefully removed with an Adson forceps or the disc fenestration excavator. The ventral venous sinuses are very close, and injury to these will result in severe bleeding. Remnants of the dorsal longitudinal ligament are removed. The slot can be filled with a small piece of subcutaneous fat or a piece of Gelfoam.

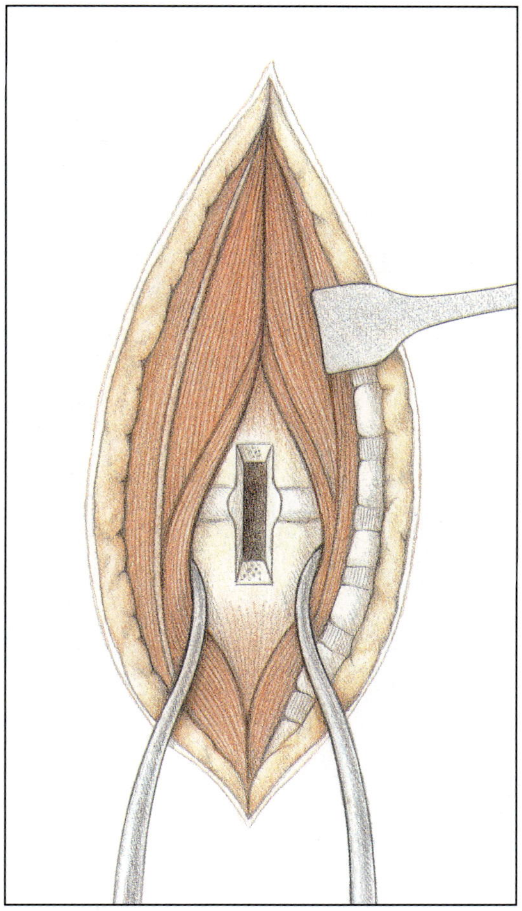

FIGURE 6.6 Tapered slot in ventral surgical slotting technique.

At closure, the trachea is replaced and the separation between the sternohyoid muscles is sutured. Routine closure of the skin and subcutaneous tissue is performed.

Postoperative pain is controlled with sedation. Although no external support is needed, confinement to a cage for a week is recommended. In most cases relief is seen within a few days.

Thoraco-Lumbar Disc

Fenestration has been thought to be of value for cases in which the collapsing disc has brought mild upward pressure to bear on the spinal cord but nuclear or annular material has not ruptured into the spinal canal. Fenestration has also long been advocated as a prophylactic procedure when more definitive surgery was done on an individual disc. However, both of these concepts have been challenged, the claim being that a laminectomy is always required and that prophylactic fenestration is useless. Proper neurologic diagnosis with radiography must be made. Surgery usually involves discs T11–12 through L3–4 (Fig. 6.7).

SURGICAL TECHNIQUE

The dog is placed in sternal recumbency, with the spine held gently arched upward by a small sandbag. A dorsal midline incision through the skin and subcutaneous tissues is made from T-8 to L-6. Subcutaneous fat is cleared from the dorsolumbar fascia, which is then incised with a scalpel just lateral to the tips of the dorsal spinous processes. By blunt dissection with the scalpel handle, the musculature can be easily distracted laterally from the dorsal spines. The blunt dissection is carried further until the articular processes are exposed. Their muscle attachments are carefully severed. Muscle attachments to the accessory processes are severed. Cranially, the heads of ribs 12 and 13 will be exposed. The transverse processes of the lumbar vertebrae are cleared of muscle tissue, and retractors are placed to maintain the exposure. The spinal nerves and vessels exit from the intervertebral foramina just craniodorsal to the discs. In the lumbar area, the tissues just cranial to the cranial edge of the lateral process at its attachment to the vertebral body are cleared to expose the disc. The vessels and nerves just cranial to the disc are gently

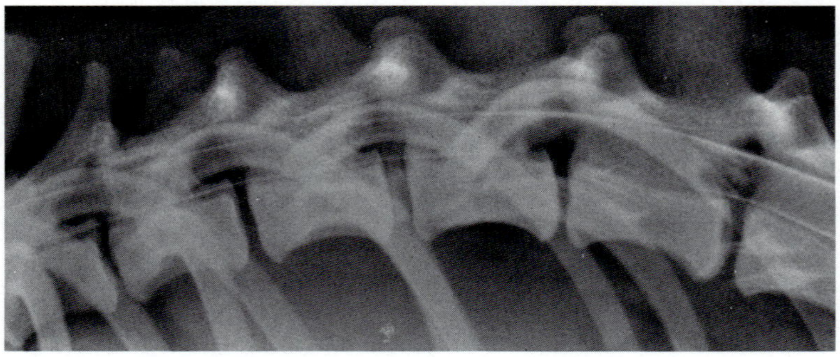

FIGURE 6.7 A narrowed disc can be seen at T-13.

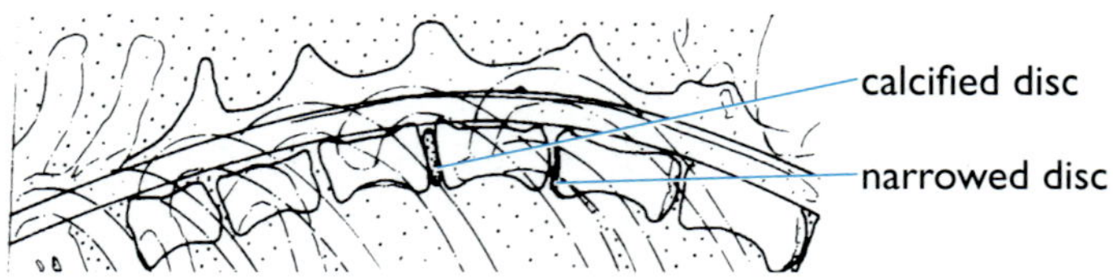

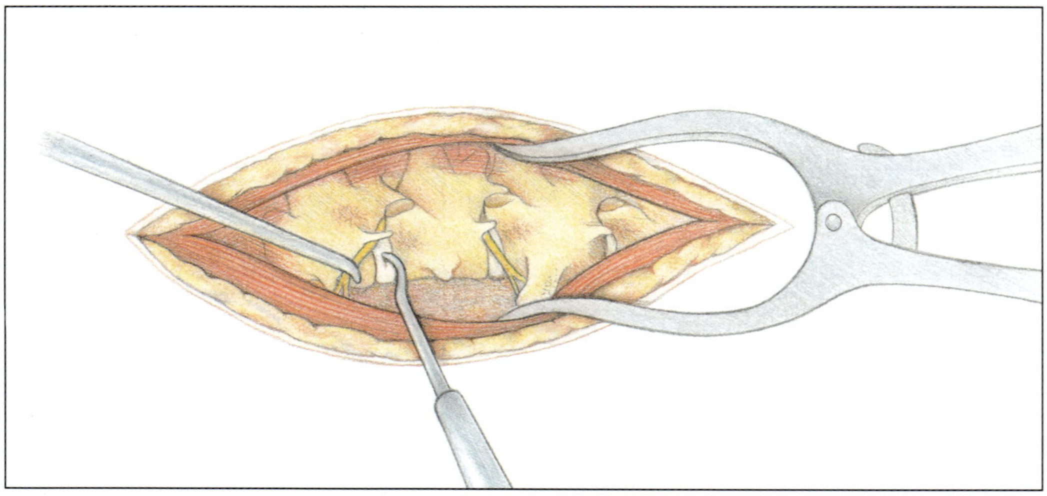

FIGURE 6.8 Removal of disc material in a thoracolumbar fenestration.

retracted. A small scalpel blade can be used to incise the anulus, or it can be cut with the disc fenestration knife, which is inserted and pulled downward to avoid penetrating the spinal cord. The disc fenestration excavator is then used in a similar fashion (Fig. 6.8). Each lumbar disc is treated similarly. The thoracic discs are located just cranial and dorsal to the head of the ribs. Too deep a ventral thrust may injure the aorta.

For closure, the muscles are allowed to resume their normal positions. The lumbodorsal fascia and subcutaneous tissue are sutured with simple interrupted sutures of 2-0 chromic catgut. The skin is closed with nonabsorbable suture material.

Rigorous postsurgical attention is needed, with special care taken to provide physiotherapy and nursing care.

CERVICAL INSTABILITY

Signs of interference with neural control of the limbs caused by cervical cord compression can have a number of causes. Among the more common are calcific disc degeneration and, in some of the larger breeds, hypertrophy of the dorsal longitudinal ligament resulting from instability caused by cervical vertebral malformation or malarticulation, usually at the level of C5–6 (Fig. 6.9). Marked vertebral malformation causes severe signs, which are usually seen in younger dogs of large breeds (e.g., Great Dane), whereas the lesser malformations may not cause signs until the animal is 6 to 8 years of age (e.g., Doberman /pinscher). The gait defect seen gives rise to the term "wobbler." Confirming diagnosis is made by radiography and myelography (Figs. 6.10 and 6.11). Surgical treatment has been directed towards stabilization of the affected vertebral joint but, because of many problems with a variety of fusion techniques, decompression by ventral slotting is recommended.

SURGICAL TECHNIQUE

The dog is placed in dorsal recumbency with the neck stabilized in an upward arched position by a sandbag. The patient is taped to the table to ensure immobility.

A ventral midline incision is made through the skin and subcutaneous tissue from the cranial tracheal region to the sternum. The muscle aponeuroses are cleared of subcutaneous fascia and fat and are incised on the midline. The median raphe between the paired sternohyoid muscles is incised and the trachea is exposed. The incision is carried caudally on the ventral midline separating the sternohyoid muscles. The trachea is isolated by blunt dissection with the fingers along the right side. Care must be taken to avoid injury to the recurrent laryngeal

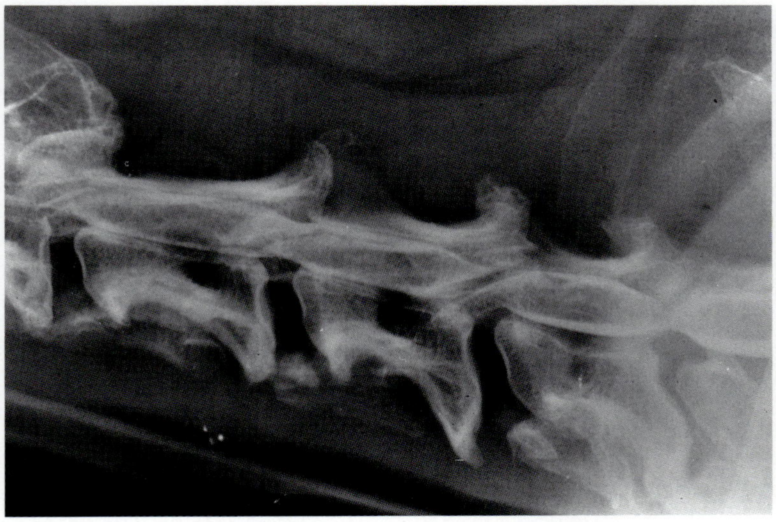

FIGURE 6.9 Radiograph shows cord compression at C5-6 in a dog with cervical instability when its neck is extended.

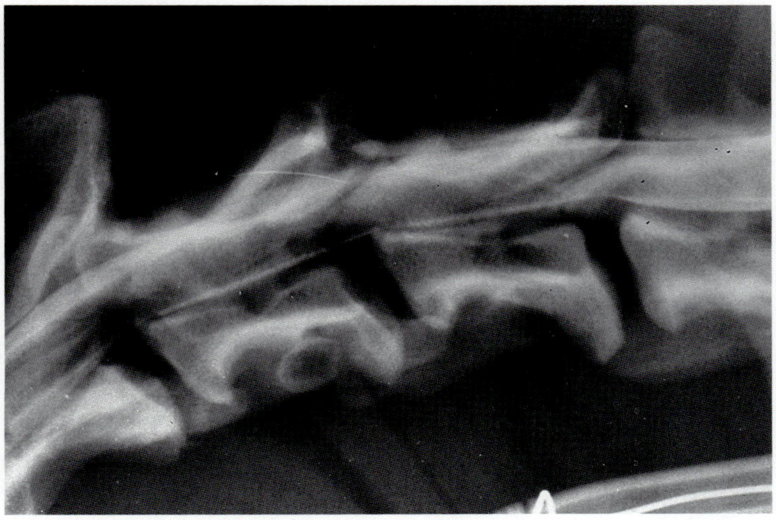

FIGURE 6.10 Radiograph of a dog with cervical instability when its neck is flexed shows relief of cord compression at C5-6.

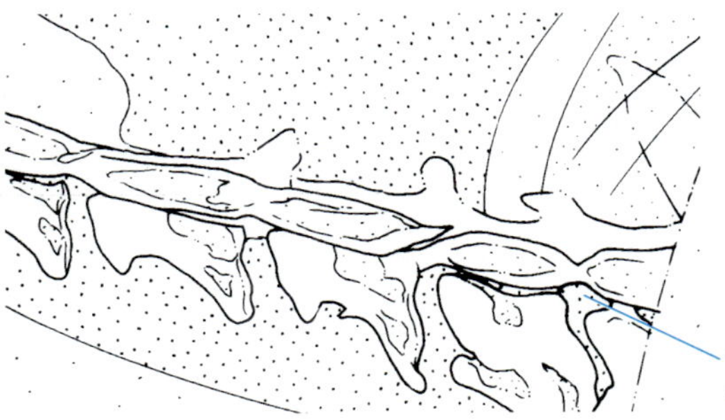

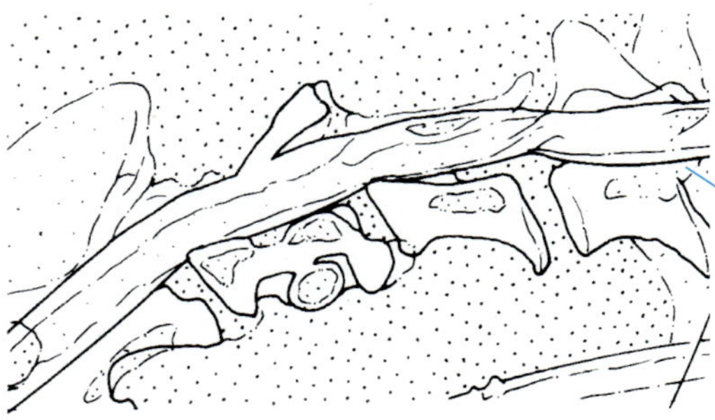

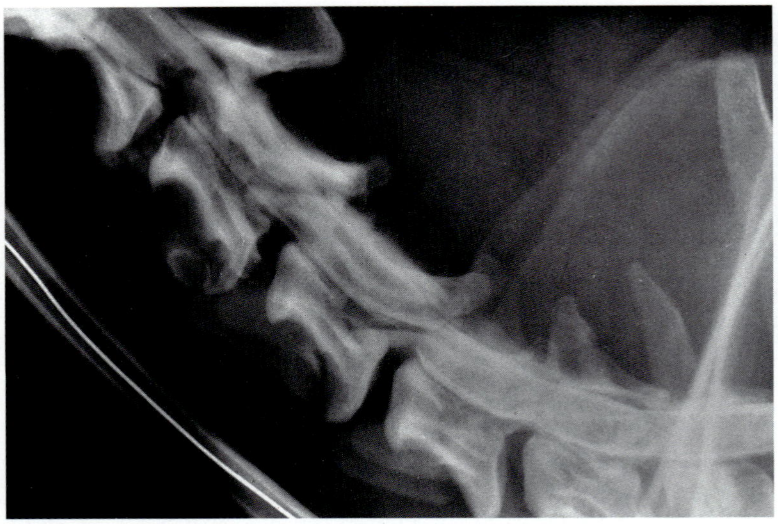

FIGURE 6.11 Myelogram of cervical instability, normal neck position.

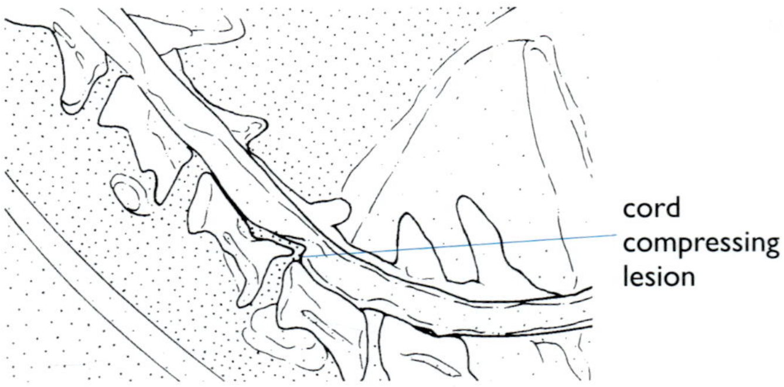

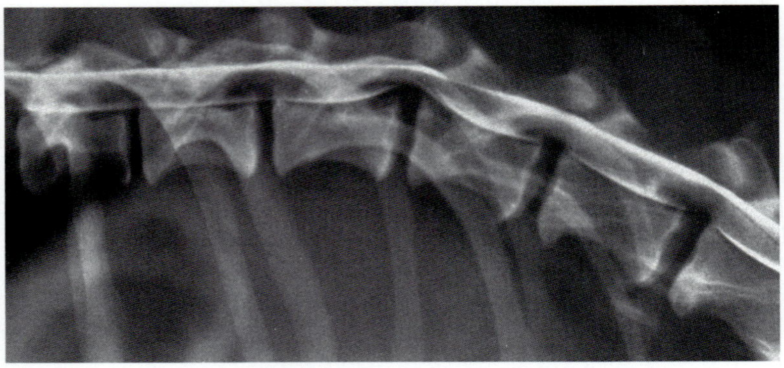

FIGURE 6.12 Radiograph showing cord compression from an intervertebral disc protrusion.

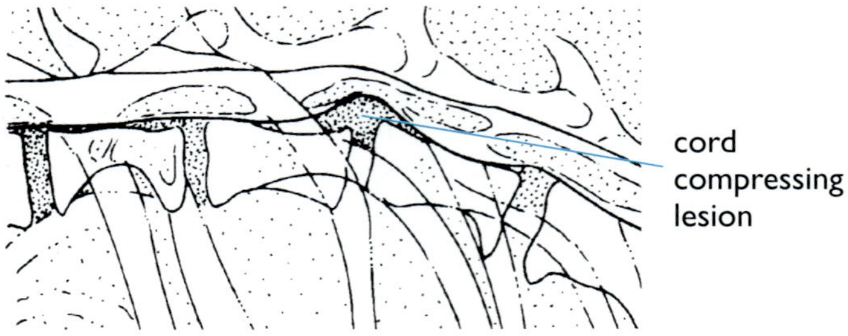

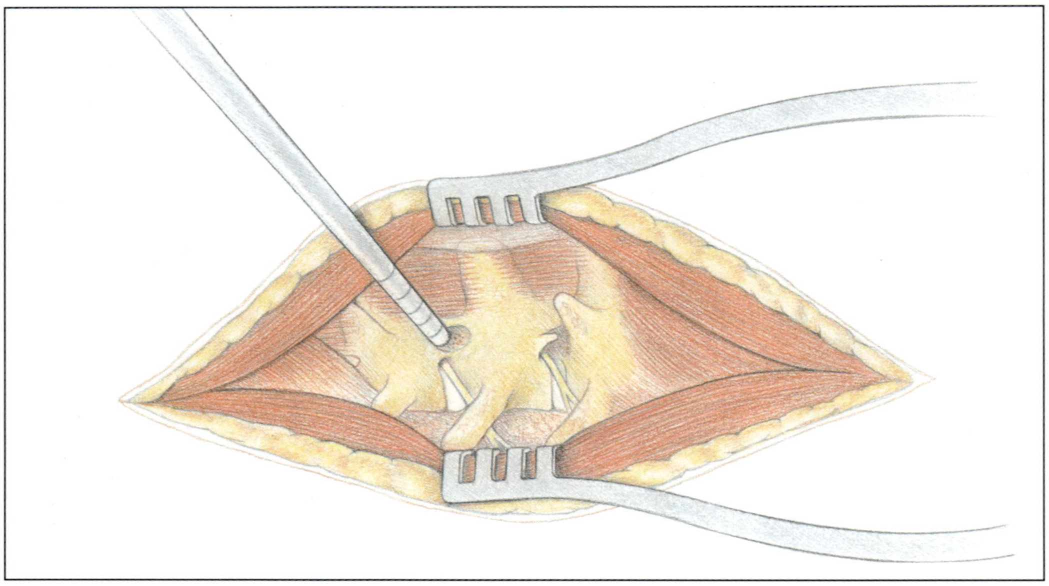

FIGURE 6.13 Michel trephine in use.

nerve or the structures in the right carotid sheath (carotid artery and associated nerves and veins). A considerable depth of muscle tissue must be separated and held laterally with retractors before the muscles that cover the ventral surfaces of the cervical vertebrae are seen. Cervical vertebra C-6 is an aid to vertebral identification because of its enlarged ventrally directed processes. The ventral tubercle is identified to locate the midline, and the longus colli muscles are bluntly dissected away to expose the ventral aspect of the vertebrae. The surgeon must be careful to avoid extending the dissection too far laterally, thus striking vessels that will hemorrhage excessively. The instability of the intervertebral articulation can often be demonstrated by elevating the cranial vertebral component of the affected disc space. The ventral tubercle is cut off with rongeurs, providing a flat cancellous surface for the burr of the high-speed air drill. The disc space is at a dorsoventral angle and the cranial aspect of the caudal vertebral component is often malformed, so care is necessary as the cord is approached. By cutting exactly on the midline, the ventrolaterally located venous sinus will be avoided. Frequent flushing and suctioning are necessary while drilling. The slot is cut square on the sides, tapering at each end. First the cortical layer of bone is removed, then the cancellous bone is removed, and finally the last cortical layer is approached. This should be cut away very carefully. Testing the depth of this layer with an 18-gauge needle is recommended. Pieces of anulus and the hypertrophied dorsal longitudinal ligament are removed. The exposed cord is covered with a bit of subcutaneous fat. Two sutures of 2-0 chromic catgut are placed to approximate the longus colli muscles over the fat to hold it in place. The Gelpi retractors are removed, and the trachea and muscles are returned to normal position. The midline incision in the muscle aponeuroses and the subcutaneous tissues are sutured with 2-0 chromic catgut. The skin is closed with nonabsorbable suture material.

Postoperative pain is controlled with sedatives, and immobilization is necessary. The skin sutures can be removed in 7 to 10 days. Recovery depends on the relief from cord pressure provided by removing the cause of the compression from within the vertebral canal. In general, the prognosis is guarded.

HEMILAMINECTOMY

When neurologic and radiographic examination have identified and localized a ruptured intervertebral disc causing spinal cord compression, decompression is imperative (Fig. 6.12). Entry into the spinal canal and removal of the offending disc material, with release of pressure, can be accomplished by a hemilaminectomy. This procedure is advantageous in that it does not require a high-speed air drill, although the use of such a drill can be very effective. Hemilaminectomy, which produces an opening that can be easily extended, does not cause a dorsal spinal defect, does not significantly interfere with spinal stability, and provides access to the cord and disc.

SURGICAL TECHNIQUE

The dog is placed in sternal recumbency. An incision is made on the dorsal midline through the skin and subcutaneous tissue from T-10 to L-5. The subcutaneous fascia and fat are cleared to expose the lumbodorsal fascia. An incision is made through the fascia with the scalpel along the midline, just skirting the ends of the dorsal spines. With the handle of the scalpel, the muscles are moved laterally away from the dorsal spines. Intervening fibrous bands of the multifidus dorsi are incised. The musculature is bluntly removed to expose the articular processes. Two vertebrae above and below the identified disc are cleared. Muscle attachments to the articular processes are severed, as are those to the accessory process above the affected disc. Hemorrhage is

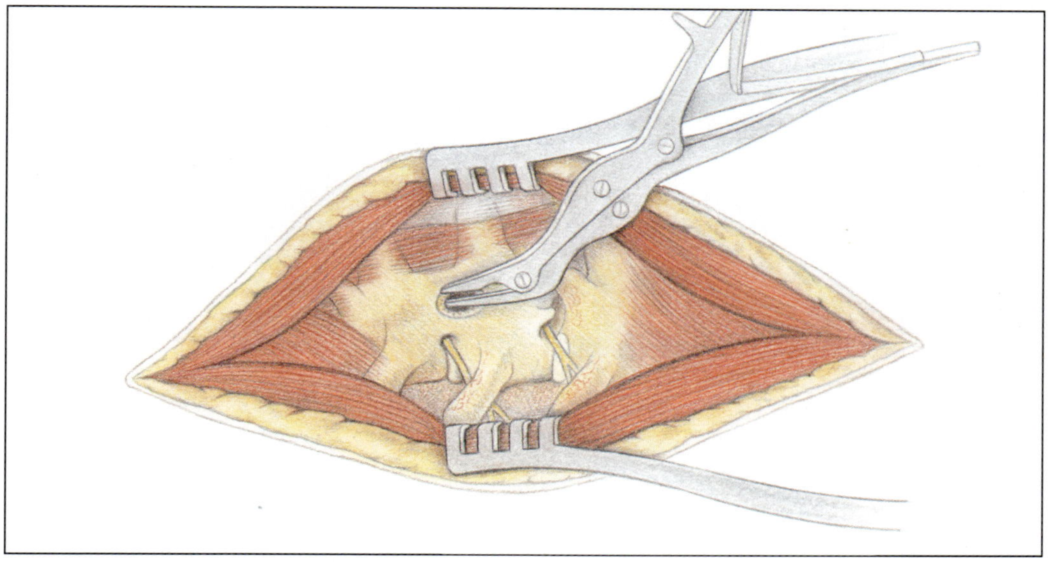

FIGURE 6.14 Double-action duck-billed rongeur.

controlled, and the dorsal surfaces of the transverse processes are exposed. Retractors are placed at each end of the incision to hold the lumbar muscles laterally.

The articular processes over the affected disc are cut off with the Liston bone cutter. The exposed flat area of cancellous bone is used as a starting point for the Michel trephine. A round plug of bone is cut away (Fig. 6.13). Care is taken not to injure the underlying spinal cord. As cutting progresses, the instrument is rocked back and forth to determine the looseness of the bone plug. When it is removed there may be underlying fat, which is carefully removed with suction or Adson forceps to expose the dura. The lamina is cut away cranially and caudally with small double-action rongeurs (Fig. 6.14). Pressure on the cord should be avoided. Small bites of bone are taken, further exposing the area above the disc. Care must be taken to avoid injury to the adjacent nerve root. Disc material will usually be found in the ventrolateral portion of the canal, and can be removed with a hook or an Adson forceps. The disc itself is removed by inserting the disc fenestration knife carefully under the cord and sweeping downward. The venous sinuses may bleed profusely when severed. This is controlled by placing pinhead-size pieces of muscle tissue at the bleeding site within the canal and closing the defect with a piece of Gelfoam. While the surgeon waits for hemostasis to be achieved, the adjacent discs are fenestrated as a prophylactic procedure. The Gelfoam is removed and a piece of subcutaneous fat is placed over the laminectomy. The retractors are removed, and closure of the lumbodorsal fascia and subcutaneous tissues with 2-0 chromic catgut is performed. The skin is closed with nonabsorbable suture.

Intravenous antibiotics are given before surgery and at 3-hour intervals until the surgery has been completed. If bladder infection is present, administration of appropriate antibiotics is continued. Careful nursing is required to prevent bedsores and cystitis. The sutures can be removed after 10 days. Depending on the progress of skin healing, active physiotherapy, such as warm baths, is begun after 5 to 7 days. In cases with early recognition, pain perception, and early removal of damaging disc material, good results can be expected.

SPINAL FRACTURES

The degree of cord damage must be determined before surgery to identify animals that have the capability for recovery. Because the degree of injury may not be commensurate with the radiographic appearance, myelography can be of considerable value (Figs. 6.15, 6.16). Extreme care must be taken in moving and examining such cases, both to protect the animal from further injury and to protect personnel from being bitten. Securing the patient to a litter is recommended. Surgical repair by vertebral body plating is possible with fractures from T-13 to L-4, a very common location for such injuries.

SURGICAL TECHNIQUE

The dog is placed in sternal recumbency and held firmly in normal spinal position with sandbags. A dorsal midline incision is made through the skin and subcutaneous tissue from T-11 to L-5. The dorsal thoracolumbar fascia is exposed and incised with a scalpel, skirting the ends of the dorsal thoracic and lumbar spines. The

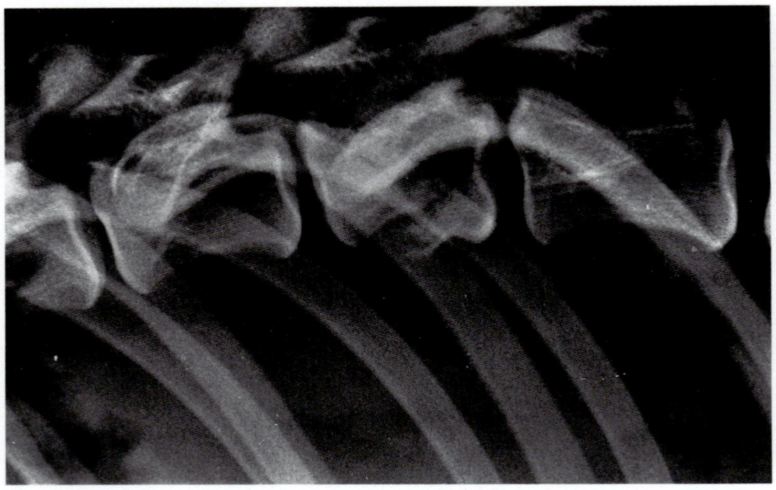

FIGURE 6.15 Radiograph of a spinal fracture.

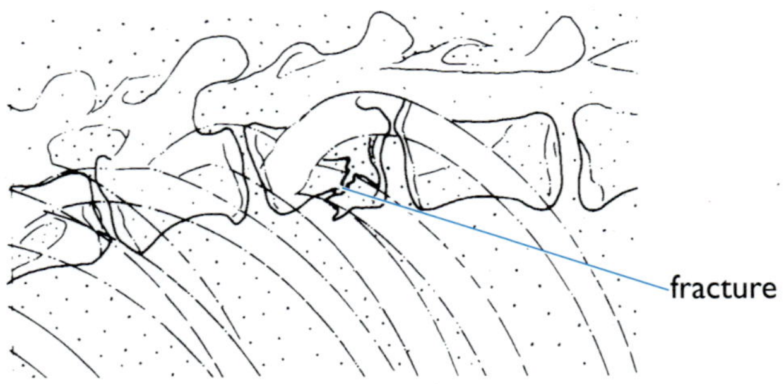

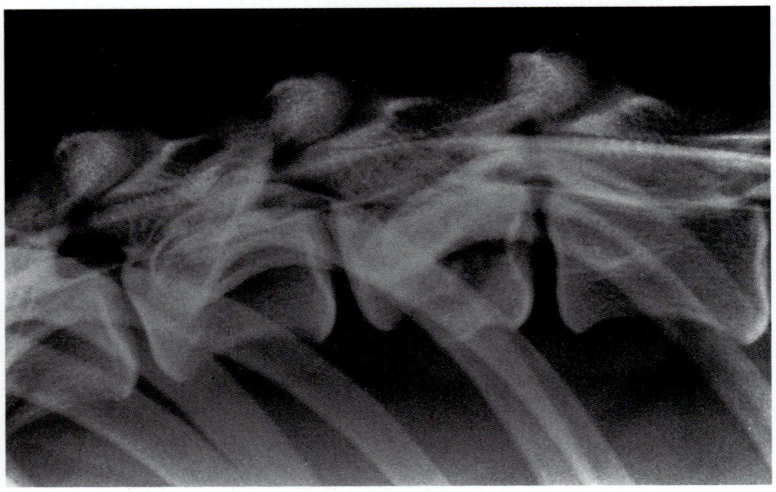

FIGURE 6.16 Myelogram of a spinal fracture.

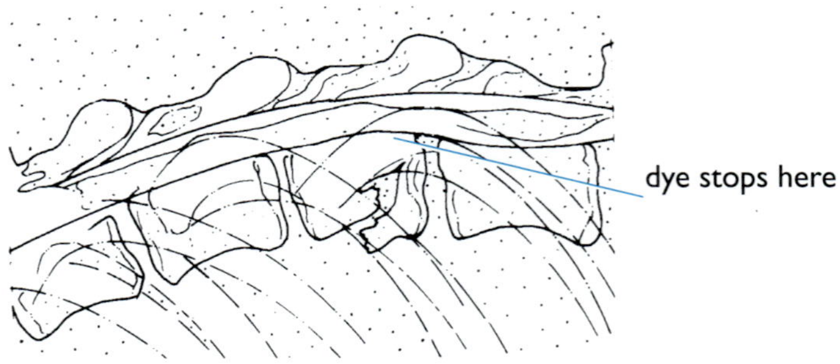

spinal muscles are separated from the dorsal spines with the handle of the scalpel. Continued blunt dissection moves the muscles laterally to expose the articular facets. Muscle attachments to these structures are cut and muscle reflection is continued; the attachments to the accessory processes are severed. The transverse processes are exposed along with the head of the last rib at T-13. Retractors are placed at each end of the incision to pull the muscles laterally. A bone plate can be fitted into the natural gutter that runs along the bodies of the vertebrae where the transverse processes attach. To seat the plate properly, it may be necessary to bend the plates slightly with plate benders, or to trim away some bone with the high-speed air drill and a burr. The exiting spinal nerves lie just under the plate. If indicated on the basis of myelography, a hemilaminectomy can be done, but excessive manipulation should be avoided. In the presence of reasonably intact neurologic signs, it is better to achieve stability than exact repositioning. Two screws are placed in each vertebral body if possible (Fig. 6.17), one located at the cranial edge of the junction of the transverse process with the vertebral body

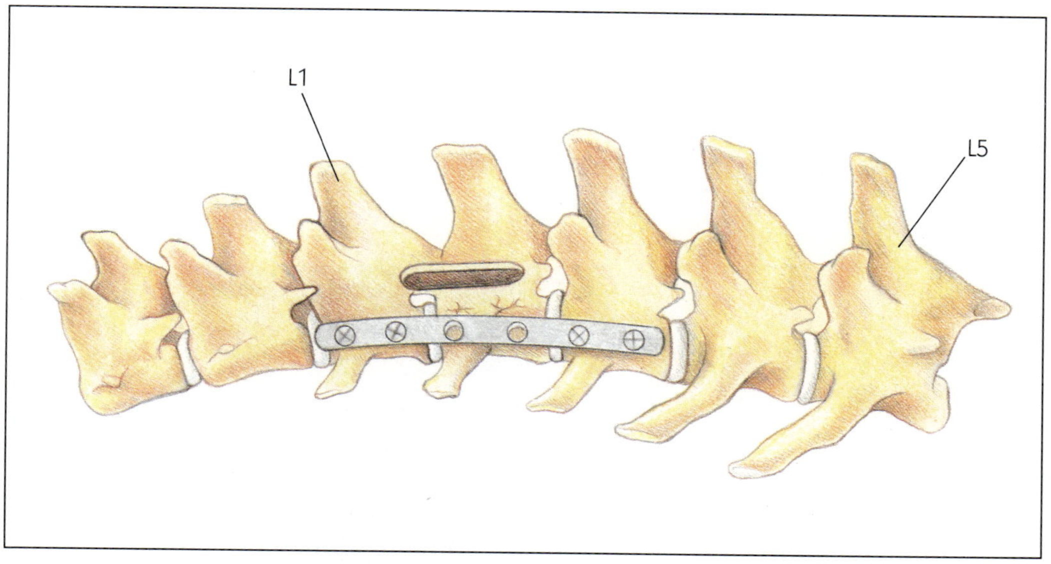

FIGURE 6.17 A bone plate on a spine.

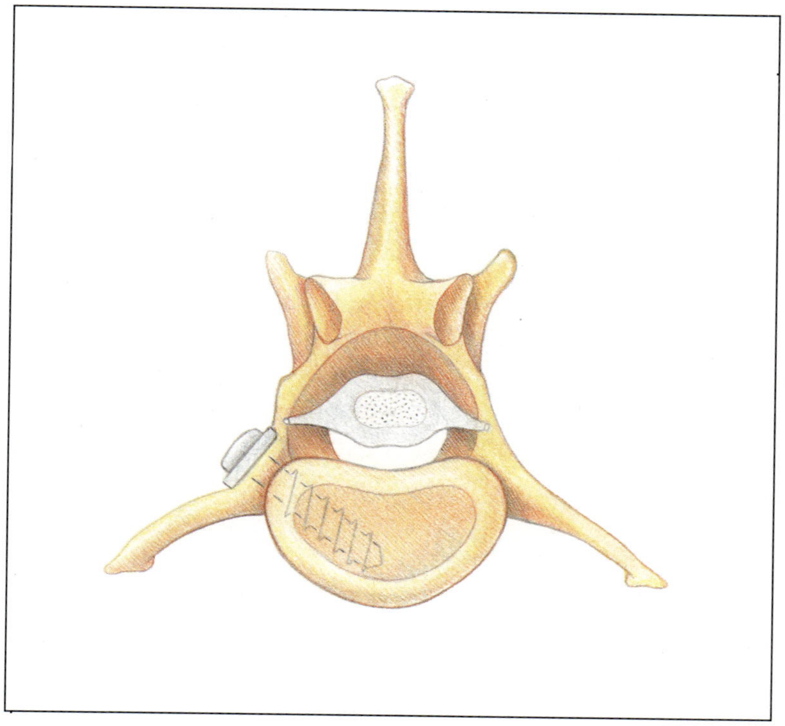

FIGURE 6.18 Screw location in spinal plating.

and one screw at the caudal edge. The screws must be directed downward and inward so that they do not enter the spinal canal, yet have a firm seat in the vertebral body (Fig. 6.18). The hole for the screw is drilled, measured for depth, and tapped, then the screw is inserted. This is done at each end of the plate. The rest of the screws are then applied and set firmly with the fingers.

Additional support is gained by bending one end of a small intramedullary pin in a "U" shape to fit on the base of the cranial aspect of one of the dorsal spines two or three vertebrae cranial to the injury. The pin is placed laterally along the base of the dorsal spines, extending caudally two or three vertebrae distal to the injury.

Small holes are drilled through the base of the dorsal spines so that orthopedic wire can be inserted through them and around the pin, which is secured firmly to the spines by twisting the wire. The support of this pin relieves stress on the bone plate (Fig. 6.19).

Closure is performed by suturing the thoracolumbar fascia and subcutaneous tissues with 2-0 chromic catgut and closing the skin with nonabsorbable suture material. The sutures can be removed after 10 days.

Postoperative care is imperative and demanding. The patient is restrained in lateral recumbency on a soft padded surface by a heavy wire mesh screen placed just above it. Every 2 hours the animal must be turned from one side to the other, always with the spine down. This must done by two people to avoid torque on the spine. The bladder is expressed every 4 hours. Perineal hair is removed to improve sanitation. Decubitus ulcers must be precluded by constant attention. This routine may be necessary for up to 6 weeks before ambulation can be permitted. The prognosis is always guarded.

CAUDA EQUINA COMPRESSION—A

This condition is an acquired or developmental abnormality that causes narrowing of the lumbosacral canal, which leads to neurologic signs resulting from compression, destruction, or displace-

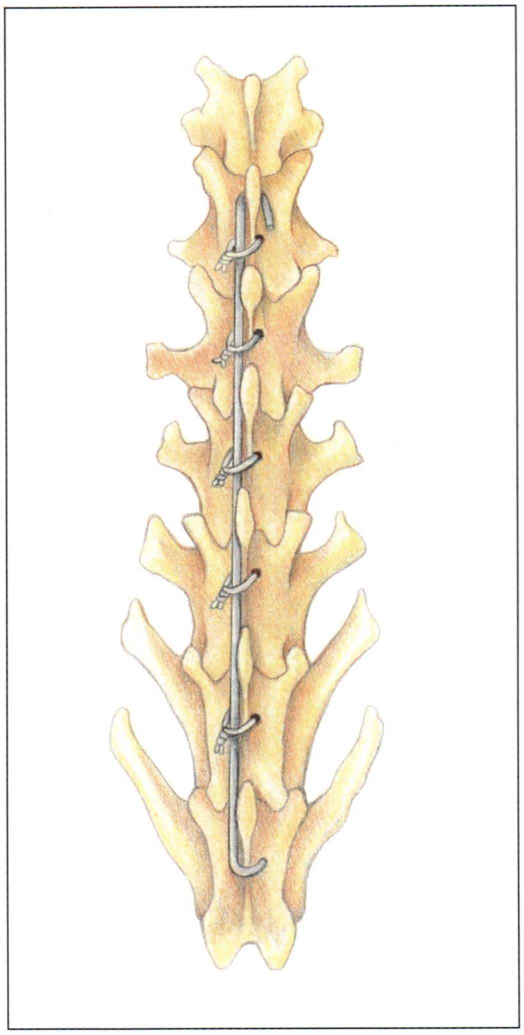

FIGURE 6.19 Small intramedulary (IM) pin locked around dorsal vertebral spine.

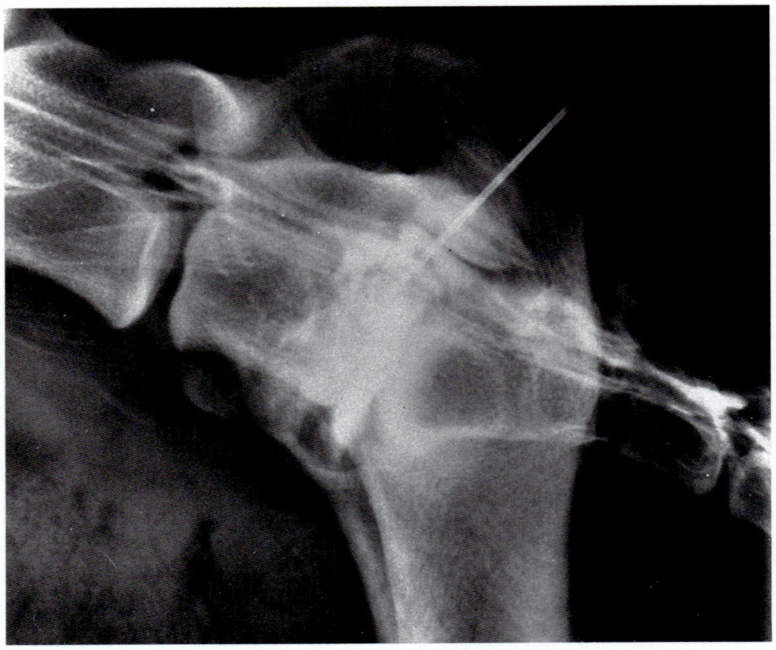

FIGURE 6.20 This cauda equina compression was caused by a herniated disc.

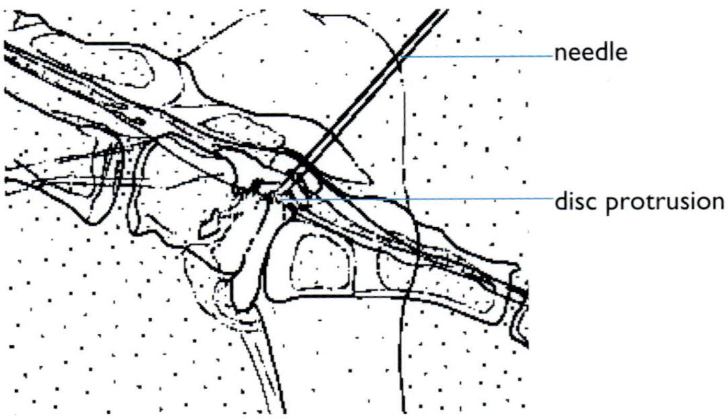

ment of nerve roots in the cauda equina. It is seen in middle-aged dogs, frequently German shepherds.

Altered soft-tissue structures, including joint capsule, dorsal anulus fibrosus, interarcuate ligament and type II disc herniations, can further narrow the canal in some cases. Marked spondylosis is often seen at the ventral lumbosacral junction (Fig. 6.20).

Neurologic findings are manifested clinically as motor and/or sensory function abnormalities of the cauda equina. Chief among these are intermittent lameness and marked pain on direct manipulation of the lumbosacral area, coupled with paraparesis, myalgesia, analgesia of the perineum and/or tail and bladder, or fecal incontinence. Treatment is dorsal laminectomy and freeing of the nerve roots, and foraminectomy when there is entrapment of the spinal nerves from L-7.

SURGICAL TECHNIQUE

Dorsal Laminectomy The dog is placed in sternal recumbency, with the hind legs drawn alongside the body, which is immobilized by sand bags. An incision is made through the skin and subcutaneous tissues directly on the midline from L-6 to the caudal edge of the sacrum. The superficial and deep fascia are incised to expose the multifidus and dorsal coccygeal muscles. Their tendinous insertions on the dorsal spinal processes are cut with the scalpel. The muscles are reflected subperiosteally to the level of the articular processes. The attachments of the lateral dorsal sacrococcygeal muscles are cut from the articular processes. A retractor is placed to hold the muscles laterally. The ligamentum flavum is incised and cut away dorsally.

The dorsal spines of L-7 and S-1 are cut away with rongeurs, leaving a cancellous bone surface for the first cut with the high-

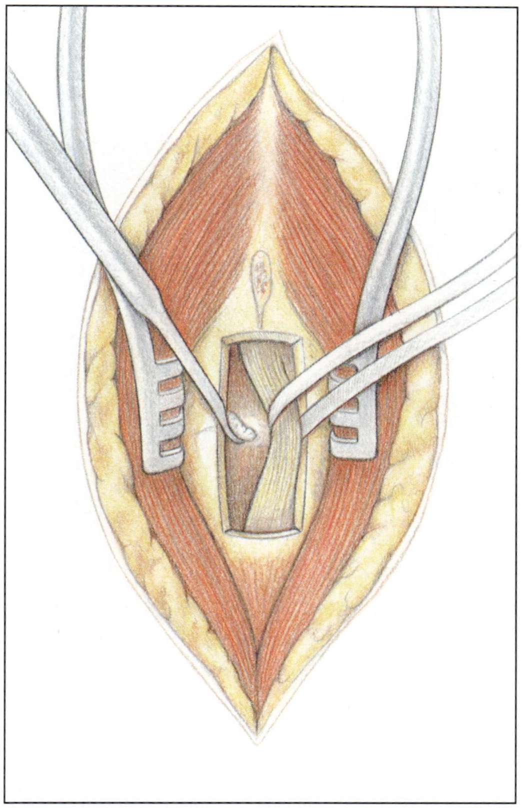

FIGURE 6.21 Dorsal laminectomy at L-7 to S-1.

speed air drill burr. A narrow laminectomy is done, leaving the articular processes intact (Fig. 6.21). The exposed nerve roots are covered with fat, which is carefully removed. The roots can be gently retracted with a loop of moistened umbilical tape. If the exposed intervertebral disc bulges into the canal, it is incised with the tip of a #11 scalpel blade and the thickened dorsal longitudinal ligament and disc are carefully removed with Adson forceps and the disc excavator in large dogs. The large venous sinuses must be avoided. A piece of subcutaneous fat from the lumbar region is placed over the laminectomy defect, and the retractors are removed. Closure of the reflected muscles is performed by suturing the heavy fascia with 2-0 chromic catgut. The subcutaneous tissues are similarly sutured, and the skin is closed with nonabsorbable suture.

Postoperative pain may require sedation for a considerable time after surgery. Exercise is restricted, and special care in nursing is required to prevent decubitus ulcers and cystitis. The sutures can be removed in 7 to 10 days.

CAUDA EQUINA COMPRESSION—B

Lumbosacral Instability

This is a condition in which the cauda equina is compressed by abnormal movement at the lumbosacral articulation. Subluxation of L-7 to S-1 can be demonstrated radiographically, especially when the sacrum is extended and flexed (Fig. 6.22). Pain and neurologic signs of compression of the cauda equina are present.

Stabilization is achieved by placing bone screws through the caudal articular process, the cranial articular process of the sacrum and the sacroiliac articulation. The dorsal spines of L-7 and the sacrum are left intact.

SURGICAL TECHNIQUE

The dog is placed in sternal recumbency, with the hind legs drawn alongside the body, which is immobilized by sandbags. An incision is made directly on the midline from L-6 to the caudal edge of the

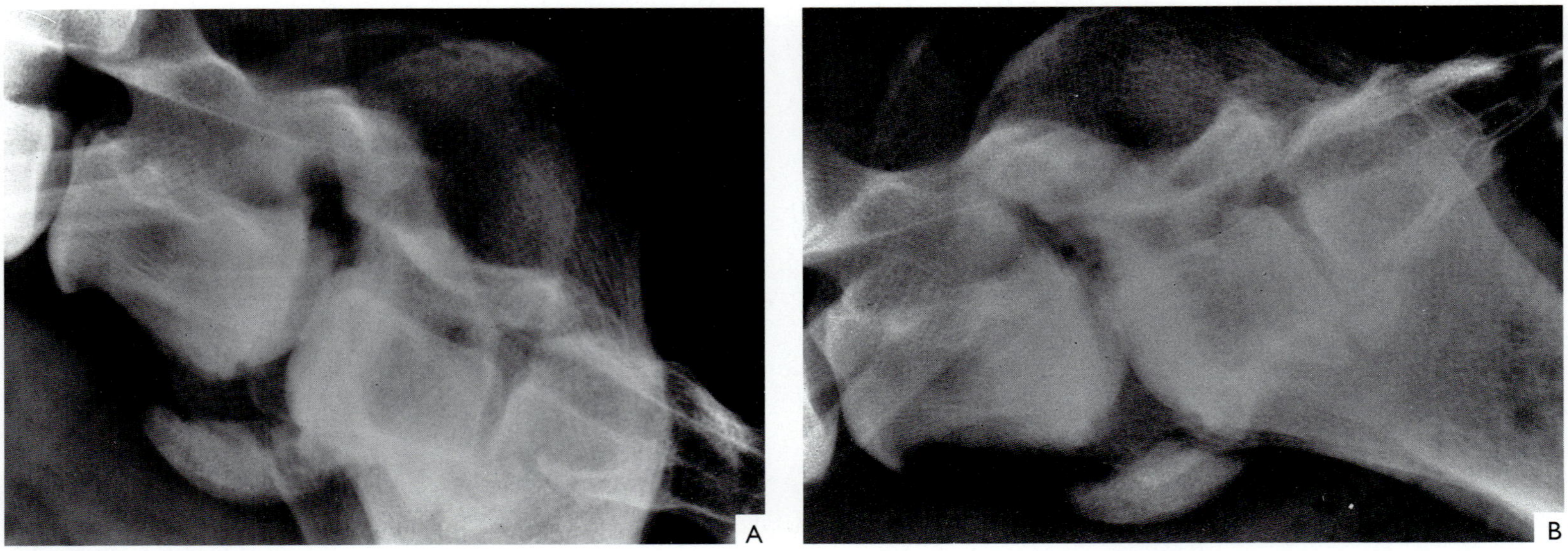

FIGURE 6.22 An unstable caudal equina compression.

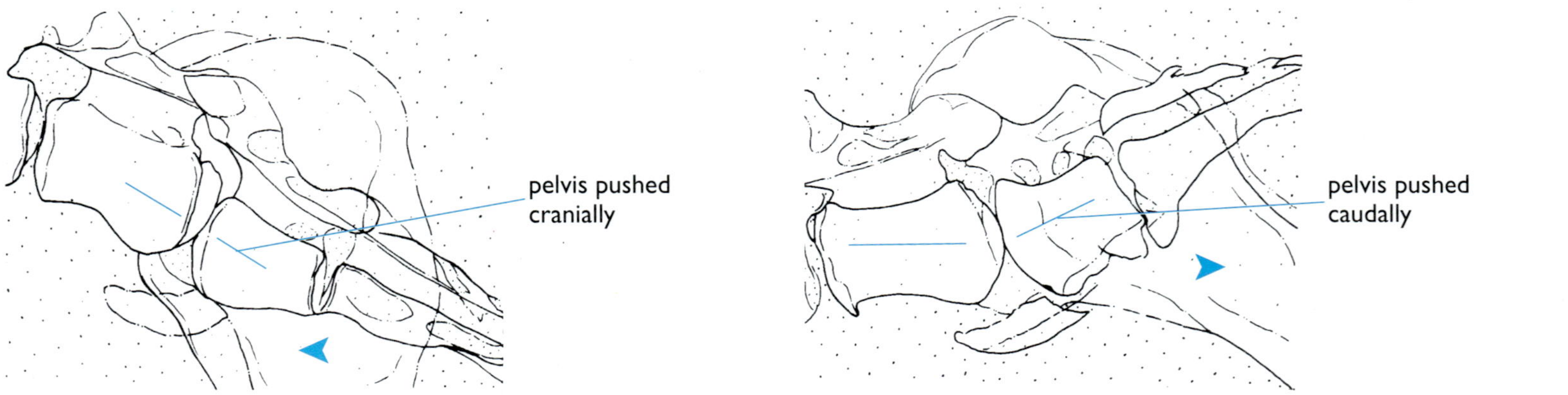

sacrum. The superficial and deep fascia are incised to expose the multifidus and dorsal coccygeal muscles. Their tendinous insertions on the dorsal spinal processes are cut. The muscles are reflected subperiosteally to the level of the caudal articular processes. The attachments of the lateral dorsal coccygeal muscles are cut from the articular processes. With the muscles retracted, it is possible to demonstrate the abnormal motion of the caudal articular processes by elevating L-7 with bone forceps clamped on its dorsal spinal process.

The location for the bone screws is identified with a small intramedullary pin. The pin is placed in a chuck handle and rested against the proximal caudal edge of the dorsal spine of L-7. The point is introduced into the center of the caudal articular process. The pin is drilled through the center of the articular surface, through the cranial articular process of the sacrum, and through the sacroiliac articulation (Fig. 6.23). The pin is removed. The length of screw required is determined with a depth gauge. A bone screw is inserted and tightened firmly. The opposite side is similarly treated.

Closure is performed by replacing the retracted musculature and suturing the deep and superficial fascia and the skin in the usual manner.

Postoperative pain is controlled with sedatives. The dog is kept confined for a week, then allowed exercise—only on a leash—for 3 weeks. Return to normal function can be expected if, indeed, the problem was confined to the instability.

FRACTURED RIB

This condition usually responds to bandaging and rest. However, motion between broken rib ends is very painful. The use of a K-wire and a figure-8 wire can immobilize the fracture, thereby reducing pain and speeding healing.

SURGICAL TECHNIQUE

An incision is made directly over the fracture area. The fascia and muscles are reflected from the outer surface of the rib. Because of the bowed shape of the ribs, a small-diameter K-

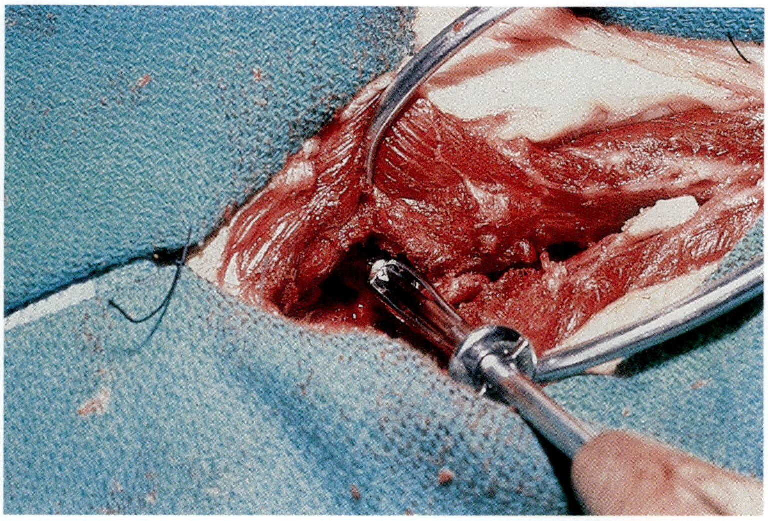

FIGURE 6.23 Placement of a screw for stabilizing the L-7 to S-1 articulation.

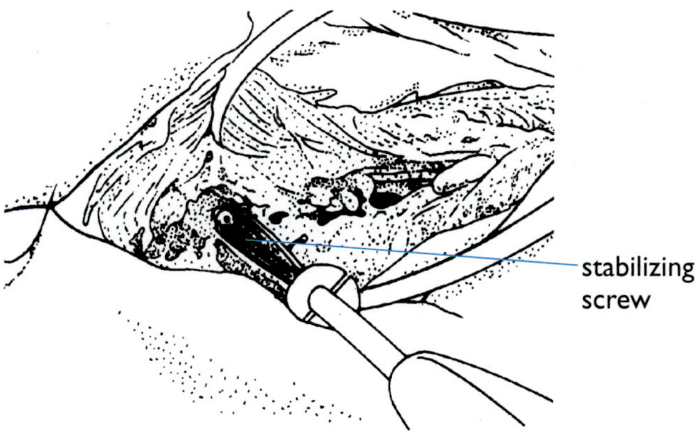

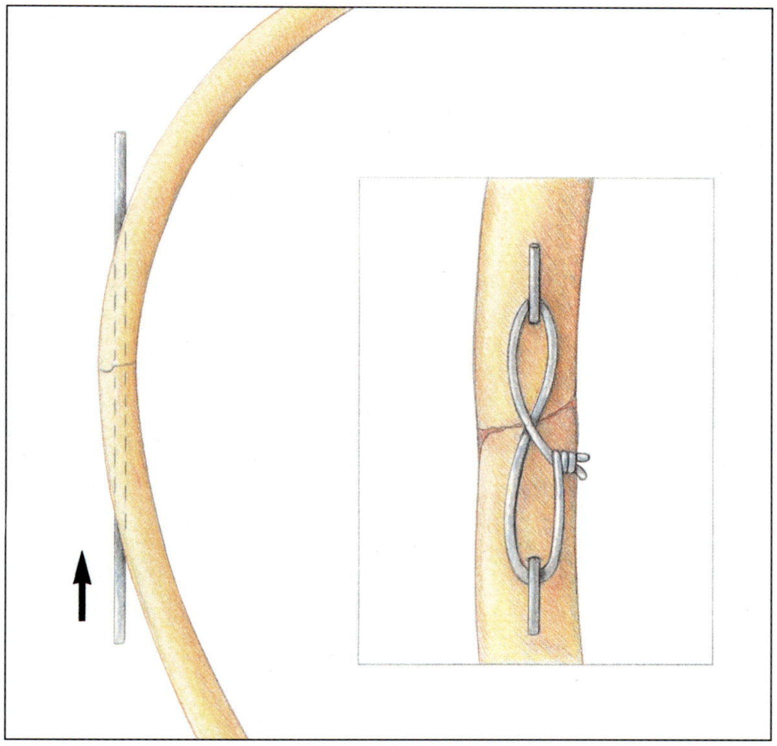

FIGURE 6.24 Placement of K-wire and figure-8 wire for treating fractured rib.

wire can be introduced from below the fracture through the fractured ends, to exit above the fracture. A figure-8 wire is placed around the projecting ends of the K-wire, which are then cut off. This compresses the fracture as the K-wire aligns it (Fig. 6.24).

Closure is performed by replacing the retracted muscles and suturing the deep and superficial fascia and the skin in the usual manner.

FRACTURE/LUXATION OF THE TAIL VERTEBRAE

Fractures of the tail vertebrae rarely heal well. Unfortunately, they are often associated with luxation and nerve damage that leaves the tail paralyzed. This subjects the tail to trauma, soilage, infection, and sometimes dry necrosis. The tail may be separated from the sacrum or nearby vertebrae, with extensive nerve damage that results in incontinence. It is not uncommon for injuries to the tip to become desiccated by a dry necrosis resulting from destruction of the blood supply. After a period of waiting, if the nerve injuries have not recovered and incontinence is not present, owners usually request amputation.

A fracture beyond the base of the tail can be immobilized by use of a cardboard tube as a splint. It is not uncommon for such injuries to heal at an angle. Attempts to wire or pin the fragments are not very successful.

PECTUS EXCAVATUM

This congenital defect is found occasionally in small and toy dog breeds and in cats. The sternum is markedly depressed into the chest, compromising the lungs and the heart (Fig. 6.25). Treatment involves surgical separation of the infolded portion and bringing the ends into a more normal position, where they are secured with longitudinally inserted K-wires.

SURGICAL TECHNIQUE

A ventral midline incision is made directly over the sternum, and the covering musculature is reflected. The malformed costal cartilages are incised at the sternal level. This involves entry into the chest, which will require assisted respiration by the anesthetist. The sternum is sectioned at its most inward point. If the diaphragm is involved, it is sectioned and resutured more distally. The sternal cartilage is fairly flexible in young animals, which permits the loosened portions of the sternum to be brought down and fitted into a more normal alignment. One or two longitudinally inserted K-wires are threaded from cranial to caudal across the separation site. The wire ends are cut off close to the sternal surface.

At closure, the reflected musculature is sutured over the midline to close the chest. Air is withdrawn from the chest, which enables the patient to begin voluntary respiration. Subcutaneous and skin closure is performed in the usual manner. The pins are left in place. The results of this procedure are usually satisfactory.

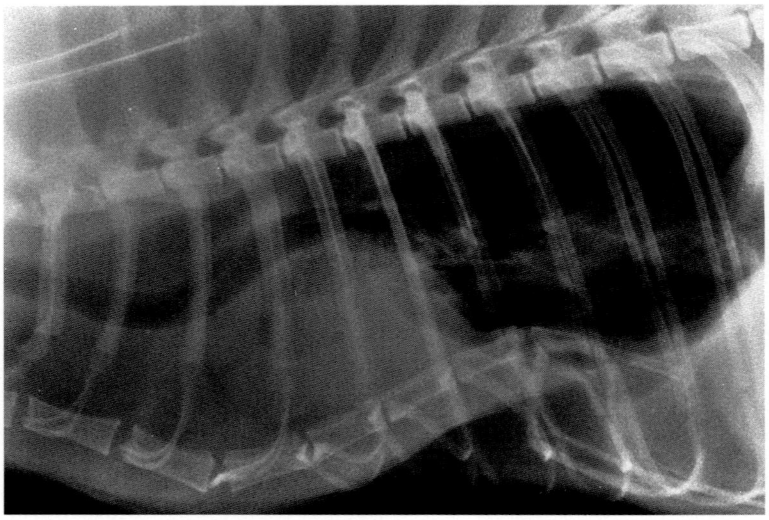

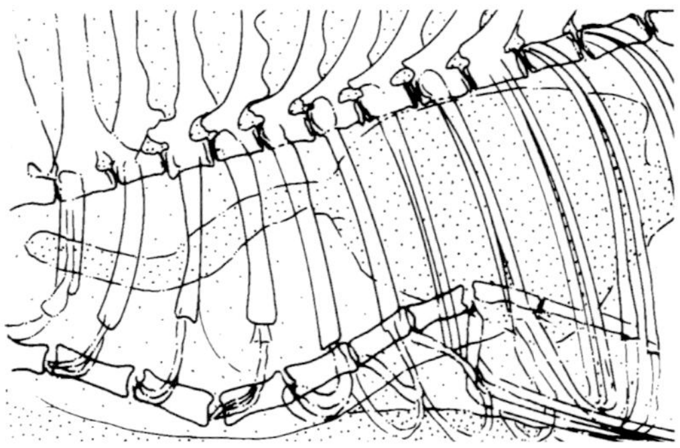

FIGURE 6.25 Radiograph of pectus excavatum.

CHAPTER 7

SPECIAL SURGERIES

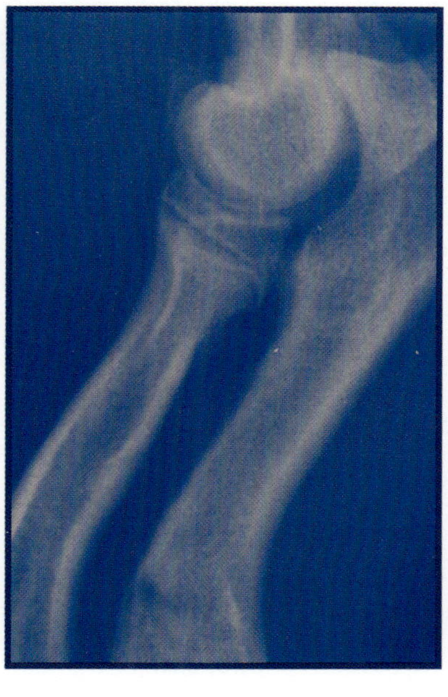
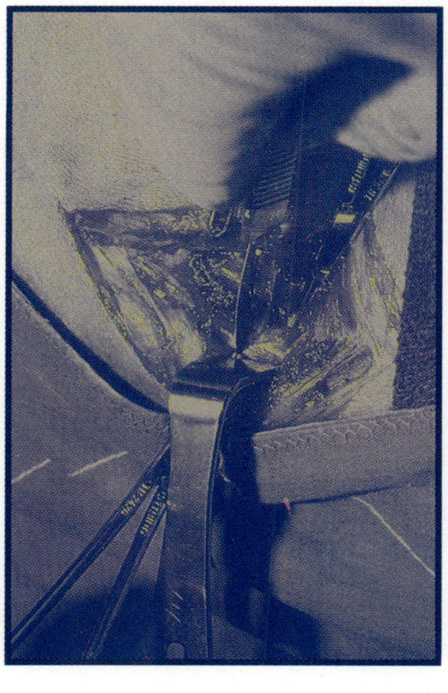
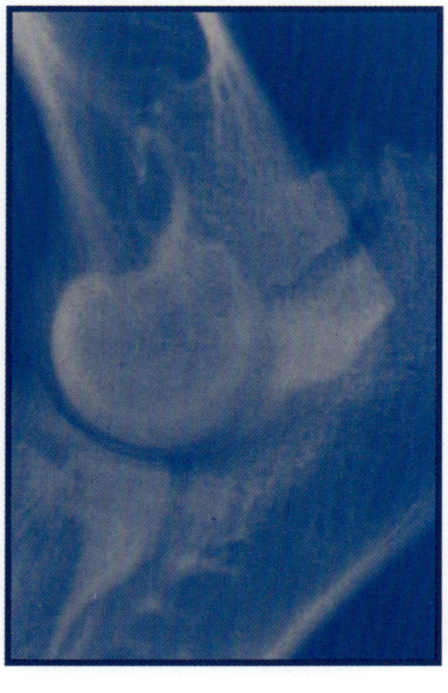
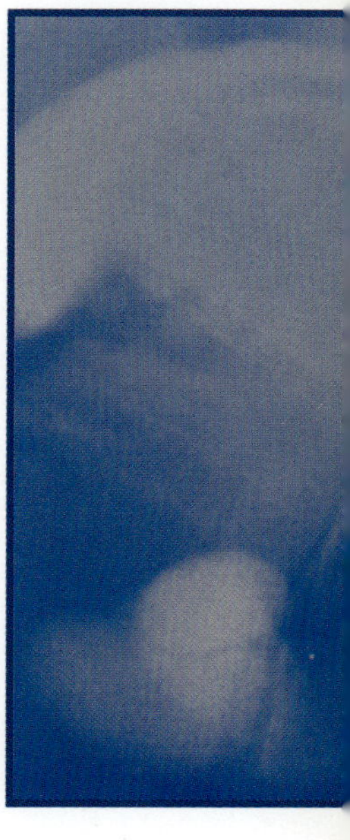

OSTEOCHONDROSIS DISSECANS OF THE JOINTS

Shoulder

The caudal aspect of the humeral head is the usual location of the loose cartilage fragment in osteochondrosis dissecans (OCD) of the shoulder joint (Fig. 7.1). Treatment consists of removing the loose fragment and curetting the lesion.

SURGICAL TECHNIQUE

The dog is placed in lateral recumbency. An incision is made through the skin and subcutaneous tissue along the distal third of the spine of the scapula, curving at the shoulder joint to end on the lateral aspect of the proximal quarter of the humerus. The underlying subcutaneous tissue is cleared with Metzenbaum scissors, exposing the fascia over the acromion deltoid muscle. The fascia is incised with scissors ventrally. The incision is carried dorsally, proceeding just caudal to the spine of the scapula and severing the attachment of the deltoid. The separation between the caudal aspect of the deltoid is developed by sharp and blunt dissection. The infraspinatus and teres minor muscles are cleared of fascia and identified. The teres minor is separated and retracted from the infraspinatus to expose the joint capsule. Further exposure is gained by a partial caudal transection of the acromion deltoid, 1 cm below its origin. The insertion of the teres minor on the humerus is transected. The exposed joint capsule is incised centrally with the scalpel following the curve of the humeral head.

The humerus is strongly abducted, exposing the caudal aspect of the humeral head (Fig. 7.2). The loose cartilage is removed and the lesion, especially the cartilage edge, is curetted. The caudal aspect of the joint capsule is inspected for cartilage fragments ("joint mice"). The joint is flushed with saline.

Closure of the joint capsule, reattachment of the teres minor and deltoid, repair of the partial incision in the acromion deltoid, and suturing of the fascia and subcutaneous tissues are done with 2-0 chromic catgut. The skin is closed with nonabsorbable suture.

Postoperative seroma can be avoided by meticulous attention to hemostasis and by keeping the dog confined to a kennel for several days. The dog's rapid recovery and a return to normal health can be expected.

Osteochondritic Lesional Material in the Shoulder Joint's Cranial Aspect

When osteochondrotic lesions have been present for some time, the cartilage tends to disintegrate and the fragments float free in the joint. They usually become located in the caudal cul-de-sac of the joint capsule. In some cases the loose fragments become located in the cranial extension of the joint capsule that acts as a sheath for the tendon of origin of the biceps brachii. Here, whether they become attached or remain loose, they cause pain by irritating the tendon. The condition is most likely to be found in large-breed dogs. Although the diagnosis may be overlooked, the pain is quite severe and the lameness is very obvious. The diagnosis is confirmed by radiography (Fig. 7.3). Surgical removal of the fragments is required.

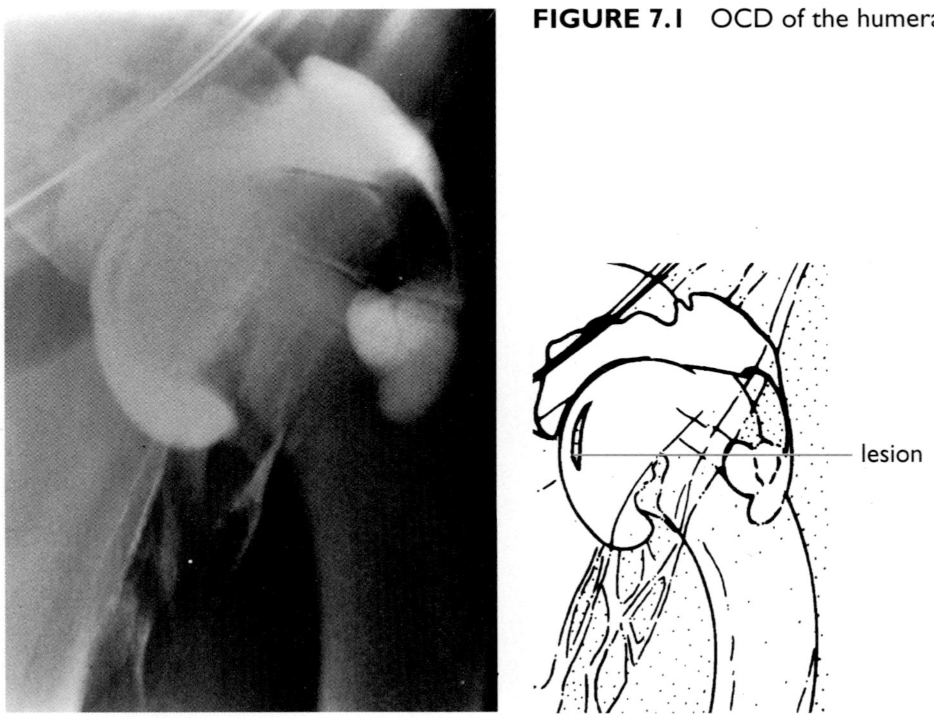

FIGURE 7.1 OCD of the humeral head.

SURGICAL TECHNIQUE

The skin and subcutaneous tissue are incised along the cranial edge of the distal scapula, over the greater tubercle and a short way over the ventral portion of the proximal humerus. The fascia of the shoulder is incised between the cleidobrachialis and the omotransversarius. The cleidobrachialis is reflected ventromedially to expose the insertion of the supraspinatus on the greater tubercle. The insertions of the superficial and deep pectorals are incised and the muscles retracted medially. The tendon of origin of the biceps brachii is exposed. The transverse humeral retinaculum is incised and the joint capsule extension covering the tendon is cut to expose the tendon and the fragments of the OCD lesion. The fragments are removed and the area is flushed with physiologic saline. The joint itself is flushed to ensure that no free-floating material is present which could later move into the tendon area.

The covering of the tendon is not closed. The transverse humeral retinaculum is closed with a fine suture. The deep pectoral and superficial muscles are replaced by suturing them to the surrounding fascia over the greater tubercle. The incision between the omotransversarius and the cleidobrachialis is closed with simple interrupted sutures, as is the subcutaneous tissue. The skin is closed with nonabsorbable suture.

The dog is confined for a week and kept on leash for another week. Dry, careful surgery and forced inactivity will help prevent the formation of a hematoma.

The results are very satisfactory, with return of function and elimination of pain within a few weeks. All of the lesional material must be removed to achieve the best results.

Elbow

The lesion of OCD of the elbow occurs on the caudal aspect of the medial humeral condyle. It may be difficult to identify by radiography (Fig. 7.4). Treatment consists of arthrotomy and curettage of the lesion. A medial approach to the elbow is used. A fragmented coronoid process may also be present.

SURGICAL TECHNIQUE

The dog is placed in lateral recumbency with the affected leg down and the upper leg drawn out of the way. A posteromedial incision is made through the skin and subcutaneous tissue midway between the olecranon and the medial humeral epicondyle. The subcutaneous tissue is cleared from the underlying fascia with Metzenbaum scissors. Care is taken not to cut the ulnar nerve, which lies above the fascia in the proximal area of the incision. It should be identified and retracted gently with a piece of moistened umbilical tape.

The fascia is incised with a scalpel and the incision is enlarged with scissors. The origins of the heads of the superficial and deep digital flexors are identified. The superficial and the deep digital flexors are transected near their origins and are reflected distally. The joint capsule is incised with the scalpel and the incision

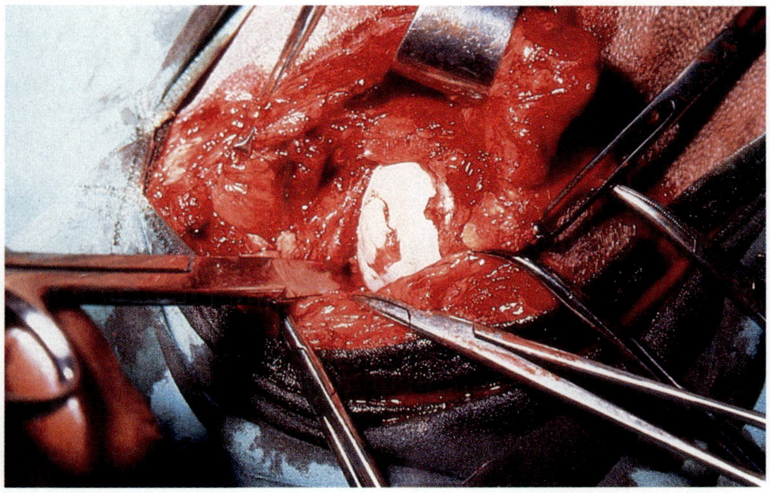

FIGURE 7.2 OCD lesion on the humeral head.

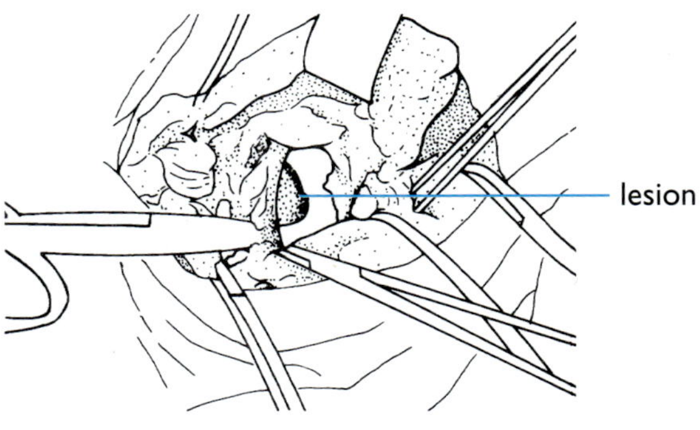

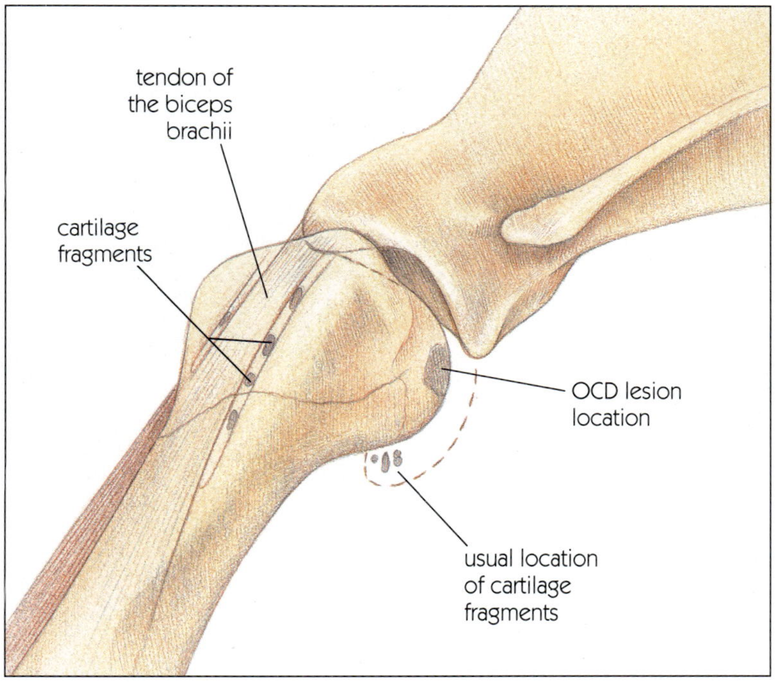

FIGURE 7.3 Cranial "joint mice" (fragments of OCD lesion) in the cranial extension of the joint capsule around the bicipital tendon.

is carried cranially to sever the medial collateral ligament, as it is integral with the joint capsule. Lateral extension of the limb will open the joint to inspection. Osteochondrotic lesions appear on the caudal aspect of the medial condylar articular surface (Fig. 7.5). Loose fragments of cartilage are removed and the lesion is curetted. Coronoid fragments may be found at the medial tip but are usually more deeply situated. The fragments are removed and the ulnar nerve is released. Closure of the joint capsule and medial collateral ligament, replacement of the transected muscles, and reapposition of the fascia and subcutaneous tissues are done with 2-0 chromic catgut. The skin is closed with nonabsorbable suture material.

Stifle

The common location of the OCD lesion in the knee of the dog is the distal medial aspect of the lateral condylar articular surface (Fig. 7.6). Surgical treatment is by arthrotomy, removal of the loose tissue, and curettage of the lesion.

SURGICAL TECHNIQUE

The dog is placed in lateral recumbency with the affected leg uppermost. A lateral parapatellar incision through the skin and subcutaneous tissue is made from the distal quarter of the femur to the head of the tibia. The superficial fascia and fat are cleared with

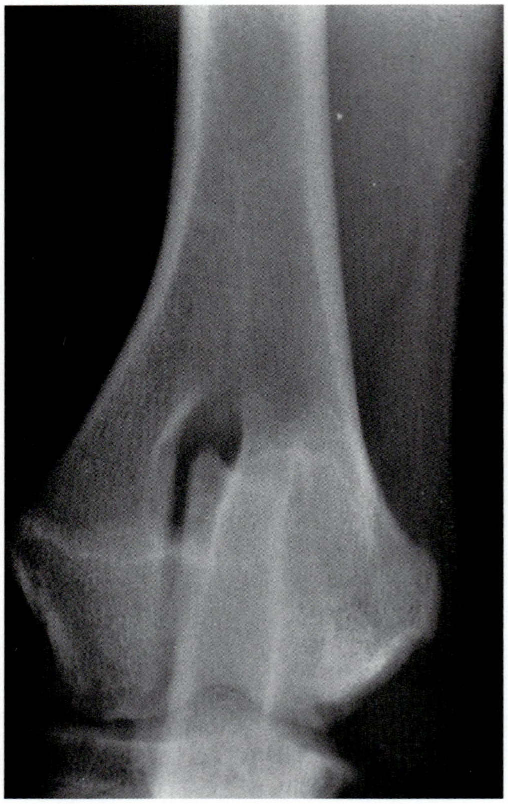

FIGURE 7.4 OCD of the elbow.

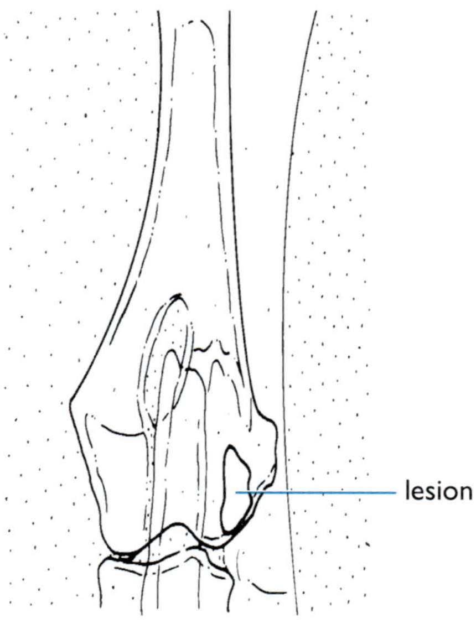

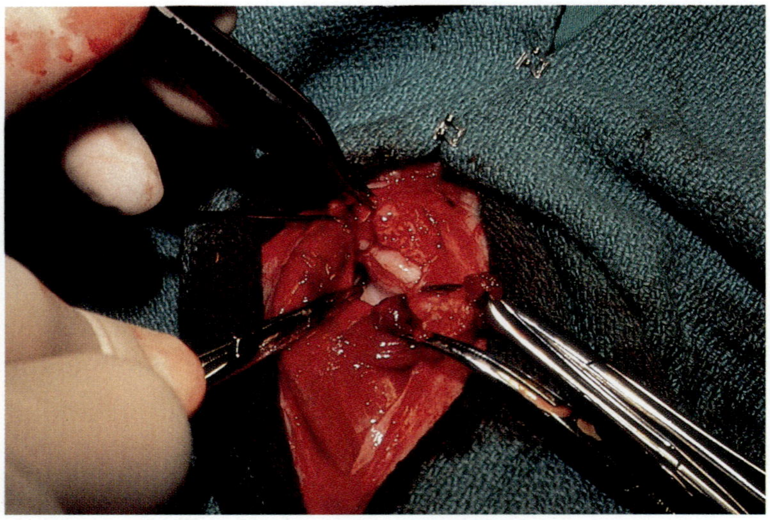

FIGURE 7.5 OCD lesion of the elbow,

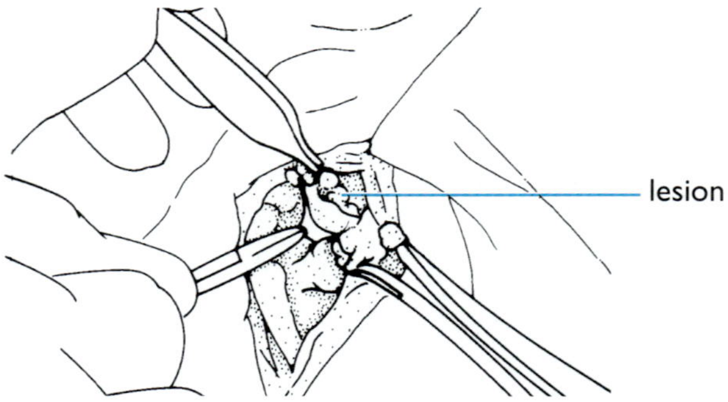

Metzenbaum scissors to expose the knee's fascia. An entry into the joint is made with the scalpel parallel to the patellar ligament just distal to the lateral condylar articular surface. This incision is enlarged with straight scissors proximally to the dorsal extent of the joint capsule and distally to the head of the tibia. A 2- to 3-mm portion of the lateral retinacular cartilage is left attached to the patella to facilitate placement of sutures at closure. The cranial membranous support to the fat pad is incised parallel to the incision to allow the fat to be retracted medially. The patella is luxated medially. The lesion is exposed by flexing the knee. The joint cartilage over the lesion may be whole but very thin, and the loose fragment underneath is easily identifiable. This fragment is removed, leaving a rather deep pocket with ragged edges (Fig. 7.7). The curette is used to smooth the edges and gently scrape out the defect. The joint is flushed with physiologic saline solution. The patella is replaced.

Closure of the incision is made by placing several nonabsorbable sutures in the retinacular cartilage. The joint capsule and the fascia of the knee, as well as the superficial fascia and subcutaneous tissue, are sutured with 2-0 chromic catgut. The skin is closed with nonabsorbable suture.

The dog will not use the leg for several days, in contrast to the earlier return of function seen in repair of shoulder and elbow lesions. The sutures are removed in 1 week. Complete recovery will require 4 to 6 weeks.

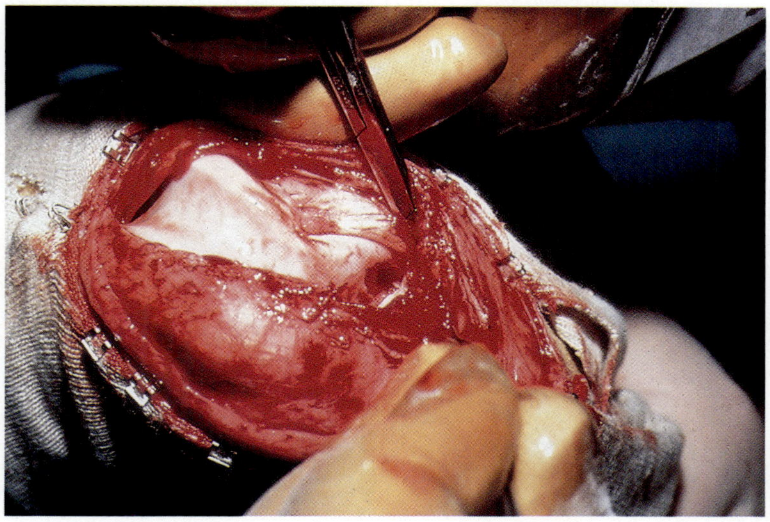

FIGURE 7.6 OCD lesion of the stifle.

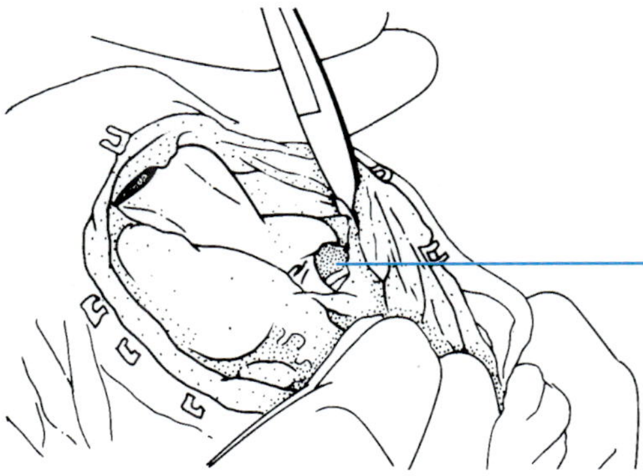

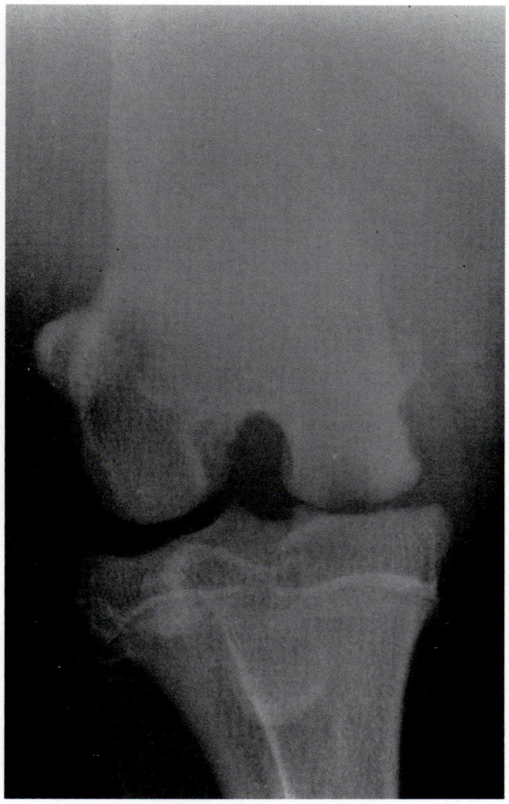

FIGURE 7.7 OCD of the stifle.

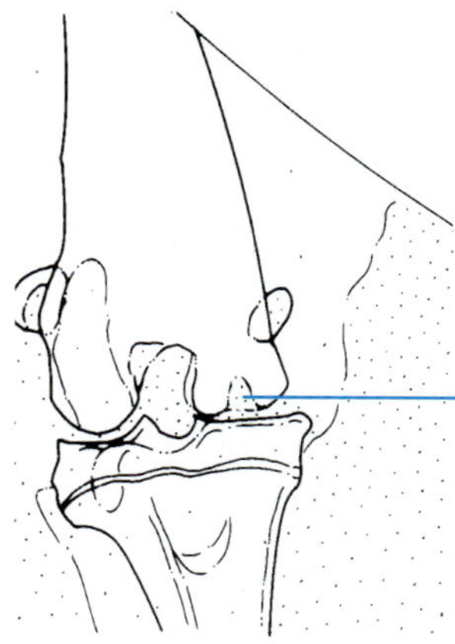

Hock

Although less common than OCD of the shoulder, this condition is often the cause of hock lameness in large-breed immature dogs. Radiographs provide the definitive diagnosis (Fig. 7.8). Treatment is surgical removal of the loose fragment and curettage of the lesion.

SURGICAL TECHNIQUE

The dog is placed in sternal recumbency with the affected leg extended caudally. An incision is made with the scalpel through the skin and subcutaneous tissue from the distal tibia to the middle of the talus, halfway between the calcaneus and the medial malleolus. Continued sharp dissection is carried through the heavy fascia and the joint capsule to expose the underlying joint space. The wound edges are retracted and the joint space is opened by flexing the hock. The loose fragment is located on the caudomedial aspect of the proximal joint surface of the talus. The small tips of Adson forceps are used to remove the fragment. The defect is curetted with a 2-mm curette. The joint is flushed with physiologic saline. Closure is done by suturing the fascia and joint capsule with 2-0 chromic catgut. The skin is closed with a nonabsorbable suture. The foot is enclosed in a modified Robert Jones splint for 5 days. This controls swelling and restricts motion without causing pressure sores. The sutures are removed in a week.

The prognosis in cases with a smaller lesion recognized reasonably early is good; otherwise, some tendency to lameness may persist.

UNUNITED ANCONEAL PROCESS

In some breeds of dog the anconeal process remains ununited to the olecranon except by a cartilaginous union, and is therefore subject to separation along this area from trauma or pressure due to unequal growth of the radius and ulna (Fig. 7.9). The loosened fragment

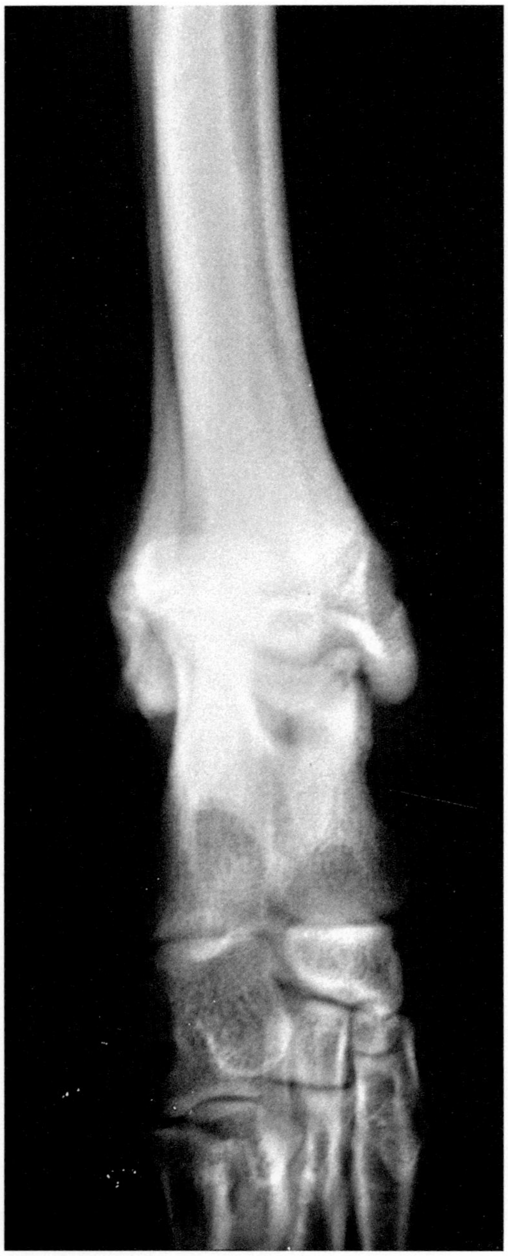

FIGURE 7.8 OCD of the hock.

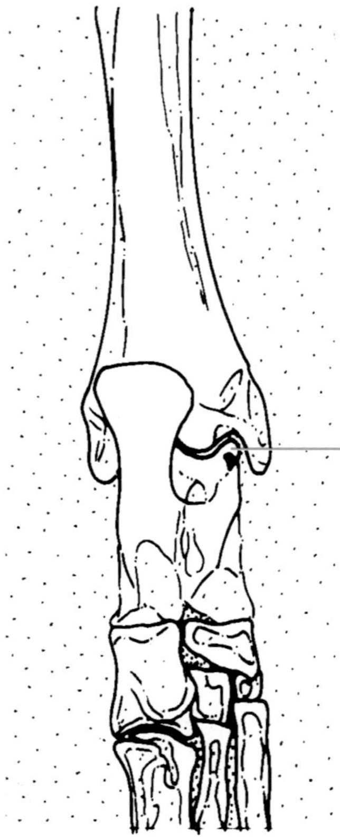

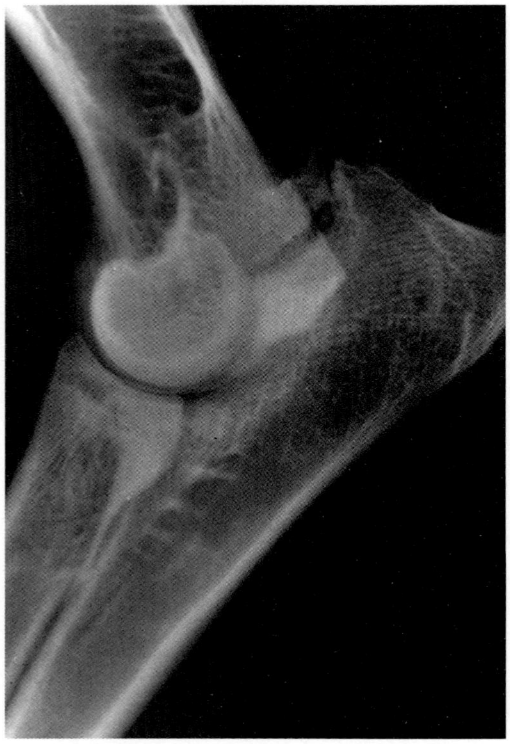

FIGURE 7.9 An ununited anconeal process.

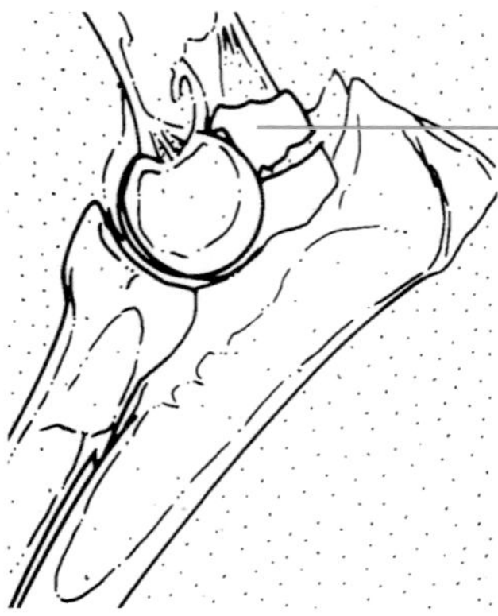

creates an osteoarthritic response and joint instability. Surgical excision offers a chance of improvement, but joint impairment in later life can be expected.

SURGICAL TECHNIQUE

With the dog in lateral recumbency, a posterolateral incision is made through the skin and subcutaneous tissue over the anconeal muscle midway between the olecranon and the lateral humeral condyle. The anconeal fascia is exposed with Metzenbaum scissors to clear the subcutaneous fascia. A scalpel is used to incise the fascia and underlying muscle to and through the joint capsule. Considerable hemorrhage can be expected and must be brought under control. The entrance into the joint is enlarged and the loosened anconeal process is identified. The fragment is grasped with small bone-holding forceps and is removed after the dorsal joint capsule attachments are cut away with scissors. The joint is flushed with saline.

Closure is done by suturing the anconeal fascia and the subcutaneous tissues with 2-0 chromic catgut. The skin is closed with nonabsorbable suture material.

The dog should be kept quiet for several days after surgery. Improvement can be expected but some joint instability will always remain, which will lead to chronic osteoarthritis in subsequent years.

CONTRACTURE OF THE MUSCLES

Infraspinatus

Contracture of the infraspinatus as a result of trauma causes a distinctive lameness with outward rotation of the forelimb and restricted motion of the shoulder joint. Treatment consists of transecting the infraspinatus tendon.

SURGICAL TECHNIQUE

The dog is placed in lateral recumbency. An incision is made through the skin and subcutaneous tissue over the distal quarter of the spine of the scapula, curving over the lateral aspect of the shoulder joint to a point on the lateral aspect of the proximal humerus several centimeters from the humeral head. The subcutaneous tissues are cleared from the underlying fascia, which is then incised to expose the underlying acromion deltoid. The incision is carried dorsally to separate the deltoid from its origin on the spine of the scapula. The separation between the acromion deltoid and the more caudal deltoid is developed by sharp and blunt dissection. The teres minor and the infraspinatus are identified. The soft, fleshy muscle tissue is removed from the lateral aspect of the tendon of insertion of the infraspinatus. The tendon is transected with the scalpel (Fig. 7.10). The heretofore immovable joint can now be freely manipulated. The attendant bursa is often destroyed. No further treatment is needed.

Closure is made with 2-0 chromic catgut in the fascia and subcutaneous tissues and with nonabsorbable suture in the skin.

Gracilis

Fibrotic contracture of the gracilis is rarely seen except in racing Greyhounds. The affected muscle contracts as it becomes fibrotic, preventing extension of the knee. It is painful and causes a defect in growth. Treatment is by excision.

SURGICAL TECHNIQUE

The dog is placed in dorsal recumbency with the medial surface of the affected limb uppermost. The opposite leg is secured laterally out of the way. The contracted gracilis muscle is easily palpated. An incision is made through the skin and subcutaneous tissue directly over the full length of the muscle's fibrotic area.

Sharp and blunt dissection with Metzenbaum scissors exposes the firm fibrous mass that has replaced the muscle tissue. The muscle is isolated down to its insertion at the knee on the tibial crest. With the insertion isolated and sectioned, the strip of fibrous tissue is dissected proximally until normal muscle tissue is present—usually above the upper third. The muscle is transected at this point and the fibrotic portion discarded (Fig. 7.11). Bleeders are ligated and the remaining muscle stump is packed away dorsally. The knee will now extend completely.

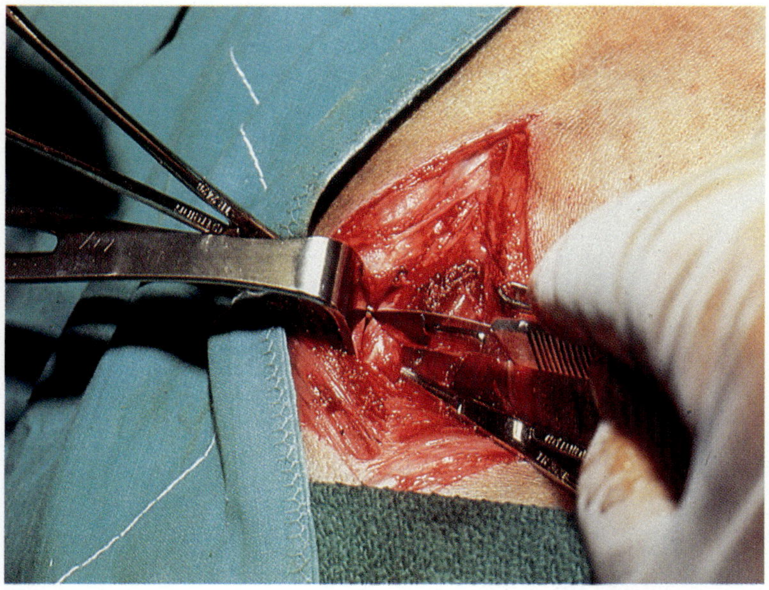

FIGURE 7.10 Cutting of the infraspinatus tendon

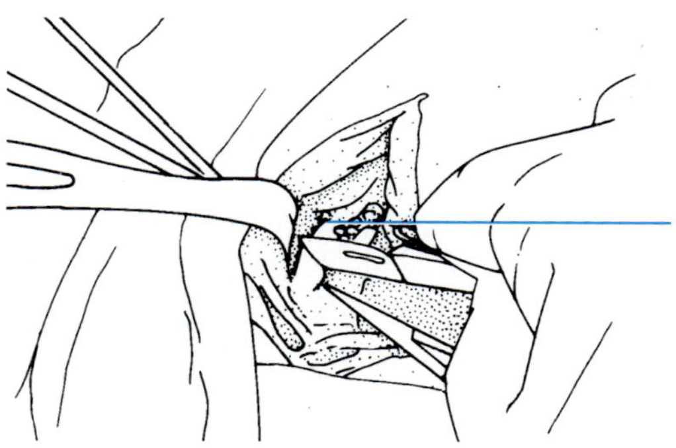

Closure is done by suturing the subcutaneous fascia with 2-0 chromic catgut. The subcutaneous tissues and the skin are closed in the usual manner. The skin sutures are removed in a week. The dog is allowed to use the leg but is restricted to a small run.

The incidence of recurrence is high unless a radical excision is done. With radical removal the prognosis is good.

Quadriceps

Fibrotic contracture of the quadriceps is usually the result of a poorly managed femoral fracture. It may occur in conjunction with a tie-down to the femur at the fracture site. The hind leg is functionless and is held in extreme extension, with the knee often caudally flexed. Z-plasty of the fibrotic quadriceps is the treatment of choice.

SURGICAL TECHNIQUE

The dog is placed in lateral recumbency with the affected leg uppermost. The firm, fibrotic mass of the quadriceps is easily palpable. An incision is made through the skin and subcutaneous tissues directly over the quadriceps mass from the proximal third of the femur to the tibial crest. The fascia lata is incised over the mass. Sharp and blunt dissection with Metzenbaum scissors separates the firm, hard fibrous mass of the quadriceps from the surrounding normal musculature. If the mass is adherent to the site of fracture, it is freed from the tie-down by use of the periosteal elevator. When the fibrotic mass is completely isolated, it is severed centrally in a Z-plasty (Fig. 7.12). The knee is flexed and any fascial structures preventing movement are incised with scissors. The leg can now be flexed and extended.

The knee is set at a physiologic standing angle and the Z-plasty is sutured end to end, which enables it to stay in this position. Although there will be no function of the knee joint, the new angle will allow use of the leg. The fascia lata and subcutaneous tissues are sutured with 2-0 chromic catgut. The skin is closed with a nonabsorbable suture.

A full K/E is applied with the proximal two pins and short bar set into the distal femoral shaft. The distal two pins and short bar are set into the shaft of the proximal tibia. A long connecting bar is secured to the short bars by double clamps. This device will maintain the knee in its cranial angulation and prevent recurrence of the hyperextension. It also allows the dog to use the leg during recovery. The K/E apparatus is left on for 2 weeks.

FRAGMENTED CORONOID PROCESS

Fragmentation of the coronoid process of the ulna is probably due to the same development of unequal growth of the radius and ulna that causes humeral osteochondritis dissecans and ununited anconeal process. The condition is somewhat difficult to identify radiologically (Fig. 7.13). Fragments should be surgically removed early for best results. An OCD-like lesion is often found on the articular surface of the medial humeral condyle.

SURGICAL TECHNIQUE

The dog is placed in lateral recumbency with the affected leg down and the upper leg drawn out of the way. A posteromedial incision is made curving midway between the olecranon and the medial humeral epicondyle. The subcutaneous fascia is cleared with Metzenbaum scissors. Care must be taken not to cut the ulnar nerve, which lies close above the fascia in the proximal area of the incision. The nerve is identified and, if necessary, is retracted gently with a piece of moistened Penrose tubing.

The fascia is incised with a scalpel and the incision is enlarged with scissors. The origins of the heads of the superficial and deep flexors and the flexor carpi radialis are identified. These muscles are

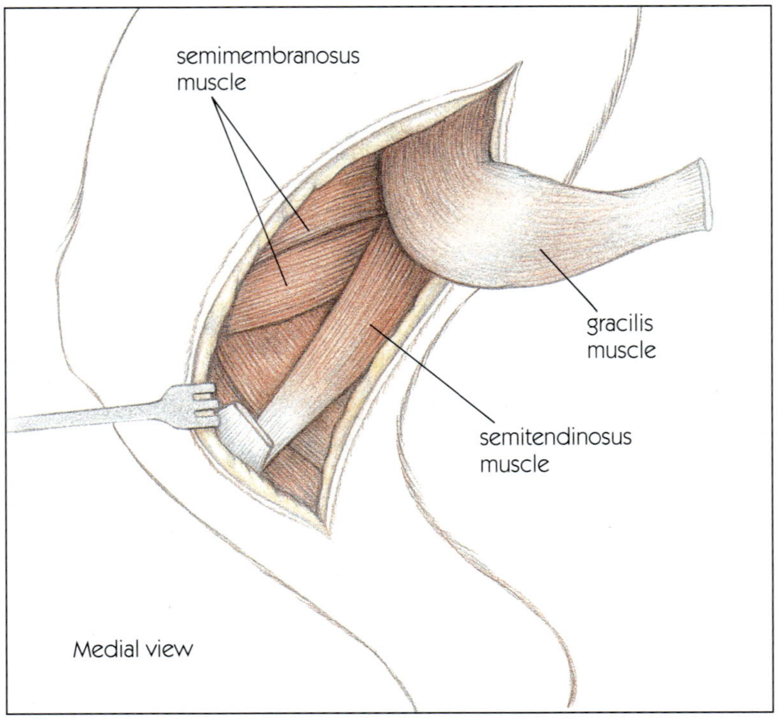

FIGURE 7.11 Excision of the fibrotic gracilis muscle.

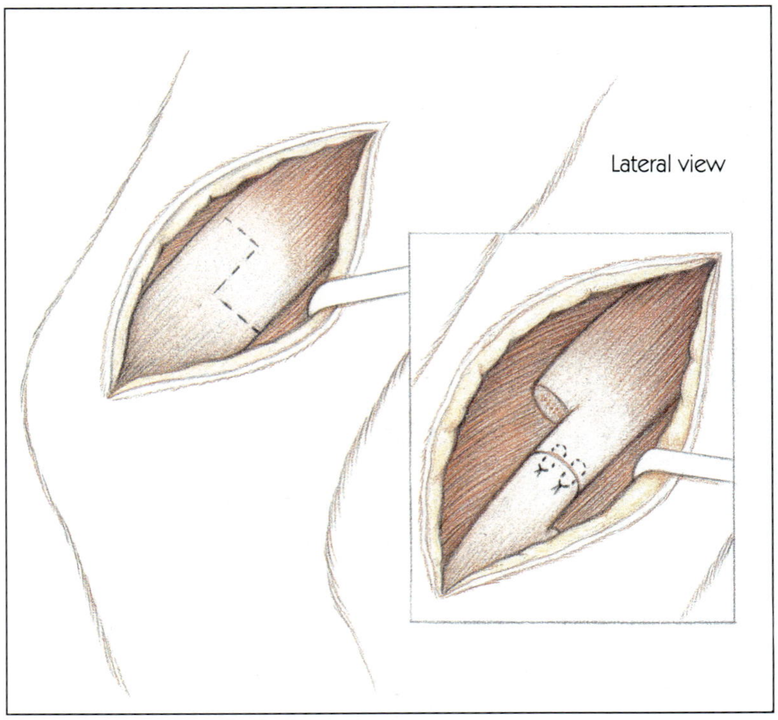

FIGURE 7.12 Z-plasty of quadriceps contracture.

transected near their origins and reflected distally. The joint capsule is incised with a scalpel. The incision is carried cranially to sever the medial collateral ligament and more cranially to expose the coronoid process. Lateral extension of the joint will give access to the lesion except when osteophytes are present. These are cut away with a small rongeur. The fragments are often deeply situated and must be pried loose. They are removed and the joint is inspected and flushed. A search is made for OCD lesions on the caudal aspect of the medial condyle of the humerus. If present, the loose cartilage is removed and the lesion is gently curetted.

Closure is performed by suturing the joint capsule and the medial collateral ligament with nonabsorbable suture. The transected muscle heads are replaced and the fascia is closed. The ulnar nerve is released. Subcutaneous and skin closure are done in the usual manner.

The dog is kept confined in a cage or run for a few days, then allowed only limited exercise on a leash for 3 weeks. The prognosis depends on the development of degenerative joint disease, which is more likely to occur in lesions of longer duration.

TENDON REPAIR

Avulsion of the Gastrocnemius Tendon

The gastrocnemius tendon is the largest of the Achilles tendon group. It and the common tendon of the biceps femoris, semitendinous and gracilis muscles attach to the tuber calcis. The superficial digital flexor, while intimately in contact with the gastrocnemius, glides over the distal end of the tuber. The gastrocnemius tendon can be torn from its attachment, often avulsing a small bone fragment. Initially severe lameness is seen, followed by partial recovery. The dog walks with increased flexion of the hock and extends the digits on weight bearing. Surgical replacement is required.

SURGICAL TECHNIQUE

A lateral paramedian incision is made over the distal tendon to the tuber calcanei. The lateral retinaculum of the superficial digital flexor is isolated and incised to allow medial luxation of the tendon. In the early stages, the end of the torn tendon can be identified. With the development of fibrous tissue, this must be cleared away to identify the end of the tendon. It is usually retracted as much as 2 or 3 cm. The end is cut cleanly across to provide a fresh surface, which will be approximated to its original insertion. The insertion area on the calcaneus is cleared of fibrous tissue. Two small tunnels are drilled from the medial and lateral sides of the calcaneus into the insertion area. Strong nonabsorbable suture (not wire) is introduced through the lateral tunnel and into the end of the tendon. A locking loop is made (Fig. 7.14), the suture is exited through the end of the tendon and the suture ends are tied. The medial side is similarly treated. The superficial digital flexor is replaced and the lateral retinaculum is resutured. Subcutaneous and skin sutures are placed in the usual manner.

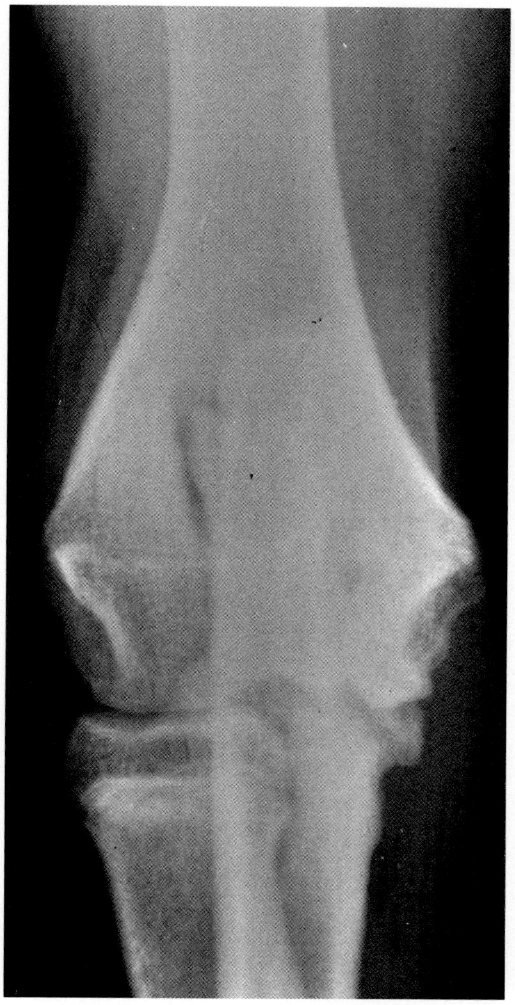

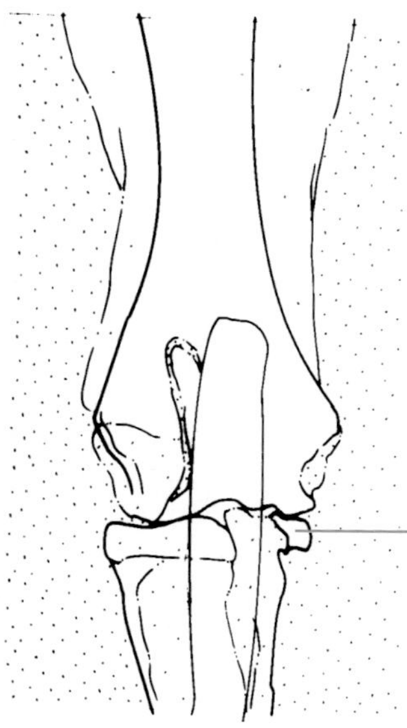

FIGURE 7.13 Radiograph of a fragmented coronoid process.

The repair must be kept from tension for a month. A lateral wood coaptation splint is used. Additional protection is given after removal of the splint with a Robert Jones splint for another week. Only light exercise is allowed for the following 3 weeks.

Transection of the Achilles Tendon

A severed Achilles tendon is most often the result of broken glass, sharp metal, or a mower blade. The dog walks in a plantigrade manner which, along with swelling above a palpable defect where the tendon would normally be, is diagnostic. Surgical repair unites the severed ends of the component structures of the Achilles group. The repair must be kept free of stress for at least 6 weeks. This is often best done with an external fixation splint.

SURGICAL TECHNIQUE

With the dog in lateral recumbency, an incision is made over the lateral surface of the tendon and the external saphenous vein is retracted. The incision must be long enough so that the proximal tendon end can be located. The tendon sheath must be slit lengthwise to reveal the cut ends. The distal end is easily found, but the proximal end will retract several centimeters in a large dog. The tip of a straight Kelly forceps is placed on the proximal tendon ends so that traction can be applied. Traction and extension of the hock will permit the approximation of the tendon ends. Each proximal end must be sutured to its respective distal end. The standard suture pattern for very large dogs is the Bunnel. The locking loop suture is preferred for most dogs. A small-diameter but very strong suture is required. Nylon or polydianone (PDS) with needles attached is recommended. For the Bunnel, sutures with needles at both ends are used. The tendon ends are trimmed just before suturing. The tendinous tissues of the insertions of the biceps femoris and the semitendinous and gracilis are sutured. No attempt is made to suture the tendon sheath. Subcutaneous and skin closure are done in the usual manner.

The greatest problem is to keep tension away from the repair until it heals. Splints and casts are often ineffective, and prolonged use may be harmful. The hock must be kept in extension to relieve any pull on the tendon. Although the placement of a screw through the calcaneus into the caudal aspect of the tibia has been recommended, it is unsatisfactory in many cases.

External fixation provides the best tolerated and most substantial support. Transfixion pins are placed horizontally through the distal tibia, calcaneus, and proximal ends of the metatarsals. Connecting bars are secured to the pins with clamps (Fig. 7.15). The medial and lateral assemblies are covered with cotton, ban

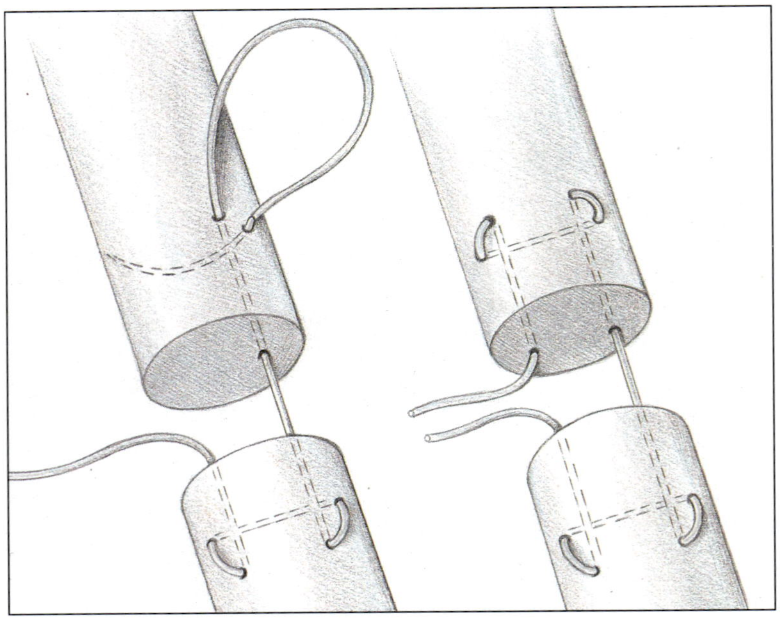

FIGURE 7.14 Locking loop suture.

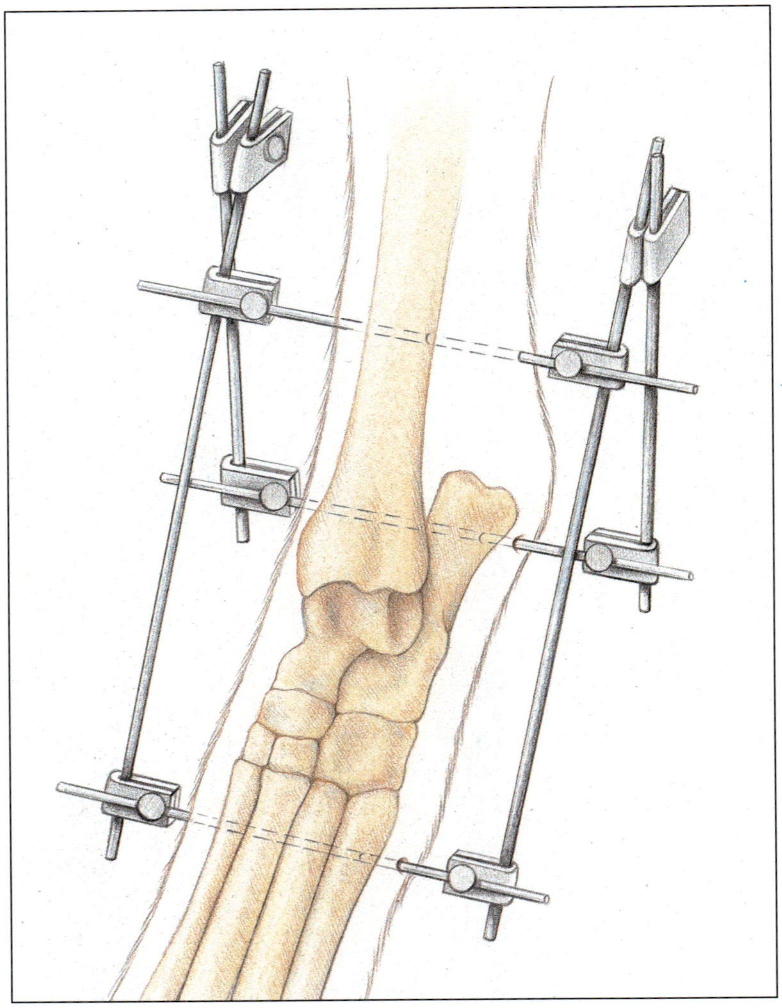

FIGURE 7.15 External fixation support for a severed Achilles tendon.

dages, and adhesive tape. All fixation splints must be checked frequently. They are removed in 6 weeks, and a modified Robert Jones splint is applied for 2 more weeks. Exercise should be moderate for a further period of a month.

GROWTH DEFECTS: PREMATURE FUSION

Distal Ulnar Physis

In young, rapidly growing dogs the distal ulnar physis is particularly susceptible to injury. Ninety percent of the growth of the ulna is from this area. In the young dog, the ulna is the larger of the foreleg's two bones (Fig. 7.16) and bears a high proportion of body weight. It is particularly vulnerable because of its conical shape, which predisposes it to compression rather than separation.

Foreleg fractures and sprains in young dogs may also cause an injury to the growth plate that is not immediately evident. With fusion the ulna ceases to grow, while the radius continues. The radius is thus trapped between the humerus and the carpus, which leads to outward bowing and pressure on the elbow and carpus (Fig. 7.17).

The earlier the onset of bowing of the radius and deviation of the paw is detected and surgically corrected, the better the chance for a more normal limb. If allowed to continue, the deformity

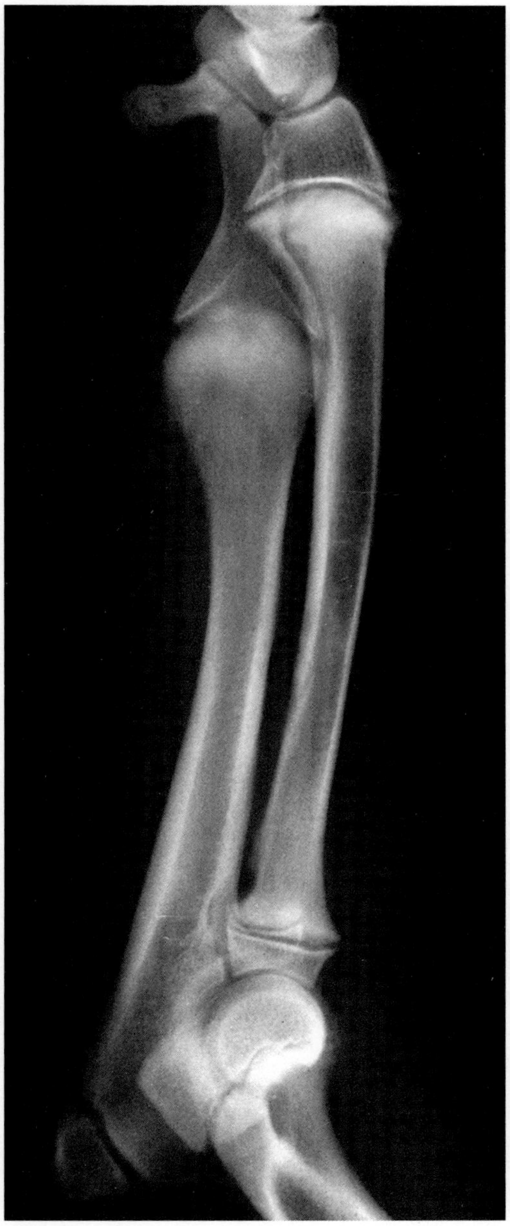

FIGURE 7.16 A normal radius and ulna in a young dog.

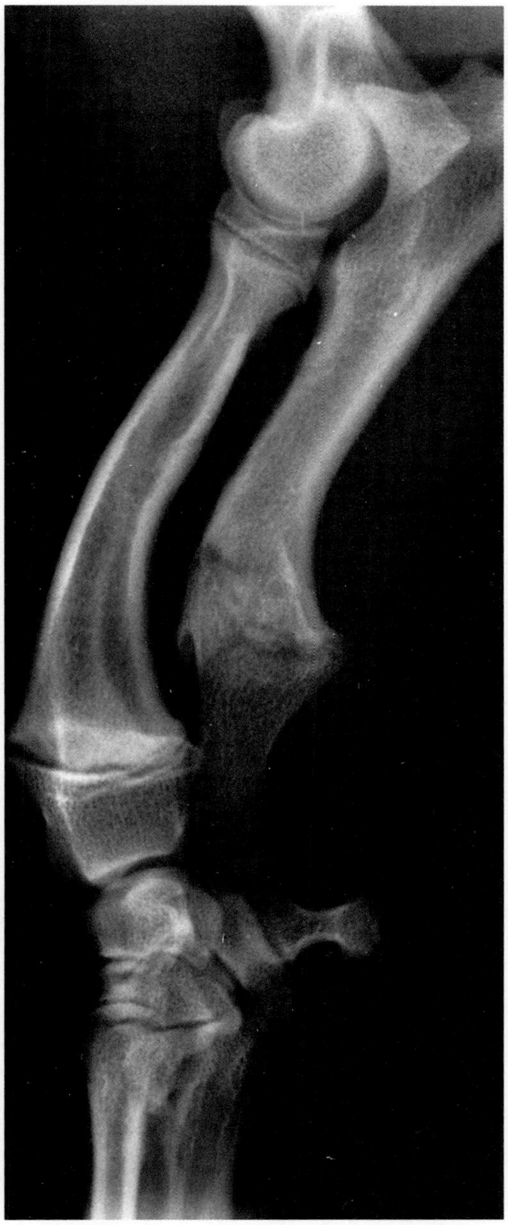

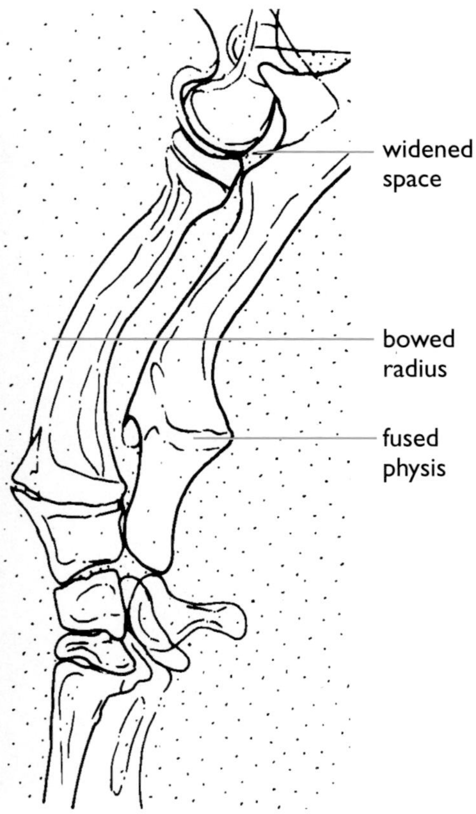

FIGURE 7.17 Premature fusion of the distal ulnar physis.

becomes more developed with subsequent injury to the elbow and carpus. Corrective surgery then becomes more difficult.

SURGICAL TECHNIQUE

Two objectives must be met: to release the bowstring effect of the ulna and to correct the bowing deformity of the radius.

The ulna is released by removing a section of the shaft; the amount depends on the estimated time for possible regrowth. Usually several centimeters are removed, along with the associated periosteum, to prevent regrowth.

An incision is made directly over the lateral surface of the ulna's shaft. The skin and subcutaneous tissues are retracted to expose the extensor carpi ulnaris caudally and the lateral digital extensor cranially. The deep antebrachial fascia is incised over the bone. The extensor carpi ulnaris is isolated and retracted. The lateral digital extensor is retracted cranially. By careful blunt dissection, a portion of the midshaft is isolated subperiosteally. The requisite section is transected with a bone saw and removed. The thick periosteum is dissected carefully away to discourage bony regrowth. Medullary bleeding is controlled with bone wax.

Closure is done by suturing the fascia, subcutaneous tissue, and skin in the usual manner. The leg is now placed in a position for a medial approach. An incision is made over the radius, preserving the cephalic vein. The deformity may have caused the radius to become twisted and flattened so that it protrudes just under the skin. The skin and subcutaneous tissues are reflected and the antebrachial fascia is incised. The most bowed section of the radius is isolated, taking care to avoid the radial artery.

Plans should be made ahead of time regarding the type of correction. The radius can be transected at an angle, preserving the length of the top of the bowed area. This pointed part is introduced into the medullary cavity of the distal fragment. This lower fragment is also rotated so that the elbow and the dorsum of the foot both face in the same direction. A medially placed K/E apparatus, consisting of a single bar with four clamps, is applied to two pins in the proximal and two pins in the distal fragments.

With very severe distortion the radius may be so flattened that it offers poor support for the pins. The rapid healing of these young animals will permit the use of a good coaptation splint.

An alternative correction is to remove a wedge of bone from the most bowed section so that there is better bone contact between the fragments. Both the lateral and cranial curves must be accounted for. Judicious use of the rongeur will make this adjustment.

Satisfactory healing takes less than a month. When correction is performed early, a return to normal can be obtained.

Proximal Radial Physis

Premature fusion of the proximal radial physis is not as common as that of the distal ulna. Stresses are placed on the elbow joint as the ulna continues to grow, resulting in increased joint space between the head of the radius and the humerus (Fig. 7.18). The medial and lateral collateral ligaments of the elbow restrain the humerus so that the ulna forces itself against it, thus increasing the humero–ulnar space. The coronoid process may be forced upward enough to be damaged. There is a variable degree of degenerative joint disease. The lameness requires surgical intervention.

This injury is treated by osteotomizing the radius to allow

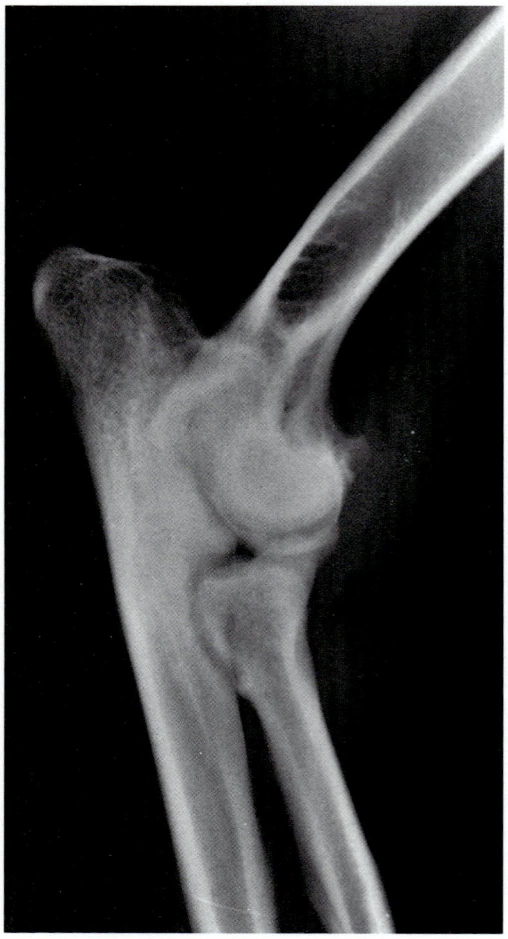

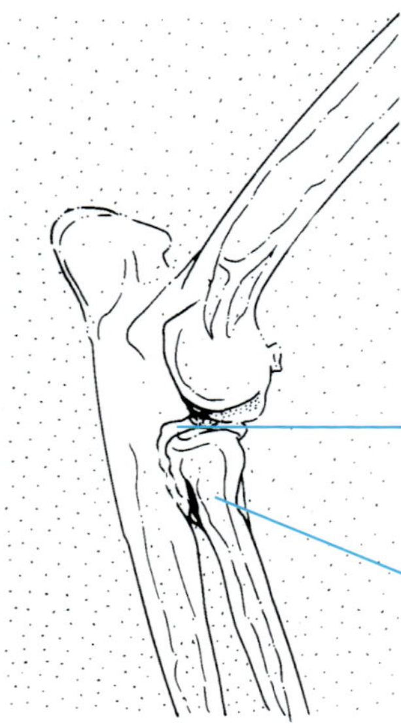

FIGURE 7.18 Premature fusion of the proximal radial physis.

the proximal portion to again contact the humeral articular surface and relieve the restraint on the humerus so that the ulna can resume its normal position. If the osteotomized area is insufficient, it may be necessary to redo the surgery at a later date to preserve the elbow.

SURGICAL TECHNIQUE

The dog is positioned for a medial approach to the leg. An incision is made from the radial head to the midshaft of the radius. The skin and subcutaneous tissues are reflected to expose the deep antebrachial fascia, which is incised between the extensor carpi radialis and the pronator teres. The median nerve, artery, and vein lie proximally. The insertion of the pronator teres is incised along the bone. By careful blunt dissection, a portion of the radial shaft is isolated and transected with a bone saw. The proximal fragment will separate slightly, and with slow, constant pressure it can be moved to force the radial head into contact with the humeral condyle. The strain on the ulna is released. The joint is returned to more normal congruency. A small bone plate is applied across the osteotomy site with two screws in each fragment.

Closure is achieved by replacing the retracted muscles, resuturing the deep fascia, and closing the subcutaneous tissue and skin in the usual manner. The leg does not require splinting.

Radiographs of the elbow are taken at monthly intervals until maturity to determine if the elbow is again affected. If this occurs the surgery is repeated.

Distal Radial Physis

Complete fusion of the distal radial physis is uncommon and is treated similarly to fusion of the proximal physis. It is more common to have a partial fusion (Fig. 7.19). Here the medial portion of the physis fuses while the lateral part continues to grow. The foot is deviated outward but the dorsum is maintained cranially. The dog is lame and the deformity is obvious. Treatment is by wedge osteotomy of the distal radius and osteotomy of the distal ulna. The latter must be done to permit repositioning of the distal radial fragment. The distal ulnar fragment will be removed from contact with its proximal portion, but this is of no consequence.

SURGICAL TECHNIQUE

An incision is made directly over the lateral portion of the distal ulna. The skin and subcutaneous tissue are retracted to expose the deep fascia. The fascia is incised and the tendons of the lateral digital extensor and the extensor carpi radialis are retracted. The distal shaft of the ulna is isolated and transected with a small saw or a Liston bone cutter. The incision is closed in the usual manner.

The dog is next positioned for a medial approach to the limb. An incision is made directly over the radius from just above the physis to the midshaft. The shaft is carefully isolated from the tendons of the extensor carpi radialis and that of the deep digital flexor. The radial artery and the cephalic vein must be avoided. The shaft of the radius is transected straight across, far enough above the physis to allow an angled cut to be made that will permit the foot to

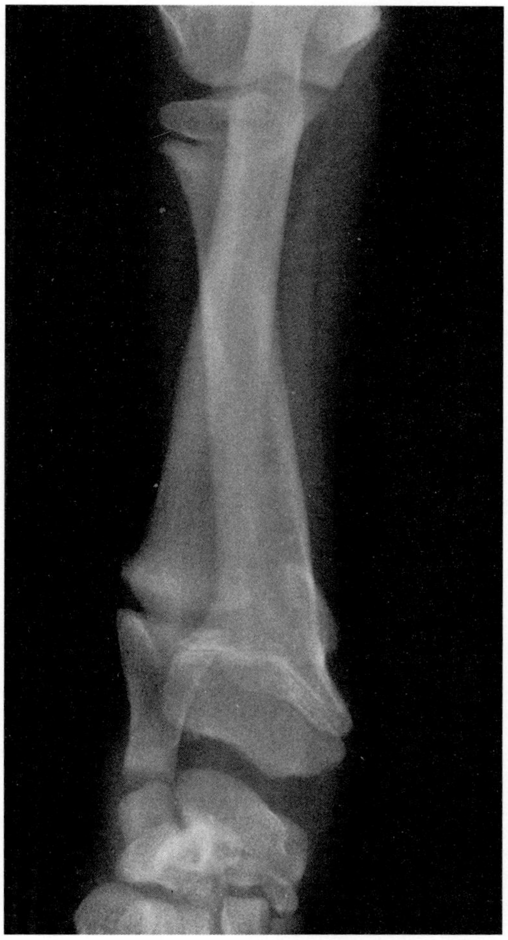

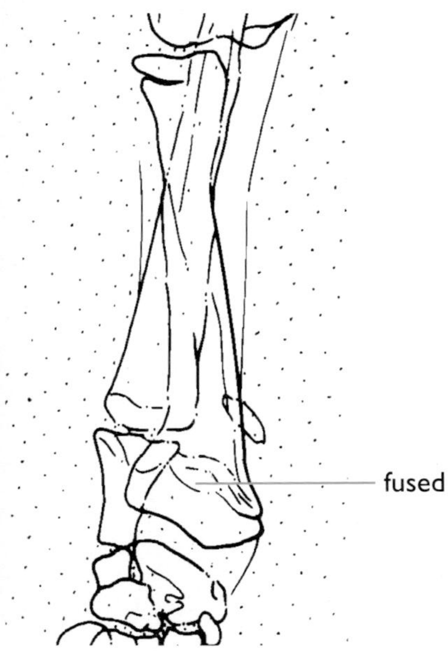

FIGURE 7.19 Partial fusion of the distal radial physis.

be at its normal position when the wedge of bone is removed. Closure is done by suturing fascia, subcutaneous tissue, and skin in the usual manner.

Smaller dogs will require only a good coaptation splint. Larger dogs must have an external fixation splint, consisting of two transfixing pins in the proximal fragment and one in the small distal fragment. The pins are connected to a single bar medially and laterally. The devices are bandaged. Healing is rapid, and the splint can be removed in less than 3 weeks. If the dog is near maturity the results are favorable.

AMPUTATIONS

Forelimb

Leg amputations may be the only alternative to euthanasia. They are well tolerated, though it may require a bit of persuasion by the veterinary surgeon to convince the owner. The health and well-being of the animal in the presence of bone and other tumors, total paralysis, intractable osteomyelitis, longstanding nonunions, loss of the paw or distal portion of the limb, and severe muscle contractures, can usually be much improved.

SURGICAL TECHNIQUE

The forelimb is best amputated completely, including the scapula. With the dog in lateral recumbency, an incision is made from the dorsal to the proximal edge of the scapula along the spine of the scapula to the shoulder joint. A second incision is made from the distal end of the first one cranially over the point of the shoulder, extending caudally through the axillary space to return on the lateral side to the starting point. The cephalic vein is ligated and sectioned. The skin and cutaneous musculature are dissected cranially and caudally from the scapula. The attachments of the omotransversarius and trapezius are severed from the spine of the scapula. The attachment of the deltoideus to the spine is cut away. Dorsocaudally the thoracic portion of the trapezius is separated from the scapula. More medially and dorsally, the rhomboid is cut away. On the medial side of the scapula, the serratus ventralis is elevated away from the facies serrata. The scapula is elevated outward and the intermuscular fascia of the rhomboideus is cut away; the intermuscular fascia of the axillary space is separated by blunt dissection. The latissimus dorsi, teres major, and cutaneous trunci muscles are separated from their insertion on the teres tubercle of the humerus above the insertion of the teres major. Careful dissection is done to isolate and ligate the thoracodorsal artery and vein. The accompanying nerve is severed sharply. The major blood vessels and nerves to the foreleg are exposed. With the scapula further abducted and rotated cranially, the axillary and lateral thoracic arteries are doubly ligated and cut. The nerves from the brachial plexus are cut cleanly across, including the median, ulnar, radial, axillary, subscapular, and suprascapular nerves. Branches of the superficial cervical and suprascapular arteries are cut and ligated. The scapula is abducted further. The deep and superficial pectorals are cut away from the humerus and the cleidobrachialis is transected. The caudal insertion of the triceps is severed, and the leg is removed (Figs. 7.20, 7.21).

All blood vessels are checked for bleeding and security of the ligatures. The muscles separated from the scapula are brought together to cover the amputation site. Distally, the deep pectoral muscle is sutured to the scaleneus, the cleidobrachialis fascia to the superficial pectoral, and the ventral border of the latissimus dorsi to the deep pectoral muscle.

Over the scapular area the trapezius and omotransversarius are sutured to the latissimus dorsi and deltoid. All dead space should be eliminated. The skin, subcutaneous tissues, and the musculocutaneous muscles are sutured together in the usual manner. The finished suture line resembles an inverted T.

With strict attention to hemostasis and a comfortable protecting bandage, the tendency towards hematoma formation is reduced. The dressing is replaced in 3 days and removed in a week. Dogs and cats adjust well to the loss of a forelimb.

Hind Limb

Dogs and cats tolerate the loss of a hind limb fairly well. Except in conditions that require removal of the entire femur, such as a bone tumor, the rear leg is amputated at mid-femur. This procedure is less stressful, leaves a protective stump, and provides a more acceptable appearance. The same reasons for amputation apply as for the foreleg.

SURGICAL TECHNIQUE

The animal is placed in lateral recumbency. A distally extending curved incision is made from the flank to the tuber ischii, extending to just above the patella. A similar curved incision is made medially, reaching to the middle of the inner thigh. Blood vessels are ligated. The skin and subcutaneous tissues are reflected distally. Beginning on the medial side, the sartorius is transected midway. The gracilis is transected at the same level. The femoral artery and vein are cleared of fascia, isolated, ligated, and cut. The saphenous artery is ligated and cut. Major vessels may require double ligation. The insertion of the pectineus is freed from the

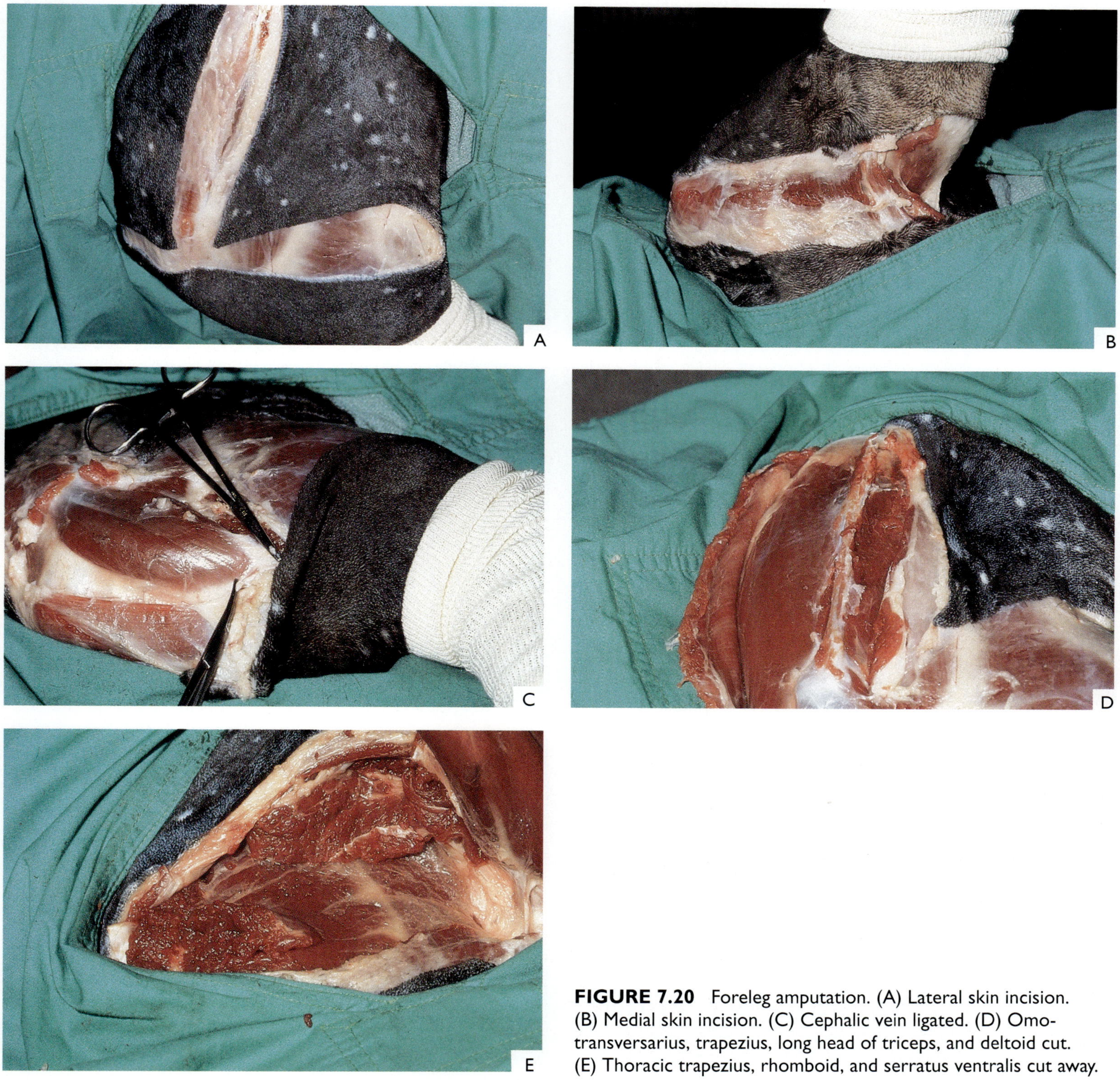

FIGURE 7.20 Foreleg amputation. (A) Lateral skin incision. (B) Medial skin incision. (C) Cephalic vein ligated. (D) Omotransversarius, trapezius, long head of triceps, and deltoid cut. (E) Thoracic trapezius, rhomboid, and serratus ventralis cut away.

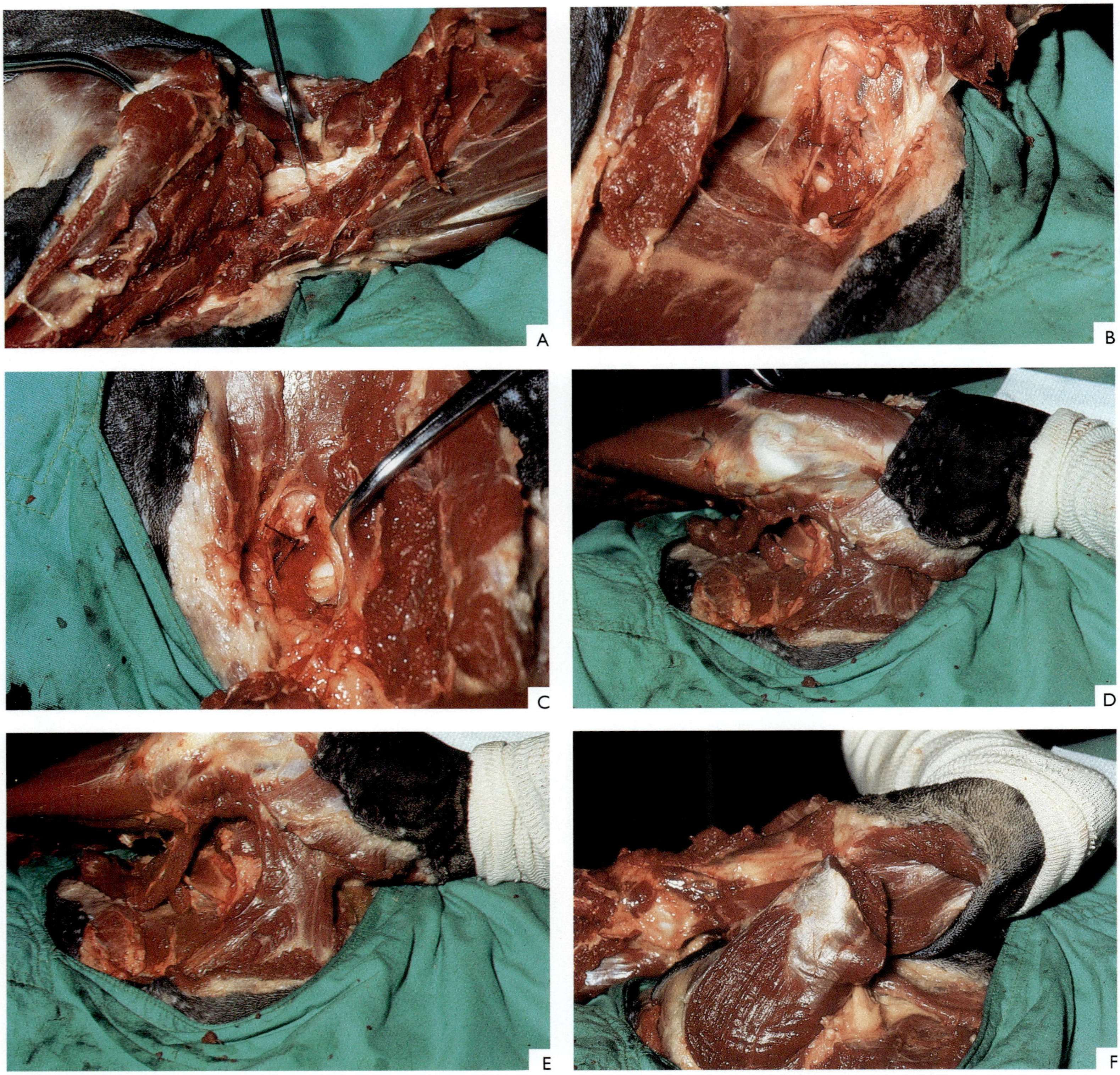
A
B
C
D
E
F

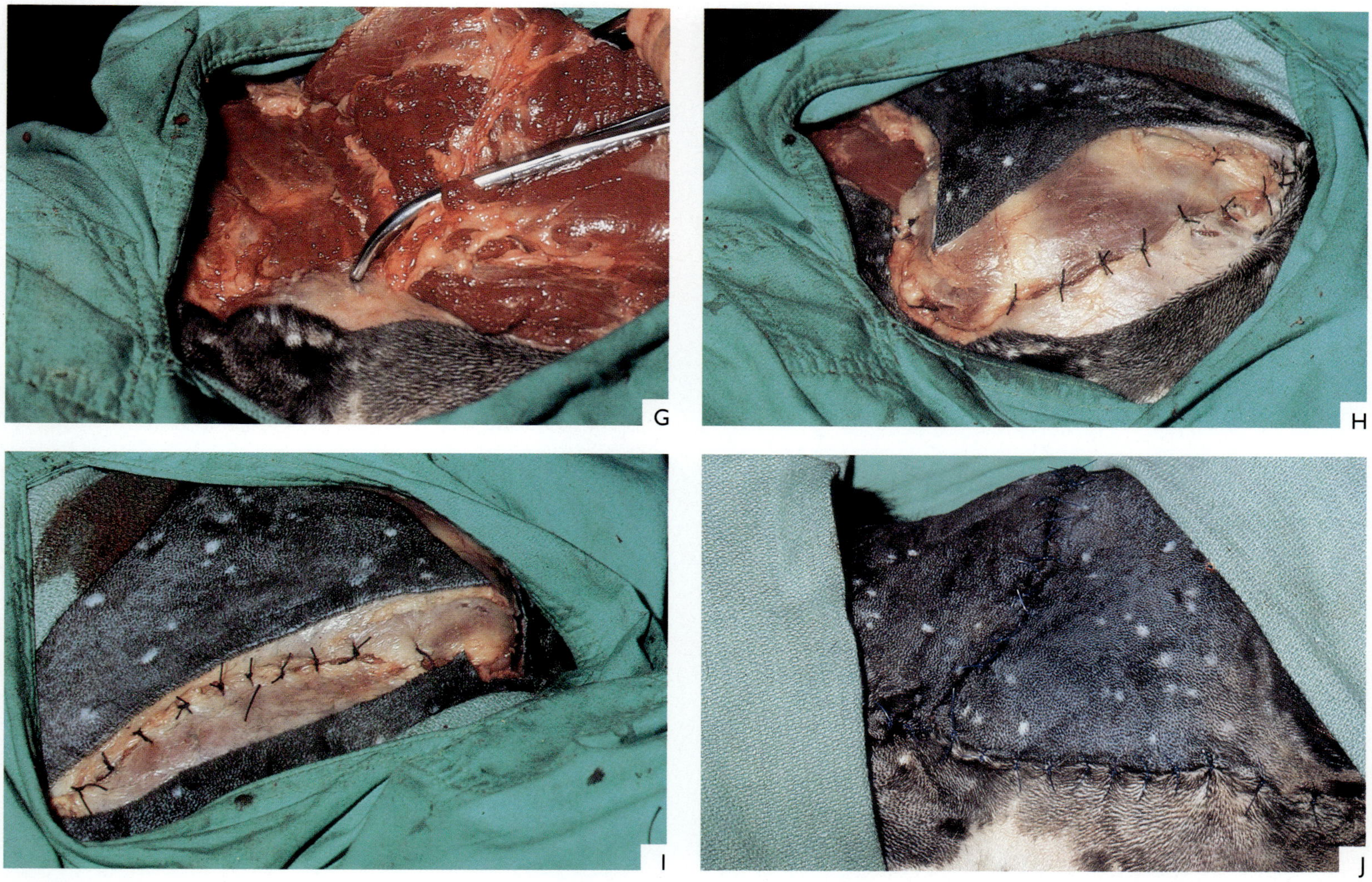

FIGURE 7.21 Foreleg amputation. (A) Insertions of latissimus dorsi, teres major, and cutaneous trunci cut. (B) Major vessels and nerves exposed. (C) Major vessels cut and ligated nerves cut. (D) Superficial pectoral cut. (E) Deep pectoral to be cut. (F) Cleidobrachialis and the distal portion of the triceps cut. (G) The leg is removed. (H) Distal incision closed. (I) Proximal incision closed. (J) Finished closure.

femoral shaft. The descending genicular artery is ligated and cut laterally. The cranial bellies of the sartorius and the quadriceps group are transected proximal to the patella. The aponeurosis of the biceps femoris, the fascia lata, and the belly of the biceps femoris are incised parallel to the skin incision. All blood vessels are clamped and ligated. The ischiatic nerve is isolated and transected several centimeters from the amputation site. The semitendinosus and semimembranosus muscles, along with the adductor magnus, are transected at the amputation level. The femur is transected with a bone saw at its upper third. The leg is removed (Figs. 7.22, 7.23).

Closure is performed by bringing the severed ends of the cranial and caudal muscle groups together to form a solid protection for the femoral stump. The quadriceps group is sutured to the adductor. The biceps femoris is sutured to the gracilis. The sartorius is sutured to the fascia lata. The skin and subcutaneous tissues are closed in the usual manner.

Every effort must be made to prevent hematoma formation. The incision is protected by a light bandage for a few days. It takes longer for dogs to adjust to the loss of a hind limb than to a front one. They do strengthen the opposite leg, and soon get along well.

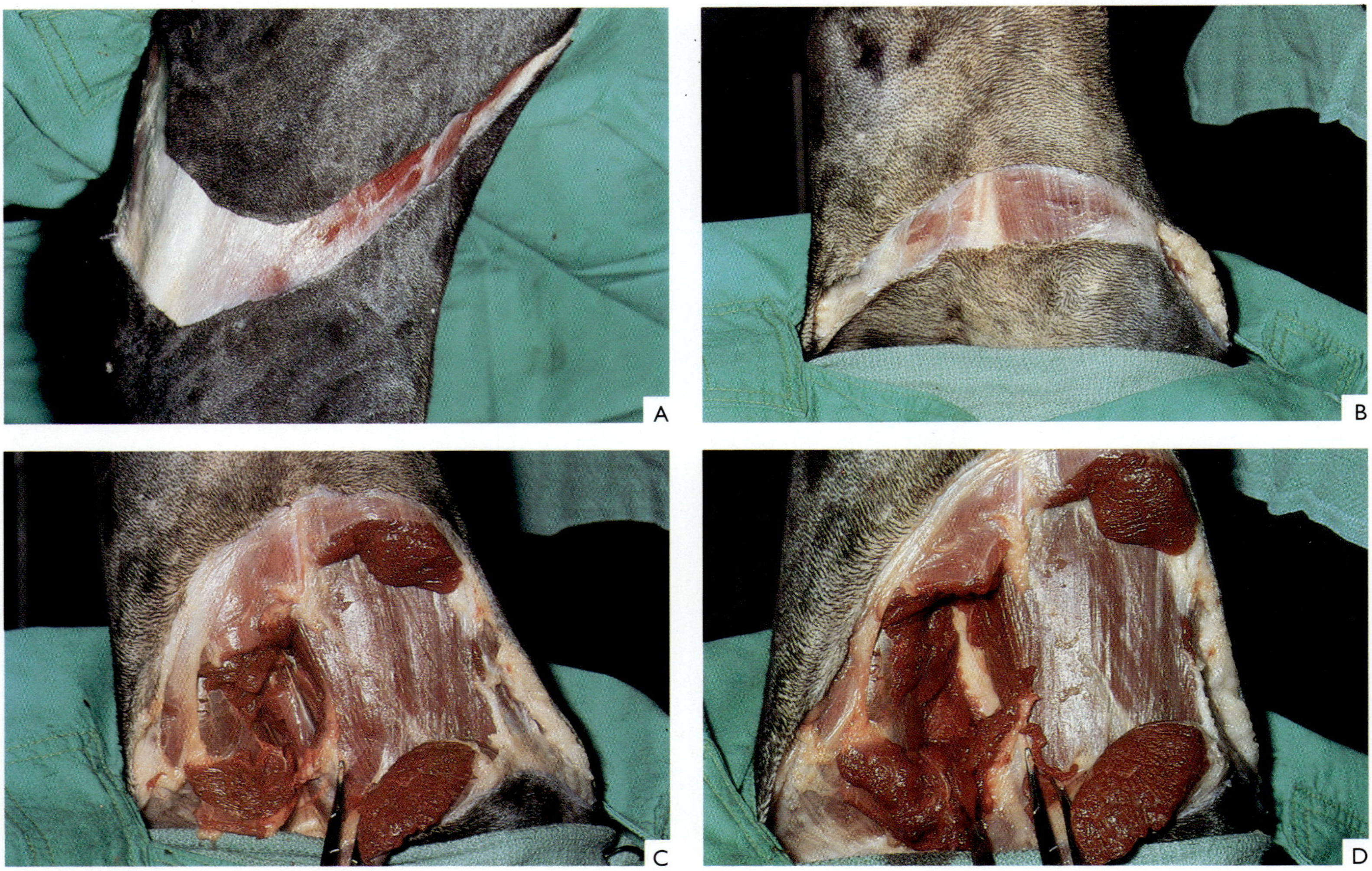

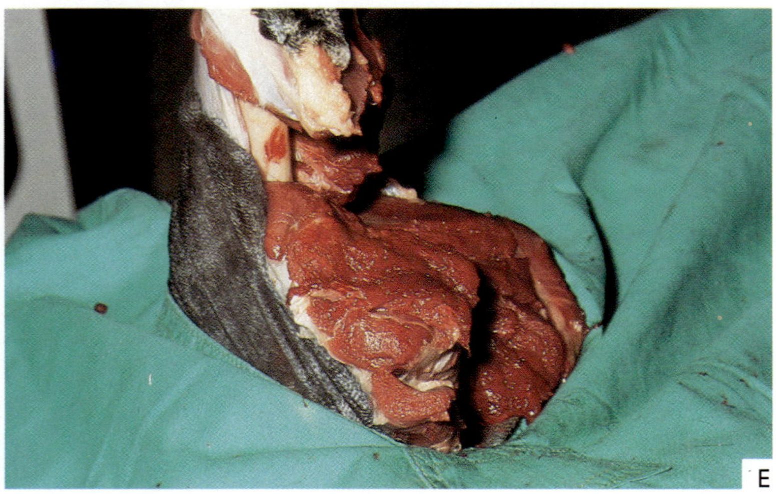

FIGURE 7.22 Hind leg amputation. (A) Lateral skin incision. (B) Medial skin incision. (C) Sartorius and gracilis transected. (D) Pectineus freed from the femur and femoral artery and vein ligated and cut. (E) The cranial bellies of the sartorius and quadriceps group cut proximal to the patella.

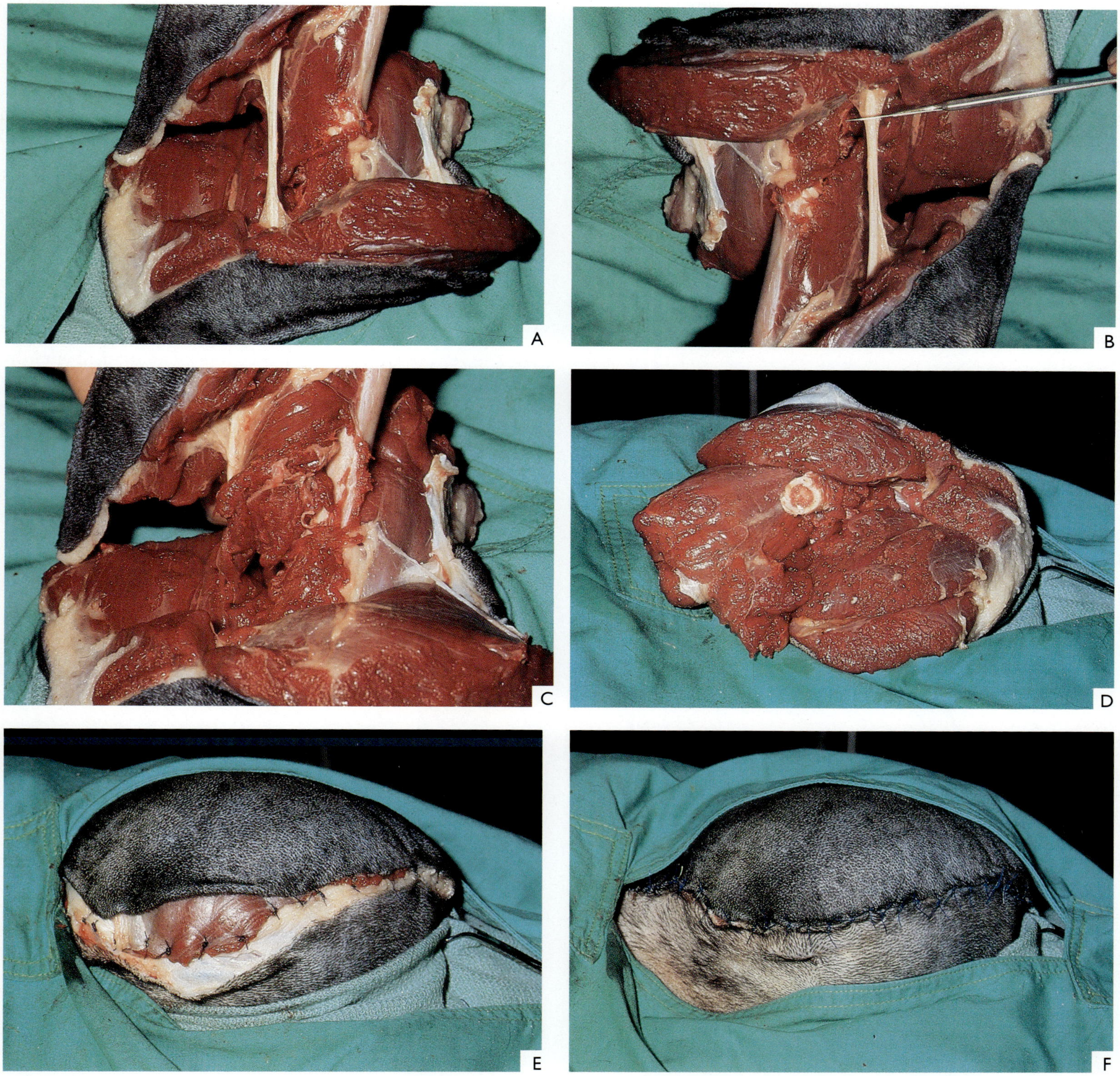

FIGURE 7.23 Hind leg amputation. (A) The fascia lata and belly of the biceps femoris cut and the ischiatic nerve demonstrated. (B) Ischiatic nerve severed. (C) Semimembranosus and semitendinosus cut. (D) Adductor cut, femur transected, and leg removed. (E) Muscle closures completed. (F) Final closure of the stump.

Toe

Occasionally it is necessary to remove a toe because of severe injury or chronic infection. Chronically infected nails are treated by removing the distal phalanx. More severe injuries may require removal of all the phalangeal bones in a toe.

SURGICAL TECHNIQUE

A lozenge-shaped incision is made that encircles the toe but preserves the pad. The skin is reflected and the tendons cut. The third phalanx is disarticulated and removed. The distal end of the second phalanx is cut off with rongeurs (Fig. 7.24).

Closure is done by bringing the pad over the stump and suturing the skin and subcutaneous tissues. Redundant skin on the sides of the incision is excised to make a smooth appearance.

Removal of All Three Phalanges

Removal of the phalanges of the inner or outer toes can be done without laming the dog. Removal of one of the central supporting toes may result in persistent lameness.

SURGICAL TECHNIQUE

A skin incision is made through the web tissues and on each side of the selected amputation site. The skin is reflected to allow the tendons to be severed and the phalanx disarticulated from the metacarpal or metatarsal bone. The distal ends of the medial or lateral metacarpals or metatarsals are cut at an angle to provide a smooth appearance. The central ends are transected above the area of the sesamoids.

Closure is by suturing the subcutaneous tissues and skin together. The foot is placed in a bandage for about a week.

Tail

Tail amputations are done for both cosmetic and necessary reasons. Legal and breed requirements should be observed. Severe injuries and paralysis to the tail will require surgical removal. The surgery is done so as to provide a covering of the stump with strong dorsal skin.

SURGICAL TECHNIQUE

The skin of the tail over the amputation site is pushed cranially with the fingers. Dorsally, a caudally curved incision is made from the midpoint of the sides of the tail. Ventrally, a similar incision is made that does not extend so far caudally (Fig. 7.25). The skin flaps are reflected and a Liston bone cutter is used to cut between the tail vertebrae. Blood vessels are clamped and ligated.

Closure is by suturing the skin and subcutaneous tissues of the dorsal and ventral flaps together. The dorsal flap should cover the end of the tail. There should be no stress on the sutures. The nerves should be clean cut to prevent neuroma formation. Usually no bandage is required.

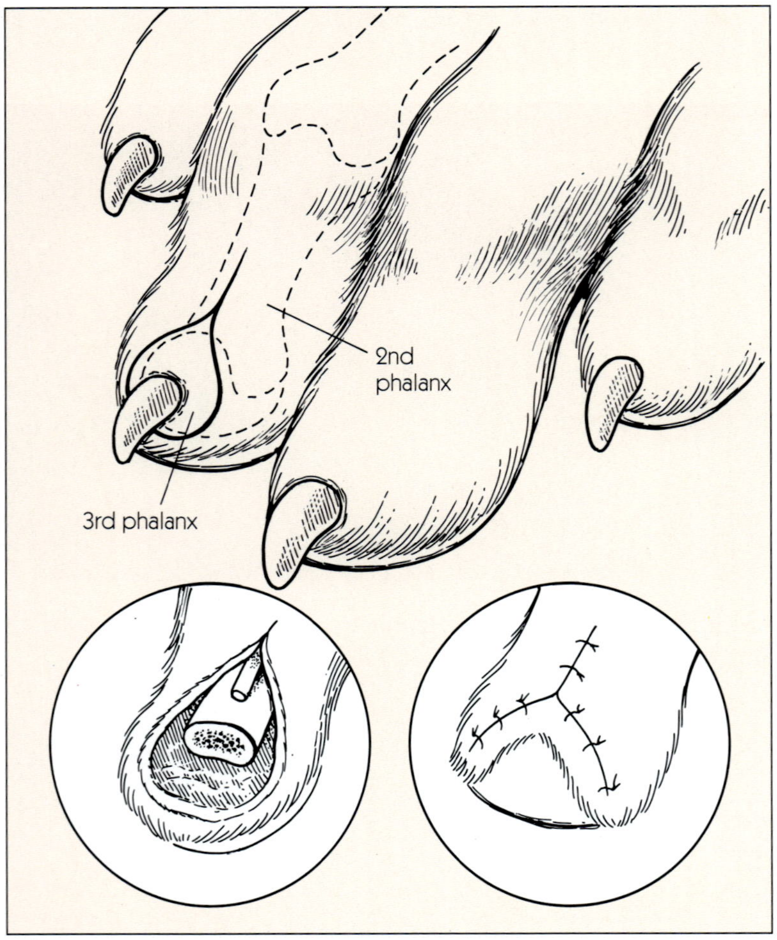

FIGURE 7.24 Incision lines for amputation of the toe.

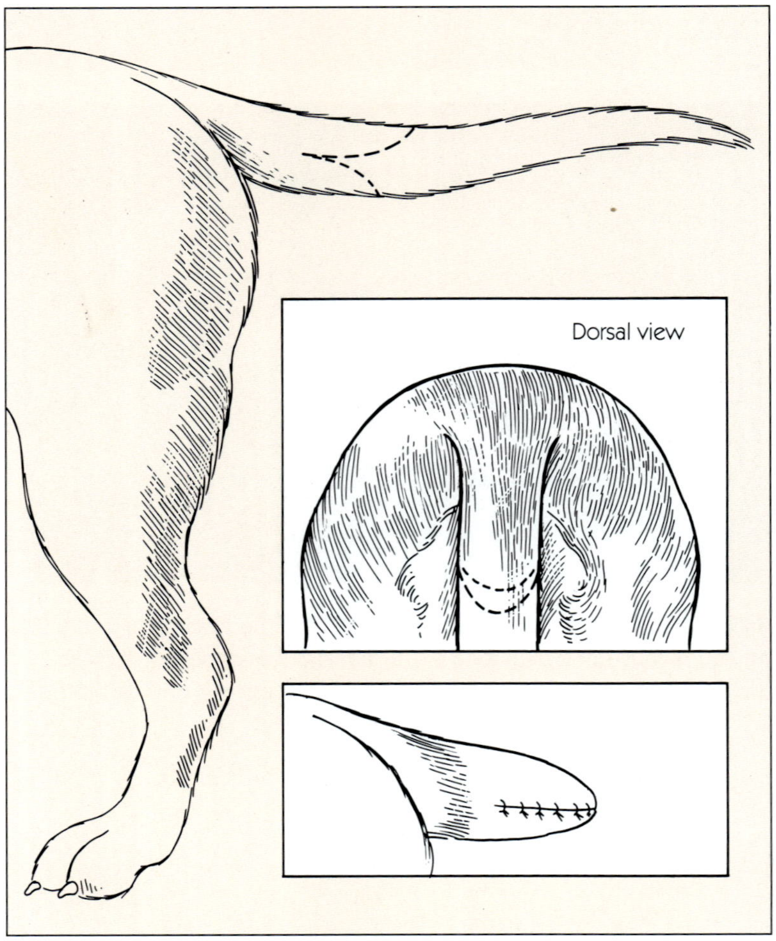

FIGURE 7.25 Incision lines for amputation of the tail.

INDEX

A

B

C

D

E

F

G

H

I

J

K

L

M

O

P

Q

R

S

T

U

V

Z